mult, arre

— think beyond ent

Layc splen

Journal of Health
Communicale. Vol 1
Issue 1) Feb 1996.

Kerr, lohie

ReimerKirkham, & Brown,
2006

F. Culum
differential   Affiliative Need

The Politics of Women's Health

Exploring Agency and Autonomy

The Politics of Women's Health

Exploring Agency and Autonomy

The Feminist Health Care Ethics
Research Network

Susan Sherwin (coordinator)

Françoise Baylis   Margaret Lock

Marilynne Bell   Wendy Mitchinson

Maria De Koninck   Kathryn Pauly Morgan

Jocelyn Downie   Janet Mosher

Abby Lippman   Barbara Parish

 Temple University Press: *Philadelphia*

Temple University Press, Philadelphia 19122
Copyright © 1998 by Temple University
All rights reserved
Published 1998
Printed in the United States of America

Text design by Susan Gutnik

⊗ The paper used in this publication meets the requirements of the American National
Standard for Information Sciences—Permanence of Paper for Printed Library Materials,
ANSI Z39.48-1984

Library of Congress Cataloging-in-Publication Data

Sherwin, Susan, 1947–
  The politics of women's health : exploring agency and autonomy/
the Feminist Health Care Ethics Research Network, Susan Sherwin . . .
[et al.].
      p.   cm.
  Includes bibliographical references and index.
  ISBN 1–56639–632–8 (cloth : alk. paper). — ISBN 1–56639–633–6
(pbk. : alk. paper)
    1. Women's health services—Political aspects.   2. Women's health
services—Social aspects.   3. Women—Health and hygiene—
Sociological aspects.   I. Feminist Health Care Ethics Research
Network.   II. Title.
RA564.85.S53   1998
362.1'082—dc21   98-16025

Contents

Acknowledgments

As we explain in Chapter 1, this book is the result of a four-year collaborative research project supported by the Social Sciences and Humanities Research Council of Canada (SSHRC). Under the auspices of a SSHRC Strategic Research Network Grant, we were able to meet regularly over the years of the project and to communicate effectively between meetings despite the distances between us. Given the geographical dispersion of Network members, it would not have been possible to produce this integrated book without such financial support.

The work of the Network was greatly facilitated by the excellent support we received from the research and administrative assistants who participated in all dimensions of this project. Peggy Spencer worked with the Network in its first year as we were finding our collective feet and direction. As a nurse with many years experience and excellent skills at promoting effective group interactions, Peggy was invaluable in helping us to gain our initial focus. In subsequent years, Ariella Pahlke, a video artist, community activist, occasional editor, and practiced "rebel," became the major assistant for the Network. Ariella brought a unique and important perspective to our meetings and newsletters. She handled the many administrative details of the project, coordinated our internal communications, fulfilled numerous requests for research support, and often shared her experiences and opinions with the Network. Jan Sutherland is responsible for the final production of the manuscript; this work involved many painful hours struggling with recalcitrant computers and pursuing uniformity and accuracy in format and structure from a range of submissions whose diversity seemed even greater than the Network encompassed. And, on occasion, Carolyn McLeod filled in with essential tasks when the regular assistant was unavailable. All four women shared our commitment to the values represented in this work and all brought to it their excellent skills, valued views, and wonderful senses of humor. We are very grateful to them. Quite honestly, we could not have produced this work without them.

Dalhousie University provided the administrative support for managing the grant and provided various important material resources we depended on (fax machines, printing services, computers, etc.). In particular, we wish to acknowledge the support offered by the Philosophy Department and the Health Law Institute at Dalhousie University. Both units provided workspace and the necessary technology to facilitate this project. Secretaries in both units pitched in to help when we ran into deadline pressures, graciously gave up their work stations when needed, and helped out if no administrative assistant was available.

Because we live in different parts of the country, it was always difficult to find times to get together. The times we did manage were precious and intense. Meetings were inevitably scheduled over weekends in order to keep costs down and reduce the pressure of other professional responsibilities. Unfortunately, this scheduling often involved a significant cost to family members. It also sometimes involved significant financial expense for Network members who had to make private childcare arrangements for those weekends. Although the Network considered child care during meetings to be an expense of participating in our research project, SSHRC guidelines prohibit the use of grant funds for child care. We did protest this restriction but did not succeed in changing this policy. So we want to pay particular thanks to caregivers who helped out on the weekends of Network meetings. We also want to acknowledge the patience of all family members and of friends for the many times that Network business cut into the "personal" time of Network members and our assistants.

The Politics of Women's Health

Exploring Agency and Autonomy

1 Introduction

Susan Sherwin
With Voices from the Network

This book is the result of four years of intense and lively conversations and debates of an interdisciplinary group of scholars and practitioners who share a primary interest in feminist approaches to women's health.[1] Our group includes physicians (Marilynne Bell and Barbara Parish), lawyers (Jocelyn Downie and Janet Mosher), philosophers (Françoise Baylis, Kathryn Morgan, and Susan Sherwin), social scientists (Maria De Koninck and Margaret Lock), a self-described "generalist" with a background in genetics (Abby Lippman), and a historian (Wendy Mitchinson). We also benefited from the insights and perspective of our research and administrative assistant, Ariella Pahlke, a community activist and video artist. Our group was organized around the theme of feminist health care ethics and feminist concerns about women's health, hence our name: the Feminist Health Care Ethics Research Network (hereafter, the Network).

Let me start with my fear of doctors—which is not a fear of physical pain but more a fear of being silenced, of being made to feel like a child, of being told directly or indirectly that I ought not to question, and that I need not understand—that's the doctor's business, not mine. A fear of not being given all the relevant information that I ought to have; a fear of loss of control to the authority and expertise of medicine. I frequently "prepare" for my visits to a physician— read all that I can—so that I will

Our interest in the subject of women's health is both professional and personal. As women ourselves, questions about women's health have particular salience for each of us. Most of the group underwent significant life changes during the course of our Network discussions. Three members gave birth to four babies (Kaila, Nicole, Sam, and Jacob), and three others entered menopause. One underwent major surgery for cancer, two experienced open-heart surgery, and others faced different sorts of serious health threats. Some helped care for their mothers and grandmothers through various stages of illnesses, and a few faced deaths of important women in their lives. At the same time, two of our members were engaged in delivering health care to women patients (one as an obstetrician-

1

be able to ask "intelligent," "informed" questions. Indeed on some occasions I've gone with a list of questions in hand and a pen to take notes about the answers. But this hasn't been received enthusiastically by most physicians whom I've encountered—they seem to prefer that I not read, and not ask questions.

—Janet

I chose nursing as my dream career when I was about three and never really wavered from that. This choice had something to do with caring and a lot to do with security and movement up the social ladder, plus I was confident that it was within my capabilities. Now I suppose that I could analyze it in terms of the three great estates of femaleness, nursing, teaching, and secretarial work, but it certainly did not feel like that then.

—Barbara

I am the eldest, but not first born, of a strong-willed West Indian woman and a reserved Englishman. From a young age, my mother taught me to be proud of my "dark" secret— though to all appearances I am of White Anglo-European descent, I am Black, or according to those who are blacker than me (of which there are many),

gynecologist, the other as a family physician), and several of our members were engaged in health-related research involving women as subject-participants. The questions we discussed concern the ways we live our own lives and conduct our professional work; we are not neutral observers of these matters.

We consider our approach to be feminist in that we understand gender to be an important feature in how individuals experience the world. We begin with a recognition that women are systematically oppressed in society, that, typically, they have less power and authority than comparably situated men and their interests are often sacrificed in favor of the interests of others.[2] We work from an understanding that women are placed in subordinate positions with respect to economic, political, legal, and social structures; we are, however, keenly aware that the nature and degree of women's oppression varies significantly depending on other features of their lives (including race, class, age, sexuality, health, and ethnicity).

Although feminism is especially concerned with the systematic oppression based on gender, it must be sensitive to other forms of oppression. For one thing, we are all not only gendered but also members of particular races and classes; all such features affect how we experience power and oppression, privilege and disadvantage; therefore, gender oppression is inseparable from other forms of oppression. Furthermore, we understand feminism to involve both the recognition that oppression of women and other groups exists and an appreciation that oppression (of all sorts) is unjust, that is, it is morally wrong. Feminism is more than just the theoretical observation of injustice. It also involves a commitment to acting to try to end existing oppression.[3]

I am Red. In my youth I learned to be both proud and fearful of this truth. For a time, I would introduce myself to others by name and by race. Far better that I should be rejected at the meeting point, than after having developed a relationship that, unbeknownst to me, was so fragile that it could not withstand the disclosure of an important fact about my heritage.

—Françoise

Although I think "oppression" captures an important political reality that demands relief, it is in itself an impoverished notion because it speaks only negatively about removing barriers. It reduces our view of the people who are oppressed to the circumstances of their oppression, defining them in terms of that political force, and excludes other important dimensions of their lives. It encourages us to think only about the value of relieving oppression as if there were no other features that distinguish the lives of those who are oppressed. The positive aspects of other ways of being may be overlooked when we focus only on the facts of oppression. The direction I want to be moving in is one that goes beyond the removal of barriers to consider also how to facilitate the

Even though we argue that oppression is an important feature of a group's experience, none of us believes that it is fully determinate of that experience. Hence, while our various analyses perceive women as "victims" of oppression, they do not portray them as *mere* victims—that is, as people who are passive and helpless in the face of oppression. Oppression typically restricts options, but it does not remove them completely; often (though perhaps not always), it leaves open the possibility of resistance and challenge against oppressive forces. We believe that systemic patterns of oppression run very deep within social expectations and relations, creating a complex network of interconnected restrictions that cannot be fully escaped. We do not view these patterns, however, as either natural or timeless. As feminists, we believe that change is possible through individual and collective actions.

Our work is grounded in a belief that a society's organization of health services has great potential to either deepen or relieve existing patterns of oppression, just as it has the potential to worsen or relieve specific health problems. We each understand health to be a key factor in women's lives and we recognize that the social and economic conditions of women's lives are major factors in their health. Because biomedicine, the technology-oriented medical model that dominates health services in the West and much of the rest of the world, is the major determinant of our health care system in North America, we are particularly interested in understanding how it operates with respect to women's health needs. As do many other feminist theorists, we see medicine as playing an active role in perpetuating some aspects of women's oppression while helping to reduce other dimensions of women's oppression. We are, therefore, committed to taking a careful

*development of empowering
political and health care systems.
No mean feat, but one worth far
more attention, I think.*

　　　　　　　—Susan

*Throughout all this, I still feel
very comfortable in saying
I am a feminist, which means
I believe in the necessity to
redefine social relations between
women and men (rapports
sociaux de sexe) but "equality"
is not a magic formula. The
challenge is to integrate in our
analysis and actions all the
necessary nuances and measure
their adverse effects. How can
we deal with inequalities
between women? To what
extent do we and should we
"share" and can we relate a
"biological" category to the
"social" category?*

　　　　　　　—Maria

*After sixteen years of medical
practice and six years of
academic teaching I entered the
Feminist Bioethics Network at a
time when I needed to take a deep
breath and reflect critically with
other women with other "points
of view" on what I had been
doing. As I started to re-examine
theory and practice outside my
discipline, I started to see my
own role in the "medicalization"
of woman abuse as a "specialist"
in the field.*

　　　　　　　—Marilynne

critical look at the values and conceptual assumptions implicit in medicine's approach to women. In particular, we explore some of the ways in which the biomedical model ignores the value of nonmedical contributions to health and we examine the tendency of medicine to take power and control over health matters away from those who are most directly affected by its interventions. We do not expect to make power differentials in health care encounters disappear or become irrelevant, but we do seek to make them more visible and, thereby, less dangerous. We seek as well to recognize women as possessing important knowledge about their own health experiences that is not readily accessible to, or accepted by, most professional "experts." As feminists, we seek to use our training and research skills to help end that oppression through critical reflections on some of the underlying concepts and values that structure contemporary health care.

The Process

Our efforts were guided not only by feminist objectives but also by feminist ideals of method.[4] In particular, we draw on work in feminist epistemology (theory of knowledge) that argues that "the knower" is not the "featureless abstraction" (or neutral, disinterested investigator) that is so commonly portrayed and assumed to be in the appropriate position for obtaining reliable, objective knowledge. Rather, the specific social location of the knower is significant (Code 1991).[5] The location of the knower influences what is observed/observable, what is known/knowable, and what each of us experiences in the world. The location of a particular knower is shaped by reference to a great many factors: gender, age, class, race, ethnicity, political orientation,

I am deeply concerned about the hierarchy in medicine, and not just as it is experienced by most nonphysicians. What is the role of the bioethicist in the clinical setting? Where does she fit in the hierarchy? How does she work to preserve the hierarchy, the title Dr., the clinical appointments in medical departments, the salary, the social peer group, etc.

—Françoise

My professional life gave me "credit." As long as I argued out of conviction (well into my thirties), I was considered as someone unsatisfied, frustrated, and even foolish. Then, being more and more recognized on a professional basis, my discourse suddenly became serious and worth listening to.

—Maria

Anthropologists, as is well known, are trained to contextualize, to take a culturally relative stance. I whole-heartedly support this position, but only on the condition that we do not exclude ourselves but contextualize discourse and practices of all kinds, including those of science, medicine, and feminism. No knowledge should be taken as epistemologically privileged. Having watched a policy designed to encourage a "culturally sensitive"

sexual orientation, and disability, as well as by the historical circumstances of one's life. And as became clearer to many of us through our involvement in the Network, one factor in the historical circumstances of our particular lives that has demonstrably shaped our ability to observe and to know is our training in particular disciplines—we learned, to paraphrase Foucault, that they don't call them disciplines for nothing. Learning to converse across and through our respective disciplinary training was a greater challenge than we first anticipated; cross-disciplinary criticism and authorship could be both painful and exhilarating, sometimes simultaneously. That location influences both what is observed and what is known suggests that inevitably there will be not only multiple but contested knowledge claims. For example, statements about the nature and harms of addictions and appropriate preventative interventions may vary significantly depending on both the perspective of the "expert" speaking and the population being discussed. But these features of knowledge claims are frequently well-hidden, if not obscured altogether. Indeed, many knowledge claims are never voiced, let alone heard and accorded the status of "legitimate" knowledge. Rather, what most often comes to be widely accepted as "knowledge" or "truth" or "fact" are those knowledge claims advanced by persons who have social power (Minnich 1990). This is so, in part, because those who occupy positions of power have much enhanced access to the vehicles and resources necessary for "knowledge" production and dissemination. Moreover, those with significant social power are also in a position to both define and enforce criteria of "knowledge." Hence, knowledge production frequently travels the circuit of what is perhaps best described as a closed

*health care system wax and
wane in Canada and been called
on, as a result of this policy, to
undertake the impossible
task of educating health care
professionals in sixty minutes
or less about "culture, health,
and illness," I continue to be
concerned about a facile ability
to locate "others" in a culture,
all the while leaving our own
assumptions unexamined.
Bioethics stands guilty on this
score, in my estimation, since
authoritative knowledge is rarely
questioned by this discipline.*

—Margaret

*As did many of my generation
of war babies, I got my
"training" in most important
things, feminism included,
from the street, not from school.
There were no women's studies
courses for us, and books which
boldly said "feminist . . ." to
learn from had not yet been
written. There were, though,
groups of women doing things,
especially community/political
"things," and I learned about
feminism, though it was
certainly not called this, in
these apprenticeships.*

—Abby

*I not only wrote but published
articles on sexuality, on
androgyny, on the horrors of
pathological romantic love, and,
later, on reproductive*

loop; a loop closed to those who do not enjoy social power. Feminist research attempts to break this loop by paying close attention to women's experiences and to the diverse and often competing knowledge claims to which these give rise, by giving voice to those who have been historically marginalized and often silenced, by revealing the partial (self-interested) nature of commonly accepted criteria of "knowledge," and by taking power itself to be a subject of inquiry.

In the collection we frequently use these insights from feminist epistemology to critique dominant knowledge claims and research practices in women's health. We tried to be attentive to these dimensions of knowledge construction as we engaged in the processes of constructing our own "knowledge" claims that we present in the collection. So, for example, we consciously reflect on our own position with respect to our interactions with the Tri-Council Working Group on the Ethics of Research with Humans and how our position affected our ability to be heard as we pointed to the absence of women as research participants (as both agents and subjects) in clinical trials. Our own position as feminists helped reveal the importance of attending to the conditions of women's lives (or others who are marginalized) in common invocations of the principle of "autonomy" and to challenge the pervasive devaluation of experience as a source of knowledge within medicine.

In our funding application, we made commitments to advance our understanding of ethical issues in women's health care and to produce a book within the broadly defined area of "feminist health care ethics." Precisely how we would honor these commitments was negotiated among us throughout the four years that we met as a Network. Questions *technologies and moral double-binds. Powerfully influenced by radical feminism's insistence that the "personal is political," I came to the awareness that my struggles might also speak to the struggles in some other women's lives and that whatever philosophical talent I might possess might lead to illumination for others as well. While specifically rejecting the arrogance of philosophy's universalizability pretenses, I simply hoped that my work might prove helpful to others.*

—Kathryn

In the context of my work I have occasion to discuss HIV testing of pregnant women with physicians. In such discussions, I have been told, "When a woman refuses an HIV test, we know why." "Why?" I ask naively. "Well, she obviously knows she is HIV positive." Why, I wonder, is it not equally plausible to conclude that the woman knows she is not HIV positive and so does not need the test? What does this tell us about what physicians know?

—Françoise

It is an exciting time for me to be able to participate in, give to, and receive from our Network. Our common work brings together my continuing interest in social justice, my commitment

such as how we would "construct" knowledge, what form authorship might take, and how we would make good on the imperative to engage in political work occupied us from the outset. Our answers evolved through dialogue and were shaped by the opportunities that our grant created for us to work in ways new to each of us, as well as by particular constraints of the grant and the much broader constraints in each of our lives.[6]

We first met as a group in spring 1993. Although we came together holding different conceptions of the problems and solutions that characterize feminist health care ethics, we shared a common interest in women's health issues and in feminist approaches to questions about values concerning health matters. We each welcomed the opportunity to explore these issues through participation in an interdisciplinary, collaborative research project. While many of us had prior experience of collaborative work, working in such an extensive interdisciplinary group with others was a new and untested experience made all the more complicated by being limited to intense twice-yearly face-to-face meetings for developing creative directions and resolving disputes. The opportunity, indeed the excitement that the Network generated seemed clear to all of us: an environment to explore ideas with other feminists; to share and learn across disciplines; to speak in a "safe" environment that might allow one to venture and experiment with ideas without fear. Nonetheless, many of us did feel nervous about exposing ourselves in such impressive company and worried that our ignorance about others' disciplines made us inadequate or incompetent relative to others. It was very important to each of us to earn (and maintain) the respect of the others and this meant it was often difficult for some members to share *to working for the health of women understood in the strongest, most comprehensive terms, my sense of and desire for the kind of mutual empowerment that happens in our best collective moments, and the heightened acuity, sadness, and sense of institutionally structured injustice I feel in relation to the voices and the women who are absent in our work.*

—Kathryn

When we were working together at the Westminster Institute, Françoise and I were warned against writing together too much—too many co-authored articles would not help our chances for tenure down the road. This advice made me carefully examine the "process" that I had simply taken for granted. I decided that co-authoring was extremely important to me, and I would continue it regardless of tenure consequences. Had this warning not been issued, I have no doubt that I would have continued writing with Françoise but I might never have made the explicit commitment to collaborative work (such as this grant). I continue to believe that undercutting the traditional "solo" academic work process

their work in progress. We had to struggle to find ways to offer constructive criticism to one another without its being experienced as painful rejection.

We are, then, especially proud that we have negotiated those tricky waters and have been able to produce this book as a truly collaborative enterprise. This book is fully interdisciplinary (and not just multidisciplinary). We jointly decided on the shape of the book, and though individual chapters have specific authors, every chapter has been discussed collectively at various stages of its evolution. Thus, all chapters have been written in consultation with the entire Network and with the knowledge of the focus of other chapters in the collection. In that sense, this book is not an edited anthology of distinct entries but rather an integrated work written from a variety of disciplinary perspectives.

We also worked to incorporate cross-cultural perspectives in various places within the book. Although the authors are all Canadian-based, we come from diverse backgrounds (Canadian, British, American, Belgian) and most have carried out research in at least two different countries. We were fortunate to include two members with important backgrounds in cross-cultural research: Margaret Lock has done extensive cross-cultural research, particularly in Japan, and Maria De Koninck has been involved in international health projects in Central and West Africa. We have all made an active effort to place our Canadian experience in an international context.

The Domains Addressed

This book falls within the intersection of two domains: a worldwide feminist (health) movement that is concerned with improving the sta-

(found at least in the humanities) is an important aspect of feminism.

—Jocelyn

My years in Japan have taught me that conflict models are not the only way of conceptualizing and taking on entrenched inequalities. Negotiation, education, a free exchange of information from bottom up and top down, and even compromise can be more effective. Furthermore, our continuing addiction to quantitative methods, to objectivity, and the creation of clearly demarcated categories of people and experiences ensures that we virtually silence those voices we as feminists seek to engage. Narrative accounts given by women themselves are valuable for many reasons, one of which is that they can and should be used as the starting point for research in epidemiology, bioethics, the social sciences, and those aspects of clinical medicine which seek to explain and better the lived reality of individuals being studied.

—Margaret

As many of us have noted, women are the keepers of their family's history, perhaps the real historians. To be invited

tus of women's health, and the field known as bioethics (or biomedical ethics or health care ethics), which is occupied with value questions associated with the delivery of health services. With respect to the first, we build on the work of other feminist researchers who have amply demonstrated the multiple ways in which health care institutions, and especially medicine, have contributed to women's oppression. For example, Western health care systems have been organized to place disproportionate burdens on women (as unpaid and underpaid caregivers for those who are young, ill, or infirm). Women, and particularly women who are multiply disadvantaged by virtue of age, race, class, sexuality, or illness, have been poorly served by a health care system that has neglected many of their important health needs and interests; at the same time, health care institutions, especially medicine, are keenly interested in monitoring and intervening in all aspects of women's fertility. We analyze how theoretical, clinical, and research health care practices can be transformed to respond to women's needs, to empower women as health care subjects, and to serve the collective goals of social justice.

In addition, we seek to intervene in the discussions that currently constitute health care ethics in order to redirect and reshape some of the critical debates about health care practices to better accommodate feminist concerns. Ethics is the exploration of values governing behaviors and policies; health care ethics is the field that explores value questions in the area of health and health care. Most discussions within ethics and bioethics assume that gender is an irrelevant factor, so it tends to be invisible in debates about appropriate patient care. Our discussions challenge the assumption that gender should be ignored in normative discussions

*into the kitchen with the women
to hear the stories was a rite of
passage. But when the men came
in to lunch, the stories would end
and it would be some time after
the men left that the stories
would resume. But all too soon it
was suppertime. After a day of
work the men had gone to the
barn to drink. It became
increasingly difficult for the
women to get them in to eat on
time. There was a struggle
between the men not coming
when called for dinner, not
wanting to be seen to be at
the command of the women and
the women who had worked so
hard to prepare dinner. The
drinking became worse over
the years, the stories did not
come as readily any more. Abuse
to children and wives emerged
and the stories stopped. The
memory stopped. The women
did not want to remember.
It is my task as a historian
to remember.*

—Wendy

*I was raised on principles
of equality (for men) in the
workplace, working-class pride
and equality amongst races
and religions. Politics was seen
as a legitimate expression of
personal ethics. I also witnessed
my mother humiliated in
having to negotiate every
domestic economic decision
with the "breadwinner." These*

concerning health care. We argue that explicit antioppression values and policies must be situated at the core of health care deliberations.

We have chosen not to follow the usual categories of constructing health care ethics problems around types of medical interventions (e.g., euthanasia, abortion, genetic testing) or around the interactions of isolated patient-physician encounters (e.g., informed consent, truth telling, confidentiality). Nor do we follow familiar feminist attempts to focus exclusively on medical interventions that uniquely or primarily affect women (e.g., reproductive matters, breast cancer, eating disorders). Instead, we have chosen to think about the nature of women's interactions with the health care system and to understand better the sorts of structural change necessary to really give women more power over their health needs. Feminist health care ethics does not only change the way we handle traditional bioethical problems; it also changes the agenda of the discipline by making visible a whole range of new ethical problems. In that spirit, this book explores some of the issues that become visible when we ask what feminist bioethics looks like if we start from women's experiences and concerns with respect to health matters. By adopting an interdisciplinary approach, we are able to explore a wide range of issues from many complementary points of view. This book does not so much modify existing bioethics discussions as argue that bioethics should begin in a different place, with a recognition that ethics is inseparable from politics: in both health care and in ethics, the details of oppression must be prominently addressed.

We did not, then, restrict ourselves to discussion of those issues that happen to fall within these two fields (women's health and health care ethics) as they are currently de-

*life lessons were not then
conscious but formative in
my "feminism."*

        —Marilynne

*I try to understand women's
experience in what originally
differentiates them from men:
the body and its specificity.
That leads me, from the
perspective of reproductive
health, to the issues of how
inequalities have been built into
a system and are maintained as
such. Ethics is a way to look at
these issues.*

        —Maria

*My training came from "grass
roots" organization in the
women's movement. When I
moved into academic medicine
in 1989 as a teacher of Family
Medicine at Dalhousie
University, I held a personal
goal to develop a curriculum on
family violence for the residency
program. Concurrently in
clinical practice, I had started
working in a counseling role
with a number of women
survivors of child sexual abuse.
Most of these women could not
afford to access therapists in the
private sector. They were often
stigmatized as "difficult" patients
or dismissed with medical labels
which essentially closed the door
to exploration of the role of abuse
or assault in their lives.*

        —Marilynne

fined but rather saw ourselves as engaged in an effort to influence and transform discussions in each field, expanding and refocusing their respective agendas by providing an alternative conceptual framework that will be of use to each. Just as we chose not to review the major themes of bioethics and add a feminist component, we also decided against trying simply to add an ethics dimension to the current major threads of feminist health research. Instead, we consider some of the issues that emerge if one begins with a concern about how best to respond to women's health needs when one's aim is both to improve health and to relieve oppression.

The Content

The book builds upon two major themes that emerged as areas of common focus in the course of our challenging, ongoing discussions. The first is the theme of autonomy and agency, two related (and easily confused) concepts that together illuminate our understanding of women and their roles with respect to health and health services. The second, related theme concerns the dominant practice of modern health care structures to adopt a medical model that ignores the role of social conditions and concentrates its attention on individuals as the locus for health-promoting interventions. Both these themes have to do with values that are at the heart of current health care discussions; they draw on insights from feminist health literature to help to reconceptualize the field of health care ethics.

From our different areas of training and our different foci of research, we all struggled with the question of how to acknowledge women's agency and decision making within an oppressive system that limits and skews

*ım—and can
I am. I'm
hanging by many strands,
and though ever changing,
the strands do seem to hang
together more often than not.
Strands in my web right now
include those from the other
women in our network and my
hope is that mine can be
interwoven with theirs, as theirs
are with mine, as we all try to
contribute something to make
health possible for others.*

—Abby

the options available to them. We recognize that women often demonstrate agency by making choices regarding their health care, but we reject the view that actively choosing in itself constitutes autonomy, especially when the choices made might be harmful to those making the choices. The problem is that autonomy, as it is most commonly understood, fails to address ways in which oppression may contribute to the range of choices available and may affect the weight an oppressed person must assign each option. We chose, then, to draw a distinction between the concepts of agency and autonomy; we use the term *agency* to capture the familiar bioethical ideal of informed choice. We reserve the term *autonomy*, however, for a more comprehensive notion of freedom where not only is the immediate choice uncoerced but the circumstances that structure that choice are also free of the coercive dimension of oppression. Toward this end we define the concept of autonomy relationally; a relational interpretation of autonomy helps explain the apparent paradox of women "freely choosing" options that reinforce oppression. (See Chapter 2 for an explanation of this concept.)

The second theme of the book concerns our understanding of health and the social institutions that are created to promote it. We analyze the hold that biomedical models have over our cultural understandings of health and health care. In particular, we argue that medicine's tendency to focus on the individual obscures attention to the role of social conditions in health and illness. In contrast, we argue, greater attention must be directed to the responsibilities of society in matters concerning the health of its citizens.

Outline of the Chapters That Follow

*Chapter 2: A Relational Approach to Autonomy in Health Care
(Susan Sherwin)*
This chapter develops the central conceptual distinction that frames our discussion throughout the book. It critiques the nonfeminist bioethics literature on the concept of autonomy and provides a feminist alternative. Rather than reject the concept outright, as many fem-

inist theorists do, Sherwin argues that autonomy is still a highly useful ideal for forming the basis of a feminist ethics of health care; she
shows how to reclaim it in a fashion that provides it with liberatory
potential. By distinguishing agency, the authority to make choices
from a limited range of options, from a relational concept of autonomy that is attentive to the presence of oppression in constructing
choices, we are able to capture this often invisible layer of moral concern. Full autonomy, she argues, requires removal of the barriers of
oppression that often structure options in ways that further perpetuate existing patterns of oppression. This chapter lays the conceptual
groundwork for the more concrete uses of these terms throughout the
book.

Chapter 3: Situating Women in the Politics of Health (Margaret Lock)
This chapter explores the ways in which Western understandings of
health have become focused on the individual. It traces the culturally
specific understandings we have of the concepts of the "individual"
and "society" and it considers how the growth of scientific medical
knowledge has concentrated attention on the individual as the locus
of health and illness. It notes how twentieth-century resistance to
medicalization has taken the form of a moralistic sort of "healthism"
where the responsibility for health shifts from the experts to the individual; while experts are no longer always central to mediate specific health matters, attention remains concentrated on the individual. Although many feminist and other progressive groups have
actively promoted a version of healthism as a response to excessive
medicalization of women's health needs, it is a move that must be approached cautiously. Emphasizing the ways in which health is pri-
vatized, though the conditions of health are largely a matter of public policy, Lock reveals some of the limits to individual-centered
health promotion messages and argues for greater attention to be
given to the responsibilities of society in connection with the health
of its citizens.

*Chapter 4: The Politics of Health: Geneticization Versus Health Promotion
(Abby Lippman)*
Lippman elaborates on many of the themes considered by Lock in the
preceding chapter, particularly its discussion of the politics of health
and the limits of the biomedical conception of health as merely the absence of pathology/disease. She explores the way in which the move to
healthism is taking a new, and worrisome, form in the context of in-

creased "geneticization" in the late twentieth century where biological reductionism is combined with normative demands on individuals to identify genetic susceptibilities and take "appropriate action." This pressure is especially targeted at women who are increasingly expected to undergo prenatal testing and selective abortion to prevent the birth of children who may develop disabilities. She describes geneticization as both an emerging ideology and a set of practices that together divert attention from the structural changes necessary for true health promotion. This ideology competes directly with a widespread public health knowledge that economic and social conditions are primary determinants of health as articulated in several influential Canadian policy statements.

Chapter 5: Contested Bodies, Contested Knowledges: Women, Health, and the Politics of Medicalization (Kathryn Pauly Morgan)
In this chapter, Morgan analyzes four dialectically related elements of medicalization: conceptualization, macro-institutionalization, micro-institutionalization, and personal micro-institutionalization. She explores the oppressive potential of medicalization for women and explains the dangers of two powerful paradigms that structure medicalized thinking in North America: the biomedical model of the human body and the view of females as suffering from a "natural pathology." She stresses the need to view these elements in the context of local and global political economies, dimensions of patriarchy, relations to an ideology of technological control, and structural alliances. She then considers the role of the Women's Health Movement in challenging assumptions inherent in medicalization strategies through efforts to help women reclaim subjectivity and epistemic power.

Chapter 6: Agency, Diversity, and Constraints: Women and Their Physicians, Canada, 1850–1950 (Wendy Mitchinson)
Mitchinson examines a selection of encounters between women and their physicians in Canada from the mid-nineteenth century to the mid-twentieth century. This careful review reveals many of the dimensions of the social context that constructs and limits the choices of both women and their doctors during this period. Even though physicians have long held more power than their women patients, their power has never been unlimited; there have always been circumstances that constrained the choices they could offer their patients. Moreover, many women have had opportunities to exercise choice and agency in their encounters with physicians; indeed, in many cases, it was the demands

of women that led to the institutionalization of medical practices that later generations of women came to criticize (e.g., twilight sleep for childbirth). Mitchinson makes clear, then, that medicalization is not a one-way street of power-hungry physicians imposing their methods on unwilling or ignorant women but rather is a dynamic process where significant numbers of women became dependent on physicians for re-production-related services and actively demanded better (safer, less painful) procedures. Once these procedures were accepted by a number of women, they often became the norm for other women in comparable situations (though available options could vary with race and class) such that other women had no other realistic options available to them.

Chapter 7: Reflections on the Transfer of "Progress": The Case of Reproduction (Maria De Koninck)
In this chapter, De Koninck reports on her experience of conducting re-search in Benin, a small, very poor African country with extremely high rates of maternal mortality and morbidity. She questions the growing global consensus that the organization of emergency obstetric care is the most efficient means to reduce maternal mortality. De Koninck engaged in field research in order to better understand the local women's own approach to the very high maternal mortality and morbidity rates in their country. She notes that Western medical practices are built around a particular understanding of and attitude toward risk as something that must be controlled through scientific management, an attitude she found to be quite foreign to the local women. Reflecting on the local women's own practices and desires with respect to reproduction, she argues that the women in Benin would be better served by global inter-ventions that improve their social position than by actions that put an emphasis on medical interventions aimed at problematic deliveries. This position is disquieting, since putting in place emergency services might appear as a quick life-saving solution, whereas social changes take time. But effectively reducing maternal morbidity and mortality ul-timately require these deeper sorts of changes.

Chapter 8: Anomalous Women and Political Strategies for Aging Societies (Margaret Lock)
Lock examines the ways in which North American and Japanese cul-tures approach the notion of middle age in women. She observes that both countries seem alarmed about the number of elderly women that are likely to be present in the near future and are very worried about the "expense" so many old women are likely to create. In North America

this translates into increasing medicalization of menopause, now widely defined as a disease of estrogen-deficiency. Pharmaceutical-sponsored medical research documents the many health hazards facing unmedicated women and stresses the cost savings to the public health system if medicine can reduce the number of heart attacks and broken bones experienced by elderly women. In the face of such discourse, some women have come to view not only menopause but the whole of their remaining life course as one in which they must ward off pathology through regular use of powerful medication. In contrast, the concern in Japan is on ensuring that the elderly will be cared for at home by family members and not become dependent on the state; this care is generally provided by women and there are active government efforts to promote a sense of duty among middle-aged women to care for their aging parents and in-laws. In such an environment, there is little notice of menopause as a significant life change and far fewer "symptoms" experienced. Lock argues that the body is understood in a cultural context and subject to different cultural interpretations, that biology is largely local. Differences in local biology mean that subjectivity and cultural discourse together create differences in the very experience of menopause. We must, then, decenter the reigning notion of a universalist biology. Her cross-cultural study helps the reader appreciate how culture and biology interact in ways that determine the options and choices available to women.

Chapter 9: (Re)fashioning Medicine's Response to Wife Abuse (Marilynne Bell and Janet Mosher)

Violence against women within their intimate relationships is a pervasive social problem. When violence results in injuries, as it often does, many women turn to physicians for assistance, though most do not disclose the cause of their injuries. The majority of physicians fail to identify abuse as the cause of the injuries, and even when abuse is identified, they often respond in inappropriate ways that can result in various sorts of harms. Protocols and guidelines have moved to the forefront of attempts to transform these practices and to bring wife abuse within the parameters of the everyday practice of physicians. Bell and Mosher evaluate this response under three broad headings: medicalization, standardization, and dichotimization. They argue that protocols and guidelines are frequently grounded in a biomedical model in which abuse is transformed from a social problem requiring fundamental redistributions of power into a medical entity requiring "treatment." While routine screening according to a standard protocol in the hands of a physician knowledgeable about abuse (including how violence, and responses to it, are constructed along various axes of oppression) will benefit women, routine approaches in the hands of untrained physicians are likely to harm many women. The authors also argue that protocols frequently draw upon the pervasive dichotimization of victim and agent, treating abused women as passive victims, incapable of making sound decisions. While abused women frequently lack full autonomy in the sense developed by Sherwin, they do exercise agency. The authors conclude by describing the responsibilities of the profession collectively and of individual practitioners to respond to a social problem with grave health consequences for women.

Chapter 10: Reframing Research Involving Humans (Françoise Baylis, Jocelyn Downie, and Susan Sherwin)
In this chapter, Baylis, Downie, and Sherwin discuss the Network's interactions with a national Working Group assigned the task of drafting a common set of ethics guidelines to cover all government-sponsored research involving human subject-participants. They provide an overview of the theoretical views that informed this engagement and a detailed account of the Network's feminist concerns regarding research involving human subject-participants (with particular attention being paid to women). The chapter reviews the Network's efforts to take these views and concerns to the policy-making process. It describes the various interventions (formal and informal) with the Working Group and explores some ways in which the Network appears to have been effective and other ways in which it appears to have been marginalized. It illustrates how Sherwin's understanding of relational autonomy structured the interventions and was translated into specific recommendations. It also self-consciously highlights some of the ways in which autonomy and agency were present in both the substance and process of the Network's efforts to reframe research involving humans.

NOTES

Acknowledgments: Our research was funded by the Social Sciences and Humanities Research Council of Canada (SSHRC) as a Strategic Research Network Grant (Susan Sherwin, Principal Investigator). We wish to thank Ariella Pahlke, who was especially helpful in selecting the quotations that appear in this chapter and in the last section ("About the Authors").
 1. All quotations that appear in sidebars in this chapter are selected from in-

ternal communications among Network members. Italicized quotations in the final section ("About the Authors") are from the same sources.

2. We follow Iris Marion Young (1990) in her definition of the faces of oppression as exploitation, powerlessness, marginalization, cultural dominance, and violence.

3. For a fuller discussion of our conception of feminism see Sherwin 1992.

4. Janet Mosher was especially helpful in drafting this section.

5. The precise significance of location for knowing is a matter of considerable debate; see for example Minnich 1990, Yeatman 1993, Bordo 1990.

6. Our SSHRC grant was in the category of Strategic Research Network Grants. This area of grant support is designed to encourage collaborative research on subjects SSHRC considers to be of important social worth (in this case, applied ethics), among academics from diverse disciplines and universities, i.e., a group of researchers who otherwise face institutional and geographic barriers to interdisciplinary research. The terms of the grant restricted support for participation to academics who are either Canadian or employed at a Canadian institution. These restrictions prohibited us from including participants with more grassroots backgrounds and limited the diversity of our Network in ways that frequently made us uncomfortable.

2

A Relational Approach to Autonomy in Health Care

Susan Sherwin

Respect for patient autonomy (or self-direction) is broadly understood as recognition that patients have the authority to make decisions about their own health care. The principle that insists on this recognition is pervasive in the bioethics literature: it is a central value within virtually all the leading approaches to health care ethics, feminist and other. It is not surprising, then, that discussions of autonomy constantly emerged within our own conversations in the Network; readers will recognize that autonomy is woven throughout the book in our various approaches to the issues we take up. It is, however, an ideal that we felt deeply ambivalent about, and, therefore, we judged it to be in need of a specifically feminist analysis.

In this chapter, I propose a feminist analysis of autonomy, making vivid both our attraction to and distrust of the dominant interpretation of this concept. I begin by reviewing some of the appeal of the autonomy ideal in order to make clear why it has achieved such prominence within bioethics and feminist health care discussions. I then identify some difficulties I find with the usual interpretations of the concept, focusing especially on difficulties that arise from a specifically feminist perspective. In response to these problems, I propose an alternative conception of autonomy that I label "relational" though the terms *socially situated* or *contextualized* would describe it equally well. To avoid confusion, I explicitly distinguish my use of the term *relational* from that of some other feminist authors, such as Carol Gilligan (1982), who reserve it to refer only to the narrower set of interpersonal relations. I apply the term to the full range of influential human relations, personal and public. Oppression permeates both personal and public relationships; hence, I prefer to politicize the understanding of the term *relational* as a way of emphasizing the political dimensions of the multiple relationships that structure an individual's selfhood, rather than to reserve the term to protect a sphere of purely private relationships that may appear to be free of political influence.[1] I explain why I think the relational alternative is more successful than the familiar individualistic interpretation at addressing the concerns identified. Finally, I briefly indicate some of the implications of adopting a relational interpretation of autonomy with respect to some of the issues discussed elsewhere in this book, and I identify some of the changes that this notion of relational autonomy suggests for the delivery of health services.

The Virtues of a Principle of Respect for Patient Autonomy

It is not hard to explain the prominence of the principle of respect for patient autonomy within the field of health care ethics in North America: respect for personal autonomy is a dominant value in North American culture and it plays a central role in most of our social institutions. Yet, protection of autonomy is often at particular risk in health care settings because illness, by its very nature, tends to make patients dependent on the care and good will of others; in so doing, it reduces patients' power to exercise autonomy and it also makes them vulnerable to manipulation and even to outright coercion by those who provide them with needed health services. Many patients who are either ill or at risk of becoming ill are easily frightened into overriding their own preferences and following expert advice rather than risking abandonment by their caregivers by rejecting that advice. Even when their health is not immediately threatened, patients may find themselves compelled to comply with the demands of health care providers in order to obtain access to needed services from health professionals who are, frequently, the only ones licensed to provide those services (e.g., abortion, assistance in childbirth, legitimate excuses from work, physiotherapy).[2]

Without a strong principle of respect for patient autonomy, patients are vulnerable to abuse or exploitation, when their weak and dependent position makes them easy targets to serve the interests (e.g., financial, academic, or social influence) of others. Strong moral traditions of service within medicine and other health professions have provided patients with some measure of protection against such direct harms, though abuses nonetheless occur.[3] Most common is the tendency of health care providers to assume that by virtue of their technical expertise they are better able to judge what is in the patient's best interest than is the patient. For example, physicians may make assumptions about the advantages of using fetal heart monitors when women are in labor without considering the ways in which such instruments restrict laboring-women's movement and the quality of the birthing experience from their perspective. By privileging their own types of knowledge over that of their patients (including both experiential knowledge and understanding of their own value scheme), health care providers typically ignore patients' expressed or implicit values and engage in paternalism[4] (or the overriding of patient preferences for the presumed benefit of the patient) when prescribing treatment.

Until very recently, conscientious physicians were actually trained to act paternalistically toward their patients, to treat patients according to the physician's own judgment about what would be best for their patients[5], with little regard for each patient's own perspectives or preferences. The problem with this arrangement, however, is that health care may involve such intimate and central aspects of a patient's life—including, for example, matters such as health, illness, reproduction, death, dying, bodily integrity, nutrition, lifestyle, self-image, disability, sexuality, and psychological well-being—that it is difficult for anyone other than the patient to make choices that will be compatible with that patient's personal value system. Indeed, making such choices is often an act of self-discovery or self-definition and as such it requires the active involvement of the patient. Whenever possible, then, these types of choices should be made by the person whose life is central to the treatment considered. The principle of respect for patient autonomy is aimed at clarifying and protecting patients' ultimate right to make up their own minds about the specific health services they receive (so long as they are competent to do so). It also helps to ensure that patients have full access to relevant information about their health status so that they can make informed choices about related aspects of their lives. For example, information about a terminal condition may affect a person's decisions to reproduce, take a leave of absence from work, seek a reconciliation from estranged friends or relatives, or revise a will.

Although theorists disagree about the precise definition of *autonomy*,[5] there are some common features to its use within bioethics. In practice, the principle of respect for patient autonomy is usually interpreted as acknowledging and protecting competent patients' authority to accept or refuse whatever specific treatments the health care providers they consult find it appropriate to offer them (an event known as informed choice). Since everyone can imagine being in the position of patient, and most can recognize the dangers of fully surrendering this authority to near strangers, it is not surprising that the principle of respect for patient autonomy is widely endorsed by nearly all who consider it. Despite different theoretical explanations, the overwhelming majority of bioethicists insist on this principle as a fundamental moral precept for health care. Support is especially strong in North America, where it fits comfortably within a general cultural milieu in which attention to the individual and protection of individual rights are granted (at least rhetorical) dominance in nearly all areas of social and political policy.[6] Both Canadian and U.S. courts have underlined the importance of protection of individual rights as a central tenet of patient-provider interactions, making it a matter of legal as well as moral concern.

Further, the principle requiring respect for patient autonomy helps to resolve problems that arise when health care providers are responsible for the care of patients who have quite different experiences, values, and world views from their own; under such circumstances, it is especially unlikely that care givers can accurately anticipate the particular needs and interests of their patients. This problem becomes acute when there are significant differences in power between patients and the health care professionals who care for them. In most cases, the relevant interactions are between patients and physicians, where, typically, patients have less social power than their physicians: doctors are well educated and they tend to be (relatively) healthy and affluent, while the patients they care for are often poor, and lacking in education and social authority. In fact, according to most of the standard dichotomies supporting dominance in our culture—gender, class, race, ability status—odds are that if there is a difference between the status of the physician and the patient, the physician is likely to fall on the dominant side of that distinction and the patient on the subordinate side. The tendency of illness to undermine patients' autonomy is especially threatening when the patients in question face other powerful barriers to the exercise of their autonomy, as do members of groups subject to systemic discrimination on the basis of gender, race, class, disability, age, sexual preference, or any other such feature. A principle insisting on protection of patient autonomy can be an important corrective to such overwhelming power imbalances.

Moreover, physician privilege and power is not the only threat to patient autonomy. Increasingly, the treatment options available to both patients and physicians are circumscribed by the policies of governments and other third-party payers. In the current economic climate, those who fund health care services are insisting on ever more stringent restrictions on access to specific treatment options; physicians find themselves asked to perform gate-keeping functions to keep costs under control. In such circumstances, where patient care may be decided by general guidelines that tend to be insensitive to the particular circumstances of specific patients, and where the financial interests of the institution being billed for the patient's care may take priority over the patient's needs or preferences, the principle of respect for patient autonomy becomes more complicated to interpret even as it takes on added importance.

The principle of respect for patient autonomy can also be seen as an attractive ideal for feminists because of its promise to protect the rights and interests of even the most socially disadvantaged patients. Feminist medical historians, anthropologists, and sociologists have documented many ways in which health care providers have repeatedly neglected and misperceived the needs and wishes of the women they treat.[7] The ideal of respect for patient autonomy seems a promising way to correct much that is objectionable in the abuses that feminist researchers have documented in the delivery of health services to women and minorities. Most feminists believe that the forces of systematic domination and oppression work together to limit the autonomy of women and members of other oppressed groups; many of their political efforts can be seen as aimed at disrupting those forces and promoting greater degrees of autonomy (often represented as personal "choice") for individuals who fall victim to oppression. For example, many feminists appeal at least implicitly to the moral norm of autonomy in seeking to increase the scope of personal control for women in all areas of their reproductive lives (especially with respect to birth control, abortion, and childbirth, often discussed under a general rubric of "reproductive freedom" or "reproductive choice").

In a world where most cultures are plagued by sexism, which is usually compounded by other deeply entrenched oppressive patterns, fundamental respect for the humanity, dignity, and autonomy of members of disadvantaged groups, though extremely fragile, seems very important and in need of strong ethical imperatives. Feminists strive to be sensitive to the ways in which gender, race, class, age, disability, sexual orientation, and marital status can undermine a patient's authority and credibility in health care contexts and most are aware of the long history of powerful medical control over women's lives. They have good reason, then, to oppose medical domination through paternalism. Promotion of patient autonomy appears to be a promising alternative.[8] Understood in its traditional sense as the alternative to heteronomy (governance by others), autonomy (self-governance) seems to be an essential feature of any feminist strategy for improving health services for women and achieving a nonoppressive society.

Problems with the Autonomy Ideal

Nonetheless, despite this broad consensus about the value of a principle of respect for patient autonomy in health care, there are many problems with the principle as it is usually interpreted and applied in health care ethics. As many health critics have observed, we need to question how much control individual patients really have over the determination of their treatment within the stressful world of health care services. Even a casual encounter with most modern hospitals reveals that wide agreement about the moral importance of respect for patient autonomy does not always translate into a set of practices that actually respect and foster patient autonomy in any meaningful sense. Ensuring that patients meet some measure of informed choice—or, more commonly, informed consent—[9] before receiving or declining treatment has become accepted as the most promising mechanism for insuring patient autonomy in health care settings, but, in practice, the effectiveness of the actual procedures used to obtain informed consent usually falls short of fully protecting patient autonomy. This gap is easy to understand: attention to patient autonomy can be a time-consuming business and the demands of identifying patient values and preferences are often sacrificed in the face of heavy patient loads and staff shortages. In addition, health care providers are often constrained from promoting and responding to patients' autonomy in health care because of pressures they experience to contain health care costs and to avoid making themselves liable to lawsuits. Moreover, most health care providers are generally not well trained in the communication skills necessary to ensure that patients have the requisite understanding to provide genuine informed consent. This problem is compounded within our increasingly diverse urban communities where differences in language and culture between health care providers and the patients they serve may create enormous practical barriers to informed choice.

There are yet deeper problems with the ideal of autonomy invoked in most bioethical discussions. The paradigm offered for informed consent is built on a model of articulate, intelligent patients who are accustomed to making decisions about the course of their lives and who possess the resources necessary to allow them a range of options to choose among. Decisions are constructed as a product of objective calculation on the basis of near perfect information. Clearly, not all patients meet these ideal conditions (perhaps none does), yet there are no satisfactory guidelines available about how to proceed when dealing with patients who do not fit the paradigm.

Feminist analysis reveals several problems inherent in the very construction of the concept of autonomy that is at the heart of most bioethics discussions.[10] One problem is that autonomy provisions are sometimes interpreted as functioning independently of and outweighing all other moral values. More specifically, autonomy is often understood to exist in conflict with the demands of justice because the requirements of the latter may have to be imposed on unwilling citizens. Autonomy is frequently interpreted to mean freedom from interference; this analysis can be invoked (as it frequently is) to oppose taxation as coercive and, hence, a violation of personal autonomy. But coercive measures like taxation are essential if a society wants to reduce inequity and provide the disadvantaged with access to the means (e.g., basic necessities, social respect, education, and health care) that are necessary for meaningful exercise of their autonomy. In contrast to traditional accounts of autonomy that accept and indeed presume some sort of tension between autonomy and justice, feminism encourages us to see the connections between these two central moral ideals.

In fact, autonomy language is often used to hide the workings of privilege and to mask the barriers of oppression. For example, within North America it seems that people who were raised in an atmosphere of privilege and respect come rather easily to think of themselves as independent and self-governing; it feels natural to them to conceive of themselves as autonomous. Having been taught that they need only to apply themselves in order to take advantage of the opportunities available to them, most learn to think of their successes as self-created and deserved. Such thinking encourages them to be oblivious to the barriers that oppression and disadvantage create, and it allows them to see the failures of others as evidence of the latters' unwillingness to exercise their own presumed autonomy responsibly. This individualistic approach to autonomy makes it very easy for people of privilege to remain ignorant of the social arrangements that support their own sense of independence, such as the institutions that provide them with an exceptionally good education and a relatively high degree of personal safety. Encouraged to focus on their own sense of individual accomplishment, they are inclined to blame less well-situated people for their lack of comparable success rather than to appreciate the costs of oppression. This familiar sort of thinking tends to interfere with people's ability to see the importance of supportive social conditions for fostering autonomous action. By focusing instead on the injustice that is associated with oppression, feminism helps us to recognize that autonomy is best achieved where the social conditions that support it are in place. Hence, it provides us with an alternative perspective for understanding a socially grounded notion of autonomy.

Further, the standard conception of autonomy, especially as it is invoked in bioethics, tends to place the focus of concern quite narrowly on particular decisions of individuals; that is, it is common to speak of specific health care decisions as autonomous, or, at least, of the patient as autonomous with respect to the decision at hand. Such analyses discourage attention to the context in which decisions are actually made. Patient decisions are considered to be autonomous if the patient is (1) deemed to be sufficiently competent (rational) to make the decision at issue, (2) makes a (reasonable) choice from a set of available options, (3) has adequate information and understanding about the available choices, and (4) is free from explicit coercion toward (or away from) one of those options. It is assumed that these criteria can be evaluated in any particular case, simply by looking at the state of the patient and her deliberations in isolation from the social conditions that structure her options. Yet, each of these conditions is more problematic than is generally recognized.

The competency criterion threatens to exclude people who are oppressed from the scope of autonomy provisions altogether. This is because competency is often equated with being rational,[11] yet the rationality of women and members of other oppressed groups is frequently denied. In fact, as Genevieve Lloyd (1984) has shown, the very concept of rationality has been constructed in opposition to the traits that are stereotypically assigned to women (e.g., by requiring that agents demonstrate objectivity and emotional distance),[12] with the result that women are often seen as simply incapable of rationality.[13] Similar problems arise with respect to stereotypical assumptions about members of racial minorities, indigenous peoples, persons with disabilities, welfare recipients, people from developing countries, those who are nonliterate, and so on. Minimally, then, health care providers must become sensitive to the ways in which oppressive stereotypes can undermine their ability to recognize some sorts of patients as being rational or competent.

Consider, also, the second condition, which has to do with making a (reasonable) choice from the set of available options. Here, the difficulty is that the set of available options is constructed in ways that may already seriously limit the patient's autonomy by prematurely excluding options the patient might have preferred. There is a whole series of complex decisions that together shape the set of options that health care providers are able to offer their patients: these can involve such factors as the forces that structure research programs, the types of results that journals are willing to publish, curriculum priorities in medical and other professional schools, and funding policies within the health care system.[14] While all patients will face limited choices by virtue of these sorts of institutional policy decisions, the consequences are especially significant for members of oppressed groups because they tend to be underrepresented on the bodies that make these earlier decisions, and therefore their interests are less likely to be reflected in each of the background decisions that are made. In general, the sorts of institutional decisions in question tend to reflect the biases of discriminatory values and practices.[15] Hence, the outcomes of these multiple earlier decisions can have a significant impact on an oppressed patient's ultimate autonomy by disproportionately and unfairly restricting the choices available to her. Nevertheless, such background conditions are seldom visible within discussions of patient autonomy in bioethics.

The third condition is also problematic in that the information made available to patients is, inevitably, the information that has been deemed worthy of study and that is considered relevant by the health care providers involved. Again, research, publication, and education policies largely determine what sorts of data are collected and, significantly, what questions are neglected; systemic bias unquestionably influences these policies. Further, the very large gap in life experience between physicians, who are, by virtue of their professional status, relatively privileged members of society, and some of their seriously disadvantaged patients makes the likelihood of the former anticipating the specific information needs of the latter questionable. While an open consent process will help reduce this gap by providing patients with the opportunity to raise questions, patients often feel too intimidated to ask or even formulate questions, especially when they feel socially and intellectually inferior to their physicians and when the physicians project an image of being busy with more important demands. Often, one needs some information in order to know what further questions to ask, and large gaps in perspective between patients and their health care providers may result in a breakdown in communication because of false assumptions by either participant.

The fourth condition, the one that demands freedom from coercion in exercising choice, is extremely difficult to evaluate when the individual in question is oppressed. The task becomes even trickier if the choice is in a sphere that is tied to her oppression. The condition of being oppressed can be so fundamentally restrictive that it is distorting to describe as autonomous some specific choices made under such con-

ditions. For example, many women believe they have no real choice but
to seek expensive, risky cosmetic surgery because they accurately perceive that their opportunities for success in work or love depend on
their more closely approximating some externally defined standard of
beauty. Similar sorts of questions arise with respect to some women's
choice of dangerous, unproven experiments in new reproductive technologies because continued childlessness can be expected to have devastating consequences for their lives. In other cases, women sometimes
choose to have abortions because they fear that giving birth will involve them in unwanted and lifelong relationships with abusive partners. Some women have little access to contraceptives and find themselves choosing sterilization as the most effective way of resisting
immediate demands of their partners even if they might want more
children in the future. Or, some women seek out prenatal diagnosis
and selective abortion of cherished fetuses because they realize that
they cannot afford to raise a child born with a serious disability, though
they would value such a child themselves. Many middle-class Western
women choose hormone replacement therapy at menopause because
they recognize that their social and economic lives may be threatened
if they appear to be aging too quickly. When a woman's sense of herself and her range of opportunities have been oppressively constructed
in ways that (seem to) leave her little choice but to pursue all available
options in the pursuit of beauty or childbearing or when she is raised
in a culture that ties her own sense of herself to external norms of physical appearance or fulfillment associated with childbearing or, conversely, when having a(nother) child will impose unjust and intolera-
ble costs on her, it does not seem sufficient to restrict our analysis to the
degree of autonomy associated with her immediate decision about a
particular treatment offered. We need a way of acknowledging how
oppressive circumstances can interfere with autonomy, but this is not
easily captured in traditional accounts.

Finally, there are good reasons to be wary of the ways in which the
appearance of choice is used to mask the normalizing powers of medicine and other health-related institutions. As Michel Foucault (1979,
1980b) suggests, in modern societies the illusion of choice can be part
of the mechanism for controlling behavior. Indeed, it is possible that
bioethical efforts to guarantee the exercise of individual informed
choice may actually make the exercise of medical authority even more
powerful and effective than it would be under more traditionally paternalistic models. In practice, the ideal of informed choice amounts to
assuring patients of the opportunity to consent to one of a limited list

of relatively similar, medically encouraged procedures. Thus, informed consent procedures aimed simply at protecting autonomy in the narrow sense of specific choice among preselected options may ultimately serve to secure the compliance of docile patients who operate under the illusion of autonomy by virtue of being invited to consent to procedures they are socially encouraged to choose. Unless we find a way of identifying a deeper sense of autonomy than that associated with the expression of individual preference in selecting among a limited set of similar options, we run the risk of struggling to protect not patient autonomy but the very mechanisms that insure compliant medical consumers, preoccupied with the task of selecting among a narrow range of treatments.

Focus on the Individual

A striking feature of most bioethical discussions about patient autonomy is their exclusive focus on individual patients; this pattern mirrors medicine's consistent tendency to approach illness as primarily a problem of particular patients.[16] Similar problems are associated with each discipline. Within the medical tradition, suffering is located and addressed in the individuals who experience it rather than in the social arrangements that may be responsible for causing the problem. Instead of exploring the cultural context that tolerates and even supports practices such as war, pollution, sexual violence, and systemic unemployment—practices that contribute to much of the illness that occupies modern medicine—physicians generally respond to the symptoms troubling particular patients in isolation from the context that produces these conditions. Apart from population-based epidemiological studies (which, typically, restrict their focus to a narrow range of patterns of illness and often exclude or distort important social dimensions), medicine is primarily oriented toward dealing with individuals who have become ill (or pregnant, [in]fertile, or menopausal). This orientation directs the vast majority of research money and expertise toward the things that can be done to change the individual, but it often ignores key elements at the source of the problems.

For example, physicians tend to respond to infertility either by trivializing the problem and telling women to go home and "relax," or by prescribing hormonal and surgical treatment of particular women, rather than by demanding that research and public health efforts be aimed at preventing pelvic inflammatory disease, which causes many cases of infertility, or by encouraging wide public debate (or private reflections) on the powerful social pressures to reproduce that are directed at women. In similar fashion, the mainstream scientific and medical communities respond to the growth of breast cancer rates by promoting individual responsibility for self-examination and by searching for the gene(s) that makes some women particularly susceptible to the disease; when it is found in a patient, the principal medical therapy available is to perform "prophylactic" double mastectomies. Few physicians demand examination of the potential contributory role played by the use of pesticides or chlorine, or the practice of feeding artificial hormones to agricultural animals. Or they deal with dramatically increased skin cancer rates by promoting the personal use of sunscreens while resigning themselves to the continued depletion of the ozone layer. In another area, health care professionals generally deal with the devastating effects of domestic violence by patching up its victims, providing them with medications to relieve depression and advice to move out of their homes, and devising pathological names for victims who stay in violent relationships ("battered woman syndrome" and "self-defeating personality disorder"), but few actively challenge the sexism that accepts male violence as a "natural" response to frustration and fears of abandonment.[17]

Some qualifications are in order. Clearly, these are crude and imprecise generalizations. They describe a general orientation of current health practices, but they certainly do not capture the work of all those involved in medical research and practice. Fortunately, there are practitioners and researchers engaged in the very sorts of investigation I call for, but they are exceptional, not typical. Moreover, I do not want to imply that medicine should simply abandon its concern with treating disease in individuals. I understand that prevention strategies will not eliminate all illness and I believe that personalized health care must continue to be made available to those who become ill. Further, I want to be clear that my critique does not imply that physicians or other direct care providers are necessarily the ones who ought to be assuming the task of identifying the social and environmental causes of disease. Health care training, and especially the training of physicians, is directed at developing the requisite skills for the extremely important work of caring for individuals who become ill. The responsibility for investigating the social causes of illness and for changing hazardous conditions is a social one that is probably best met by those who undertake different sorts of training and study. The problem is that medicine, despite the limits of its expertise and focus, is the primary agent of health care activity in our society and physicians are granted significant social authority to be the arbiters of health policy. Hence, when medicine makes the treatment of individuals its primary focus, we must understand that important gaps are created in our society's ability to understand and promote good health.

In parallel fashion, autonomy-focused bioethics concentrates its practitioners' attention on the preferences of particular patients, and it is, thereby, complicit in the individualistic orientation of medicine. It asks health care providers to ensure that individual patients have the information they need to make rational decisions about their health care, yet it does not ask the necessary questions about the circumstances in which such decisions are made. The emphasis most bioethicists place on traditional, individualistic understandings of autonomy reinforces the tendency of health care providers and ethicists to neglect exploration of the deep social causes and conditions that contribute to health and illness. Moreover, it encourages patients to see their own health care decisions in isolation from those of anyone else, thereby increasing their sense of vulnerability and dependence on medical authority.

The narrow individual focus that characterizes the central traditions within both medicine and bioethics obscures our need to consider questions of power, dominance, and privilege in our interpretations and responses to illness and other health-related matters as well as in our interpretations of the ideal of autonomy. These ways of structuring thought and practice make it difficult to see the political dimensions of illness, and, in a parallel way, they obscure the political dimensions of the conventional criteria for autonomous deliberation. As a result, they interfere with our ability to identify and pursue more effective health practices while helping to foster a social environment that ignores and tolerates oppression. In both cases, a broader political perspective is necessary if we are to avoid the problems created by restricting our focus to individuals apart from their location.

Feminism offers just such a broader perspective. In contrast to the standard approaches in bioethics, feminism raises questions about the social basis for decisions about health and health care at all levels. Here, as elsewhere, feminists are inclined to ask whose interests are served and whose are harmed by the traditional ways of structuring thought and practice. By asking these questions, we are able to see how assumptions of individual-based medicine help to preserve the social and political status quo. For example, the current taxonomy in Canada designates certain sorts of conditions (e.g., infertility, cancer, heart disease, anxiety) as appropriate for medical intervention, and it provides grounds for ensuring that such needs are met. At the same time, it views other sorts of conditions (e.g., malnutrition, fear of assault, low self-esteem) as falling beyond the purview of the health care system and, therefore, as ineligible to draw on the considerable resources allocated to the delivery of health services.[18] In this way, individualistic assumptions support a system that provides expert care for many of the health complaints of those with greatest financial privilege while dismissing as outside the scope of health care many of the sources of illness that primarily affect the disadvantaged. A more social vision of health would require us to investigate ways in which nonmedical strategies, such as improving social and material conditions for disadvantaged groups, can affect the health status of different segments of the community.[19]

None of the concerns I have identified argues against maintaining a strong commitment to autonomy in bioethical deliberations. In fact, I have no wish to abandon this ideal (just as I have no desire to abandon patient-centered medical care). I still believe that a principle of respect for patient autonomy is an important element of good patient care. Moreover, I believe that appeal to a principle of respect for autonomy can be an important instrument in challenging oppression and it can actually serve as the basis for many of the feminist criticisms I present with respect to our current health care system.[20]

What these criticisms do suggest, however, is that we must pursue a more careful and politically sensitive interpretation of the range of possible restrictions on autonomy than is found in most of the nonfeminist bioethics literature. We need to be able to look at specific decisions as well as the context that influences and sometimes limits such decisions. Many of the troublesome examples I review above are entirely compatible with traditional conceptions of autonomy, even though the patients in question may be facing unjust barriers to care or may be acting in response to oppressive circumstances; traditional conceptions are inadequate to the extent that they make invisible the oppression that structures such decisions. By focusing only on the moment of medical decision making, traditional views fail to examine how specific decisions are embedded within a complex set of relations and policies that constrain (or, ideally, promote) an individual's ability to exercise autonomy with respect to any particular choice.

To understand this puzzle it is necessary to distinguish between agency and autonomy. To exercise agency, one need only exercise reasonable choice.[21] The women who choose some of the controversial practices discussed (e.g., abortion to avoid contact with an abusive partner, cosmetic surgery to conform to artificial norms of beauty, use of dangerous forms of reproductive technology) are exercising agency;

clearly they are making choices, and, often, those choices are rational under the circumstances.[22] They also meet the demands of conventional notions of autonomy that ask only that anyone contemplating such procedures be competent, or capable of choosing (wisely), have available information current practice deems relevant, and be free of direct coercion. But insofar as their behavior accepts and adapts to oppression, describing it as autonomous seems inadequate. Together, the habits of equating agency (the making of a choice) with autonomy (self-governance) and accepting as given the prevailing social arrangements have the effect of helping to perpetuate oppression: when we limit our analysis to the quality of an individual's choice under existing conditions (or when we fail to inquire why some people do not even seek health services), we ignore the significance of oppressive conditions. Minimally, autonomous persons should be able to resist oppression—not just act in compliance with it—and be able to refuse the choices oppression seems to make nearly irresistible. Ideally, they should be able to escape from the structures of oppression altogether and create new options that are not defined by these structures either positively or negatively.

In order to ensure that we recognize and address the restrictions that oppression places on people's health choices, then, we need a wider notion of autonomy that will allow us to distinguish genuinely autonomous behavior from acts of merely rational agency. This conception must provide room to challenge the quality of an agent's specific decision-making ability and the social norms that encourage agents to participate in practices that may be partially constitutive of their oppression.[23] A richer, more politically sensitive standard of autonomy should make visible the impact of oppression on a person's choices as well as on her very ability to exercise autonomy fully. Such a conception has the advantage of allowing us to avoid the trap of focusing on the supposed flaws of the individual who is choosing under oppressive circumstances (e.g., by dismissing her choices as "false consciousness"), for it is able to recognize that such choices can be reasonable for the agent. Instead, it directs our attention to the conditions that shape the agent's choice and it makes those conditions the basis of critical analysis.

The problems that I identify with the conventional interpretation of patient autonomy reveal a need to expand our understanding of the types of forces that interfere with a patient's autonomy. On nonfeminist accounts, these are irrationality, failure to recognize that a choice is called for, lack of necessary information, and coercion (including psychological compulsion). Since each of these conditions must be reinterpreted to allow for the ways in which oppression may be operating, we must add to this list recognition of the costs and effects of oppression and of the particular ways in which oppression is manifested. But we must do more than simply modify our interpretation of the four criteria reviewed above. We also need an understanding of the ways in which a person can be encouraged to develop (or discouraged from developing) the ability to exercise autonomy. For this task, we need to consider the presence or absence of meaningful opportunities to build the skills required to be able to exercise autonomy well (Meyers 1989), including the existence of appropriate material and social conditions. In addition, our account should reflect the fact that many decision makers, especially women, place the interests of others at the center of their deliberations. Such an analysis will allow us to ensure that autonomy standards reflect not only the quality of reasoning displayed by a patient at the moment of medical decision making but also the circumstances that surround this decision making.

A Relational Alternative

A major reason for many of the problems identified with the autonomy ideal is that the term is commonly understood to represent freedom of action for agents who are paradigmatically regarded as independent, self-interested, and self-sufficient. As such, it is part of a larger North American cultural ideal of competitive individualism in which every citizen is to be left "free" to negotiate "his" way through the complex interactions of social, economic, and political life.[24] The feminist literature is filled with criticism of such models of agency and autonomy: for example, many feminists object that this ideal appeals to a model of personhood that is distorting because, in fact, no one is fully independent. As well, they observe that this model is exclusionary because those who are most obviously dependent on others (e.g., because of disability or financial need) seem to be disqualified from consideration in ways that others are not. Many feminists object that the view of individuals as isolated social units is not only false but impoverished: much of who we are and what we value is rooted in our relationships and affinities with others. Also, many feminists take issue with the common assumption that agents are single-mindedly self-interested, when so much of our experience is devoted to building or maintaining personal relationships and communities.[25]

If we are to effectively address these concerns, we need to move away from the familiar Western understanding of autonomy as self-defining, self-interested, and self-protecting, as if the self were simply some special kind of property to be preserved.[26] Under most interpretations, the structure of the autonomy-heteronomy fram (governance by self or by others) is predicated on a certain view (per- sons and society in which the individual is thought to be somehow sep- arate from and to exist independently of the larger society; each person's major concern is to be protected from the demands and en- croachment of others. This sort of conception fails to account for the complexity of the relations that exist between persons and their culture. It idealizes decisions that are free from outside influence without ac- knowledging that all persons are, to a significant degree, socially con- structed, that their identities, values, concepts, and perceptions are, in large measure, products of their social environment.

Since notions of the self are at the heart of autonomy discussions, al- ternative interpretations of autonomy must begin with an alternative conception of the self. Curiously, despite its focus on individuals, stan- dard interpretations of autonomy have tended to think of selves as generic rather than distinctive beings. In the traditional view, individu- als tend to be treated as interchangeable in that no attention is paid to the details of personal experience. Hence, there is no space within stan- dard conceptions to accommodate important differences among agents, especially the effects that oppression (or social privilege) has on a per- son's ability to exercise autonomy. In order to capture these kinds of so- cial concerns, some feminists have proposed turning to a relational con- ception of personhood that recognizes the importance of social forces in shaping each person's identity, development, and aspirations.[27] Fol- lowing this suggestion, I now explore a relational interpretation of au- tonomy that is built around a relational conception of the self that is ex- plicitly feminist in its conception.

Under relational theory, selfhood is seen as an ongoing process, rather than as something static or fixed. Relational selves are inherently social beings that are significantly shaped and modified within a web of interconnected (and sometimes conflicting) relationships. Individuals engage in the activities that are constitutive of identity and autonomy (e.g., defining, questioning, revising, and pursuing projects) within a configuration of relationships, both interpersonal and political. By in- cluding attention to political relationships of power and powerlessness, this interpretation of relational theory provides room to recognize how the forces of oppression can interfere with an individual's ability to ex- ercise autonomy by undermining her sense of herself as an autonomous agent and by depriving her of opportunities to exercise autonomy. Thus, it is able to provide us with insight into why it is that oppressed people often seem less autonomous than others even when offered a comparable range of choices. Under a relational view, autonomy is best understood to be a capacity or skill that is developed (and constrained) by social circumstances. It is exercised within relationships and social structures that jointly help to shape the individual while also affecting others' responses to her efforts at autonomy.[28]

Diana Meyers (1989) has developed one such theory of personal autonomy. She argues that autonomy involves a particular competency that requires the development of specific skills. As such, it can be either enhanced or diminished by the sort of socialization the agent experiences. Myers shows how the specific gender socialization most (Western) women undergo trains them in social docility and rewards them for defining their interests in terms of others, thereby robbing them of the opportunity to develop the essential capacity of self-direction. Such training relegates most women to a category she labels "minimally autonomous" (as distinct from her more desirable categories of medially autonomous and fully autonomous). Relational theory allows us to appreciate how each relationship a person participates in plays a role in fostering or inhibiting that individual's capacity for autonomous action by encouraging or restricting her opportunities to understand herself as an autonomous agent and to practice exercising the requisite skills. Such a conception makes clear the importance of discovering the ways in which oppression often reduces a person's ability to develop and exercise the skills that are necessary for achieving a reasonable degree of autonomy.

For instance, relational theory allows us to see the damaging effects on autonomy of internalized oppression. Feminists have long understood that one of the most insidious features of oppression is its tendency to become internalized in the minds of its victims. This is because internalized oppression diminishes the capacity of its victims to develop self-respect, and, as several feminists have argued, reduced (or compromised) self-respect undermines autonomy by undermining the individual's sense of herself as capable of making independent judgments (Meyers 1989; Dillon 1992; Benson 1991, 1994). Moreover, as Susan Babbitt (1993, 1996) has argued, these oppression-induced barriers to autonomy cannot necessarily be rectified simply by providing those affected with more information or by removing explicit coercive forces (as the traditional view assumes). When the messages of reduced self-worth are internalized, agents tend to lose the ability even to know their own objective interests. According to Babbitt, in such cases transformative experiences can be far more important to autonomy than access to alternative information. Feminist theory suggests, then, that women and members of other oppressed groups can be helped to increase their autonomy skills by being offered more opportunities to exercise those skills and a supportive climate for practicing them (Meyers 1989), by being provided with the opportunity to develop stronger senses of self-esteem (Benson 1994; Dillon 1992; Meyers 1989), by having the opportunity for transformative experiences that make visible the forces of oppression (Babbitt 1993, 1996), and by having experiences of making choices that are not influenced by the wishes of those who dominate them (Babbitt 1993, 1996).

Autonomy requires more than the effective exercise of personal resources and skills, however; generally, it also demands that appropriate structural conditions be met. Relational theory reminds us that material restrictions, including very restricted economic resources, on-going fear of assault, and lack of educational opportunity (i.e., the sorts of circumstances that are often part of the condition of being oppressed), constitute real limitations on the options available to the agent. Moreover, it helps us to see how socially constructed stereotypes can reduce both society's and the agent's sense of that person's ability to act autonomously. Relational theory allows us to recognize how such diminished expectations readily become translated into diminished capacities.

The relational interpretation I favor is feminist in that it takes into account the impact of social and political structures, especially sexism and other forms of oppression, on the lives and opportunities of individuals. It acknowledges that the presence or absence of a degree of autonomy is not just a matter of being offered a choice. It also requires that the person have had the opportunity to develop the skills necessary for making the type of choice in question, the experience of being respected in her decisions, and encouragement to reflect on her own values. The society, not just the agent, is subject to critical scrutiny under the rubric of relational autonomy.

It is important, however, to avoid an account that denies any scope for autonomy on the part of those who are oppressed. Such a conclusion would be dangerous, since the widespread perception of limited autonomy can easily become a self-fulfilling prophecy. Moreover, such a conclusion would be false. Many members of oppressed groups do manage to develop autonomy skills and, thus, are able to act autonomously in a wide variety of situations, though the particular demands of acting autonomously under oppression are easily overlooked (Benson 1991). Some feminists, such as bell hooks (1990) and Sarah Hoagland (1992), have observed that the marginality associated with being oppressed can sometimes provide people with better opportunities than are available to more well-situated citizens for questioning social norms and devising their own patterns of resistance to social convention. Because those who are especially marginalized (e.g., those who are multiply oppressed or who are "deviant" with respect to important social norms) may have no significant social privilege to lose, they are, sometimes, freer than others to demand changes in the status quo. They may be far more likely to engage in resistance to the norms of oppression than are those who derive some personal benefits from oppressive structures (e.g., middle-class, able-bodied, married women).

Still, we must not make the mistake of romanticizing the opportunities available to the oppressed. An adequate conception of autonomy should afford individuals more than the opportunity to resist oppression; it should also ensure that they have opportunities to actively shape their world. A relational conception of autonomy seems better suited than the traditional models to handle the complexities of such paradoxes because it encourages us to attend to the complex ways in which the detailed circumstances of an individual's social and political circumstances can affect her ability to act in different kinds of contexts.

When relational autonomy reveals the disadvantage associated with oppression in terms of autonomy, the response should not be that others are thereby licensed to make decisions for those who are oppressed; this response would only increase their powerlessness. Rather, it demands attention to ways in which oppressed people can be helped to develop the requisite autonomy skills. The best way of course to help oppressed people to develop autonomy skills is to remove the conditions of their oppression. Short of that, long-term social projects can help to provide educational opportunities to counter the psychological burdens of oppression. In the short term, it may be necessary to spend more time than usual in supporting patients in the deliberative process of decision making and providing them with access to relevant political as well as medical information when they contemplate controversial procedures (e.g., information about the social dimensions of hormone replacement therapy).

Relational autonomy is not only about changing the individual, however. It also demands attention to ways in which the range of choices before those who belong to oppressed groups can be modified to include more nonoppressive options, that is, options that will not further entrench their existing oppression (as often happens, for example, when women choose cosmetic surgery or the use of many reproductive technologies). Whereas in traditional autonomy theory only the mode and quality of specific decisions are evaluated, feminist relational autonomy regards the range and nature of available and acceptable options as being at least as important as the quality of specific decision making. Only when we understand the ways in which oppression can infect the background or baseline conditions under which choices are to be made will we be able to modify those conditions and work toward the possibility of greater autonomy by promoting nonoppressive alternatives.

As in health matters, it is important in relational discussions not to lose sight of the need to continue to maintain some focus on the individual. Relational autonomy redefines autonomy as the social project it is, but it does not deny that autonomy ultimately resides in individuals. Our attention to social and political contexts helps deepen and enrich the narrow and impoverished view of autonomy available under individualistic conceptions, but it does not support wholesale neglect of the needs and interests of individuals in favor of broader social and political interests. Rather, it can be seen as democratizing access to autonomy by helping to identify and remove the effects of barriers to autonomy that are created by oppression. A relational approach can help to move autonomy from the largely exclusive preserve of the socially privileged and see that it is combined with a commitment to social justice in order to ensure that oppression is not allowed to continue simply because its victims have been deprived of the resources necessary to exercise the autonomy required to challenge it.

Implications of a Relational Interpretation of Autonomy for Health Care

Let us now consider what a relational interpretation of autonomy offers when we consider some of the subjects explored elsewhere in this book. Many of the concerns we raise in Chapter 10 regarding the ethics of research with human subjects stem from the fact that ordinary criteria of informed consent are often insufficient to ensure that proper attention is paid to all the morally relevant circumstances; we seek ethical norms that will be concerned with relational autonomy and not merely individual consent to some predetermined research project. Whereas traditional bioethics relies on the familiar individualistic understanding of autonomy, and, hence, focuses on the ability of potential research subjects to refuse to participate in a proposed project, our relational conception leads us to a variety of broader concerns. Rather than just asking whether research subjects truly understand all relevant details

involvement (a question we still consider important), we ar-
 juestions must also be asked about who is invited to partici-
, who is not and how the specific research questions were se-
lec. Our recommendations that new research ethics guidelines
provide members of oppressed groups a larger say in the planning,
structure, and conduct of research are intended to counteract the ways
in which existing power relations foster research that selectively serves
the interests of those with privilege at the expense of those who are oppressed.

Margaret Lock's discussion of how women's aging bodies are culturally constructed in North American and Japanese societies (Chapter
8) helps to make vivid the limitations of traditional autonomy conceptions when evaluating women's personal choices regarding the use of
hormone replacement therapy at menopause. She explains how different cultural expectations about women's aging bodies seem to produce
important differences not only in medical practices but also in the experience of aging for women in these two cultures. Women in North
America are far more likely than their Japanese counterparts to be offered hormone replacement therapy as either relief from menopausal
symptoms or as prevention of heart disease or osteoporosis (or, perhaps, Alzheimer disease). Most women, however, find the decision extremely difficult to make. The problem is not merely one of insufficient
data—there is an overwhelming amount of data available, but much of
it is inconclusive or contradictory and, very frequently, the data come
from studies sponsored by the pharmaceutical companies that market
these products and do not address questions of significance to women.
Nor is it a problem of coercion—even though some women feel quite
strong pressure from their physicians, most doctors are themselves sufficiently ambivalent about the risks and benefits of long-term hormone
use that they are happy to leave the decision to their patients. Rather,
the problem women face is trying to weigh up their discomfort about
the visible signs of aging in a culture that prefers its women young
against the uncertain risks of long-term artificial hormone use, their lifelong training to avoid being a burden on others as background to their
fears of becoming disabled, their lack of experience in evaluating competing and incommensurable risks, and the background condition of
having their whole prior reproductive lives subject to medical surveillance and intervention. What makes hormone replacement therapy a
difficult choice for the mostly middle-class, middle-aged Western
women who are wrestling with this decision are the social expectations
(both external and internal) that women confront as they approach

menopause, combined with their own habits of deferring to medical expertise to monitor and regulate their bodies' changes.[29] Relational autonomy makes visible the importance of considering how such social factors affect women's decision making, and it invites us to consider how the burden of unjust social demands might be made explicit so that it can be separated out of the calculations. It allows us to help reshape the considerations that should be operative in this type of choice and to seek political changes that will challenge those influential factors that are discriminatory; at the same time, it warns us of the need to help ensure that women have the necessary autonomy skills before confronting such decisions. And it makes clear the need to ensure that if hormone replacement therapy is of benefit to some women, it be made available to all who can be expected to benefit from it and not simply to those who can afford it or who find themselves in a society that considers medical intervention an appropriate response to women's aging.

Wendy Mitchinson invites us to consider the complexity of the relationships between women and their doctors in Canada between 1850 and 1950 (Chapter 6). She reminds us that power is seldom a straightforward relation where one party holds it all and the other is fully subservient. In the past, as in the present, physicians enjoyed a great deal of social and personal power relative to most of their women patients. But they have never been in full control. Women patients always make choices and thereby exercise agency. Further, patients often make demands and pressure physicians into offering services (e.g., twilight sleep at childbirth) that the physicians might initially resist. Perhaps the modern equivalent is the tendency of many women to demand access to reproductive technologies in order to try to fulfill their reproductive aspirations. As patients, women demand as well as comply; when sufficient numbers make similar demands, they may well affect the course of medical practice. But, for the reasons reviewed above, it is not clear that we should count such influence as full autonomy as long as the conditions of choice are restricted and oppressive.

Both patients and physicians recognize that the options they may reasonably consider are limited by economic and legal restrictions and by the force of professional standards of acceptable practice. Evaluating autonomous decision making in medical encounters, then, requires us to attend to the circumstances of particular physicians and patients and to the nature of their interactions. Increasing autonomy for patients is a matter not just of increasing their power relative to their physicians but of increasing patients' social power more broadly and restructuring the health care system to ensure that it is responsive to an appropriate range of women's needs by removing discriminatory attitudes and barriers and by promoting the necessary knowledge base. It is necessary to avoid simplistic understandings of the patient–physician (or, more generically, the patient-health care worker) relationship as a contractual agreement between two fully independent parties (as is often suggested in the nonfeminist bioethics literature). We need to attend to ways in which those involved in delivering health care participate in social understandings of women, and of specific groups of women, when offering women a predefined set of treatment options. Relational autonomy invites us to appreciate that both physicians and patients are socially situated and the options each considers, like the choices each makes, are a reflection of social expectations that may well be oppressive.

Consider also what a relational ideal of autonomy might mean in some of the concrete circumstances of health care services. First, under relational as under individualistic conceptions of autonomy, it is important for health care workers to continue their efforts to explore the needs, interests, and concerns of their patients at all stages of treatment—to seek informed choice in the fullest sense possible. Under both relational and individualistic understandings, informed consent must be understood as an ongoing process; a relational interpretation can make it clearer that the pursuit of informed consent is also an interactive process in which both parties may be transformed. Also, both interpretations provide support for insisting that, apart from emergencies, health care providers should not presume to know what is best for their patients because they cannot have access to all of the relevant facts and values associated with the complexities of their patients' lives and interests.

A relational view helps us to understand how the specific social location of patients can affect their autonomy status. It explains why requiring health care providers to disclose relevant information and seek the permission of patients is a necessary, but not a sufficient, criterion for protecting patient autonomy. Because oppressive norms can undermine a patient's opportunities to develop the experience and skills necessary to practice autonomy, we need to explore ways of reversing such deficiencies and fostering greater autonomy skills. Clearly, this task extends far beyond the boundaries of health care and calls for social changes that will provide the oppressed with opportunities to develop autonomy skills that are comparable to the opportunities of the more privileged. Within health care, it is important to keep in mind that patients who have had little opportunity to exercise autonomy in other areas of their lives may need more time and more counseling than others before they are asked to give their decisions on health matters, in order to be sure that the patient understands that a choice is genuinely in her hands.

Moreover, a relational interpretation of autonomy should call into question health care orientations that view health-related services simply as consumer options, to be made available to anyone who chooses them. Policy questions about what health care procedures are developed and what services health professionals are trained to provide and encouraged to offer involve social and political values that should be subject to public debate and widespread ethical reflection. For example, each society needs to determine if it wants its medical researchers and practitioners occupied with the full range of emerging new reproductive technologies or if it wishes to set some restrictions;[30] each must also decide whether it supports massive genetic screening and testing efforts to reduce health problems associated with genetic variations, or whether it will focus its resources on other sorts of preventative initiatives and on strategies for relieving the burdens of genetic variations that now fall on individuals. It should not be the sole responsibility of physicians and researchers to determine whether to meet the demands of individuals who seek such procedures as assisted reproduction, cosmetic surgery, organ transplants, prenatal genetic testing, or diet aids.

The need for more sophisticated analyses and public policy is especially urgent when the services in question reflect and reinforce oppressive social norms that are difficult for those who are oppressed to resist. Individualistic interpretations of autonomy seem to suggest that medical consumers should be provided with whatever services are voluntarily chosen (i.e., in the absence of explicit coercion), but a relational understanding of autonomy requires that we raise questions about the context of those choices. It encourages us to explore whether the growth of practices such as cosmetic surgery and prenatal diagnosis contribute to a climate in which these practices become so normalized that future patients may find themselves unable to refuse such services. Just as home births became virtually impossible to arrange once the majority of women in North America chose hospital births, there is a real risk that the current wide acceptance and popularity of prenatal genetic testing may soon make it nearly impossible for pregnant women to refuse. Because the autonomy of some may well be affected by the choices of others, we need to recognize the interpersonal implications of current practices on the autonomy of future patients.

In addition, because a relational conception highlights rather than obscures the roles played by social and material conditions, it helps us see the importance of ensuring that material constraints do not unduly re-

˛ options that are actually available to socially disadvantaged pa-
This implies a duty on the part of each citizen to join the political
to retain a commitment to the principles of universality and equal
access in the Canadian health care system and other countries where
these principles are now threatened and to seek to have such principles
endorsed in the United States. It also suggests that we consider broadening the definition of health services to make certain that nonmedical services that improve health are also covered by public funding.

And, finally, a relational theory can show the importance of demanding that health care providers become sensitive to their own biases
and assumptions so that they can better resist the common tendency to
deny authority to patients with less social status. By disrupting norms
that validate the experiences and perceptions of the powerful while dismissing those of the oppressed, relational ideals reveal the need for
health care workers to listen carefully to the concerns and priorities of
patients who belong to groups that are systematically oppressed.
Health professionals must learn to stop assuming total expertise on
health matters. They must broaden their understanding of their responsibilities; rather than seeing their task as simply one of educating
and persuading patients to accept their learned advice, they need to develop the skills necessary to try to find out how the condition in question is experienced by the patient and what constraints on treatment options face the patient. Such a shift in orientation should lead to more
effective, patient-centered health care. It may also help to transform the
historical pattern in which health-related research and practice have focused on the specific needs and experiences of privileged members of
society at the expense of less advantaged people whose distinctive
health needs are largely neglected.

If we are truly to respect patient autonomy, we, as a society, need to
develop a health care system that is more attentive to the actual needs
of the diverse variety of citizens who depend on its services. That task
will require that policy makers and providers learn to respond more appropriately to patients who are differently situated. A relational approach to autonomy allows us to maintain a central place for autonomy
within bioethics, but it requires an interpretation that is both deeper and
more complicated than the traditional conception acknowledges—one
that sets standards that involve political as well as personal criteria of
adequacy. It examines patient autonomy in the social and political dimensions within which it resides and provides us with the theoretical
resources that we need for restructuring health care practices in ways
that will genuinely expand the autonomy of *all* patients.

NOTES

Acknowledgments: This chapter has evolved over the course of the Network interactions and has benefited enormously from Network discussions. I am grateful to all Network members for careful readings of many earlier drafts and stimulating comments. In addition to input from Network members, I have also benefited from the generous attention paid by Keith Burgess-Jackson, Sue Campbell, Richmond Campbell, Carmel Forde, Jody Graham, Carl Matheson, Barbara Secker, and Eldon Soifer.

1. Some Network members prefer the terms "contextual" or "situated" as a way of avoiding all confusion with those feminists who reserve the term "relational" to refer exclusively to interpersonal relations. I feel that this usage perpetuates the misleading sense that interpersonal relations are themselves "apolitical." I have, therefore, chosen to insist on a thoroughly political reading of the term "relational" that applies to both interpersonal and more public sorts of relations.

2. While questions of patient autonomy arise in interactions with all health care providers, North American health care delivery is largely structured around provision of medical services; moreover, physicians control most of the decision making that determines provision of health care services. Hence, much of the subsequent discussion focuses explicitly on patient autonomy in relation to physician authority, even though many of the concerns raised also extend to other (nonmedical) types of health care practice.

3. The most vivid examples appear in the distressing history of medical research with human subjects. See, for example, Katz 1972.

4. I deliberately retain the gendered term in this particular instance since it accurately reflects the connection to the traditional gendered role of patriarchal father who presumes authority to make decisions on behalf of all other family members. Traditional stereotypes of mothering and gender-neutral parenting do not retain this hierarchical flavor.

5. For a review of most of the common interpretations, see Dworkin 1988.

6. Interest in respect for patient autonomy is hardly unique to North America, however. See note 20.

7. See, for example, Corea 1985a; Ehrenreich and English 1979; Fisher 1986; Perales and Young 1988; and White 1990. This is not a straightforward history of constant abuse or one-sided power, however; as Wendy Mitchinson documents in Chapter 6, the relationship between women and their doctors has long been complex and ambiguous.

8. At the very least, we need a more complex analysis of the options for decision making than is provided by the familiar dichotomous structure of patient autonomy versus medical paternalism. See Mahowald 1993 for development of the idea of maternalism as an alternative that is aimed at capturing both these aspects of medical responsibility; see also Sherwin 1992 for a brief proposal of "amicalism."

9. *Informed choice* suggests a wider scope for patient autonomy than *informed consent* in that it includes the possibility of patients' initiating treatment suggestions, where *informed consent* implies that the role of the patient is merely to consent to the treatment proposed by the physician; further, *informed choice* makes more explicit that patients ought also to be free to refuse recommended treatments as well as to accept them.

10. Many of these concerns are not exclusive to feminists; several have also been raised by other sorts of critics. I call them feminist because I came to these concerns through a feminist analysis that attends to the role in society of systems of dominance and oppression, especially those connected with gender.

11. This reduction may be a result of a tendency to collapse the ideal of personal autonomy central to bioethics discussions with the concept of moral autonomy developed by Immanual Kant.

12. It is often taken as a truism in our culture that emotional involvement constitutes irrationality, that emotions are direct threats to rationality. It is hard to see, however, how decisions about important life decisions are improved if they are made without any emotional attachment to the outcomes.

13. Susan Babbitt (1996) argues that the traditional conception of rationality is defined in terms of propositional understanding in ways that obscure the experiences and needs of oppressed people.

14. For example, research priorities have led to the situation where birth control pills are available only for women and this increases the pressure on women seeking temporary protection against pregnancy to take the pill even when it endangers their health.

15. See Chapter 10.

16. I focus primarily on medicine since it is the dominant health profession and is responsible for organization of most health services in developed countries. Most health professions involve a similar bias toward treatment of individuals, though some (e.g., social work) pride themselves on attending to social structures as well as individual need, and most health professions, including medicine, include subspecialties concerned with matters of public health.

17. See Chapter 9.

18. Because health care is a provincial responsibility, there are differences in the precise services offered from province to province and from one administration to the next within provinces. The examples here are broad generalizations.

19. Such considerations do play a role in health care planning at a governmental level where the focus shifts from medical interventions to the idea of *health determinants*, but here, too, there is excessive attention paid to what the individual can and should be doing ("healthism") and insufficient concern about promoting egalitarian social conditions. See Chapters 3 and 4.

20. When I read an early version of this section of the paper to the Second World Congress of the International Association of Bioethics in Buenos Aires, Argentina, in November 1994, I was struck by how passionately committed local feminists were to retaining a version of the respect for autonomy principle.

They felt that most women in their country had very little authority over decisions about their health care, and so they were struggling to reverse a strongly paternalistic bias on the part of physicians by appeal to the principle of respect for autonomy. While they acknowledged that this principle was not as well-entrenched in their society as it is in North America, they considered it very important to their own feminist health agenda. They see respect for patient autonomy as having profoundly liberatory potential in their own society; this perspective provides clear reason not to dismiss this principle lightly, flawed though it may be.

21. The language of agency and autonomy is quite varied within feminist (and other) discourse. For example, the term *agency* is used throughout the collection *Provoking Agents: Gender and Agency in Theory and Practice* (Gardiner 1995) in ways that sometimes appear to overlap with my usage of *relational autonomy*. Susan Babbitt (1996), on the other hand, seems to use the two terms in ways analogous to the use here.

22. The notion of agency is itself highly contested within current feminist theory. Postmodern accounts seem to deny the possibility of subjectivity in any familiar sense; since agency is traditionally assigned to a single subject, once the subject is eliminated, the possibility of agency seems to disappear as well. I do not address this complex theoretical issue here but continue to rely on common sense understandings of both subjectivity and agency. Readers interested in understanding the feminist debates around agency may consult Gardiner 1995.

23. In addition, we need the conceptual space to be able to acknowledge that restrictive definitions of health sometimes preempt autonomy analysis by limiting the opportunity of some people even to enter the relatively well-funded health care system for assistance with problems (e.g., poverty) that affect their health.

24. The agent imagined in such cases is always stereotypically masculine.

25. Feminist discussion of these and other critiques can be found in Gilligan 1982; Baier 1985b; Code 1991; and Held 1993.

26. See Nedelsky 1989 for discussion of this view and its limitations.

27. For example, Baier 1985b; Code 1991; and Held 1993.

28. An alternative feminist conception of a relational view of autonomy is provided by Anne Donchin (1998). I see her account as complementary to, not competitive with, this one.

29. This cohort includes half of our research Network, so it is a question whose urgency we feel strongly.

30. For example, Canada funded the four-year Royal Commission on New Reproductive Technologies (1989–93) to advise on public policy regarding these technologies. In June 1996, Bill C-47, which involves restrictions on commercialization of any aspects of human reproduction, including the buying or selling of gametes or embryos, prohibits human cloning and other sorts of technologies on the horizon and restricts the use of prenatal sex selection to medical conditions, was introduced to the House of Commons in Canada.

3

Situating Women in the Politics of Health

Margaret Lock

The pursuit of individual health is an occupation taken very seriously by large numbers of people around the world today. Moreover, it is an activity fostered by all levels of government and the medical profession alike. But health is a difficult concept to pin down. Despite efforts to define it in contemporary health policy circles as well as in medical and popular literature, the idea of health continues to take on meaning primarily through the absence of disease. Such an interpretation tends to place it within the purview of the medical profession, as something that can best be sustained through a systematic, technologically sophisticated monitoring of individual bodies. Routine use of mammography and of ultrasound examinations during pregnancy are examples of this approach.

In recent years, in part as a result of the efforts of activist women responding to what they perceived to be excessive medicalization of their bodies, and in part as a result of cutbacks in health care expenditure, a perceptible shift has occurred. Individuals, more and more, are being encouraged to be active in the pursuit of their own health. Large segments of the population now take primary responsibility for the monitoring and improvement of their health, with the technological assistance of their physicians when appropriate. The media has played a significant role in promoting such activities.

The premise of this chapter is that the idea of health is not self-evident; its meaning has changed historically and differs cross-culturally. The assumption that health is signified by the absence of disease, that it is limited to the condition of individual bodies, and, moreover, that its preservation is primarily the responsibility of individuals is, I argue, a product of the social times in which we live. Social, cultural, and political meanings are inevitably implicated in how health is conceptualized. This concept depends in part on one's viewpoint, whether it be that of a politician, a health care professional, a patient, or a relatively wealthy or an economically deprived member of society. It also depends on the shared assumptions in any given society about what constitutes health, how health can best be "preserved" or "restored," and who is allocated responsibility for its fostering and preservation.

The dominant assumption in contemporary North America is that health is an individual state or condition, readily subjected to measurement and management (see Frenk et al., 1991, for example). By confining attention to individual bodies, this type of judgment inevitably has moral and political consequences, the result of tacit judgments about the causes of illness and loss of health, and what is normal and abnormal among patient populations. Moreover, because in the practice of biomedicine a reductionistic style of reasoning is frequently dominant, medicalization[1] and geneticization[2] are often the end results of visits to physicians.

To think of health as sustained almost exclusively through the monitoring of bodies by individuals, reinforced and backed up by the services of health care professionals, is to take a dangerously reductionistic position. Locating responsibility with women for the birth of healthy infants and for good health throughout life is the product of a moral discourse, one that, although it may appear innocent, is politically motivated. S. N. Tesh, in her book *Hidden Arguments* (1988), insists that a health policy that consists mainly of exhorting individuals to change their behavior not only is shortsighted but, more ominously, indirectly protects those institutions that threaten individual health through discrimination, exploitation, pollution, or iatrogenesis. In the increasingly conservative climate of North America, epitomized by managed care, the privatization of public services, and decreased government spending for social welfare and policies that coincides with increased profits by the biomedical and pharmaceutical industries, Tesh's argument has special pertinence.

The World Health Organization (WHO) set out a definition of health in 1981 that is much cited. The idea of health, it says, should include physical, mental, social, and spiritual well-being. WHO's position is that health-related issues should not fall primarily into the medical domain; that limited resources for health care should be better distributed, and, further, that the individual is not necessarily the basic unit around which the concept of health should be organized. WHO recognizes that health cannot be conceptualized without reference to politics.[3] I am in full agreement with this position, but in this chapter I go further and show how in contemporary North America (and to a slightly lesser extent in Europe) a dominant ideology has become one in which the ideas of being healthy, being in control of one's health, and maintaining health are internalized as part of individual subjectivity (Crawford 1994, 1348; Foucault 1991). Moreover, I argue, the embrace of such an ideology has put the concept of health in danger of being depoliticized.

In problematizing the concept of health in this way, my objective is to contribute a broad, political perspective to feminist and social science commentary on medicalization and geneticization, and to what has come to be termed "health maintenance." Feminist critiques of a range of biomedical practices have been and continue to be indispensable in promoting the rights and interests of women with respect to health care, one result being the proliferation of community-based action and self-help groups. Efforts by women to achieve increased autonomy in connection with decision making about health and illness have often been successful. In this chapter, however, the hope is to move the debate into a larger arena in which discourse is dislodged from an exclusive focus on individual agency and responsibility and moved to one in which the social and political origins of distress and illness, together with the responsibilities of the state for insuring the possibility of health for all individuals, are made central.

My purpose, therefore, is to challenge an approach that limits its attention to the materiality of the body and fails to pay sufficient attention to the politics of health. As Tesh argues, "If advocates of personal prevention hope for really effective disease prevention, they do have a responsibility to prescribe *social prevention* as preeminent and to put individual action in a context that indicates its surrogate role" (1988, 82, emphasis added).

Historical and Cultural Constructions of Health

Historical and anthropological research suggests that all societies have a shared concept of what constitutes a well-functioning social, political, and moral order, one that is intimately associated with the physical health and well-being of individuals who constitute any given society (Janzen 1981). A notion of a "sick society," one in which the moral order is under threat, is also widespread. Etiological explanations for the origins of disease and distress vary through time and space and often depend on the particular circumstances and form in which a disease manifests itself. Such explanations range from theories of contagion or of supernatural retribution to theories about diseases transmitted over generations (whether by spirits, blood, or genes) to environmental destruction. Allocation of responsibility for the occurrence of illness and disease, whether it be with the sick individual, society, or the supernatural, is intimately associated with specific etiological explanations and usually includes a moral dimension, although in theory, in biomedicine, illness causation is isolated and decontextualized and thus removed from the realm of morals.

Despite the availability of complex etiologies to buffer feelings of helplessness in the face of illness, the question why some people become sick while others remain healthy, even when the sickness is widespread, or why some babies die at birth while others do not is always of concern. In attempting to quell such concerns, governments, communities, and individuals must either assume that chance is at work or, much more frequently, undertake practices, ranging from divination to epidemiology and genetic testing and screening, to locate reasons and allocate responsibility for the unequal occurrence of distress and sickness.

Explanations used in contemporary scientifically oriented societies are inclined to focus on "final" causes, that is, specific identifiable factors that can be located *inside* the body, such as viruses, prions, or bacteria, genes, organic changes, or chemical and physiological malfunction, all of which produce detectable changes in the condition of the material body that are then labeled as disease. Currently, vast amounts of funding are directed toward research in which attention is focused on pinpointing genetic predispositions and genetic abnormalities as causal or contributing to the occurrence of numerous diseases. As noted above, such an approach encourages the idea that diseases are isolable entities, universal, amoral, and asocial.

In contrast, certain researchers, for the most part trained in the social sciences and epidemiology, although their effects are less well recognized, both politically and among the public, than those of biomedicine, have devoted considerable energy to the fundamental question why some people stay healthy and others do not. In order to construct suitable arguments, less attention is paid to final common pathways within the body and more attention is paid to "proximate" causes located outside the body, that is, to hierarchy, exploitation, relationships of power, the meanings attributed to illness, the environment in which individuals are situated, and access to the fundamentals of life and to health care. The focus of this approach is the relationship of individuals to the larger social and political organizations of which they are a part, and hence questions about the moral order and inequalities in human relationships cannot easily be avoided. However, such research is usually more concerned with human populations or communities than with individual clinical cases. The relationship between epidemiological and social science research findings and clinical medicine, with its focus on individuals, is always problematic.

It is important to recognize that the very concepts of "individual" and "society" cannot be taken for granted. The interpretation of these ideas, which varies historically and cross-culturally, and their relationship to each other, has a profound effect on debates about allocation of responsibility for health and illness. While some form of both these concepts are apparently recognized universally, one or the other tends to be given priority throughout history and in differing locations. Moreover, an inherent tension exists between the interests and concerns of individual people and the social groups in which they participate, in addition to tensions among social groups. These tensions may be manifest in a variety of ways. When, for example, powerful men call for a "return to traditional order," something we are witnessing in many parts of the world today, very often in part as a reaction to economic exploitation by the so-called developed countries, women in such societies are often required to forgo educational opportunities and free access to public life.

Today we assume that society is self-evident, but the idea of "a society" did not exist in the English language until the fourteenth century and originally indicated a "fellowship" of people living together. By the eighteenth century, society had come to mean a system of common life, and then a second, more abstract meaning emerged somewhat later, in which society is generally assumed to be synonymous with the state, often regarded today as in opposition to individual interests, and far removed from earlier ideas of a fellowship or community.

Carolyn Walker Bynum (1980) has argued that in medieval Europe people probably did not think of themselves as autonomous individuals. Rather, women understood their existence primarily as part of economic units, usually that of the household, while men belonged to elective communities in addition to households. Medievalists are currently of the opinion that as early as the twelfth century the idea of respect for individuals can be discerned, but that this respect was tempered and constrained by immersion in communities of various kinds; the twelfth-century notion of an individual bears little resemblance to the nineteenth-century independent individual central to our debates today (Morris 1980). Similarly, anthropological research reveals that the idea of the individual as someone in whom respect, rights, and interests are invested does not translate well across cultures, and that with few if any exceptions outside of Euro-America, social, political or supernatural domains are understood as prior to individuals and their interests. Two examples must suffice in this brief chapter.

The concept of health widely used by the majority of indigenous peoples of North America prior to colonization was one in which the health of a person is understood as being intimately related to her relationship to the land. For example, "being-alive-well," the Cree concept, suggests that individuals must be correctly situated or "balanced" with respect to the land; a "sense of place" is inherent to the continuance of health in both the family and the community, and by extension to individual health (Adelson 1991). This concept is, of course, an ideal, one currently being self-consciously rethought among the Cree, in part as a response to the massive disruptions caused in their communities by, most recently, the building of the James Bay hydroelectric dam, followed by the threat for many years of the building of a second dam. The Canada-wide movement among aboriginal peoples to take full control of their own communities and to eradicate the postcolonial situation of forced dependence and discrimination so evident for many years has also contributed to a revitalization of indigenous concepts of health (see Malloch 1989; Kaufert and O'Neil 1990).

At present Cree identity—understood in opposition to the world of "whites"—rather than gendered differences *among* Cree is of prime concern in these communities. The relationship of women and men to the land as a resource is not the same, and health is therefore gendered but nevertheless reciprocally interconnected. As the Cree battle with widespread anomie both within their communities and in their dealings with the outside world, a politicized concept of health has been mobilized to assist in reinstating a sense of order within the community. The Cree example is illustrative of the way in which a commitment to health as a communitywide sociopolitical concept may dominate the gendered concerns of women either as a group or as individuals.

A second example is provided by Confucian East Asia, where the macrocosm of the social and political order, and not the individuals it comprises, was recognized as the fundamental unit of social organization. Historically, society as a whole was understood as constituting more than the sum of its individual parts and provided the ultimate meaning of human life. This type of thinking is still very evident today in post-Maoist China. The dominant metaphor for over two thousand years in China, and for many hundreds of years in Korea and Japan, has been and remains that of harmony, implying the self-conscious maintenance by individuals of a harmonious social and political order. Health is understood in the East Asian philosophical and medical system as being in a continuum with illness, and not diametrically opposed to it. Moreover, individuals are recognized as having *relative* amounts of health, depending on such factors as the season of the year, their occupation, their age, and so on, as opposed to a finite presence or absence of health. Thus health can be understood only with respect to the location of the microcosm of the individual in the macrocosm of the social order, and the physical and mental condition of individuals is conceptualized as inextricable from that of their surroundings, social and environmental (Lock 1980).

East Asian medicine is often described by its aficionados as "holistic," by which is usually meant that attention is paid to more than the physical body. In practice, individual bodies are manipulated so that they adjust, often to their detriment, to the social order. Thus in early Chinese history, the health of the entire polity, for which the emperor's body was a living synecdoche, was dependent on the moral and healthy behaviors of his subjects. Individual concerns and interests are by definition suppressed in a Confucian ideology for the sake of society, and this attitude extends to the management of bodies. People are expected to "bend" to fit society and, should illness occur, they resort to herbal medication, acupuncture, and other therapies to bring the mind/body back into harmony with the macrocosm, with the objective of returning to active participation in society.

This system is, therefore, inherently conservative and locates responsibility for the occurrence of health and illness firmly with individuals; even though the demands posed by society on individual health are freely acknowledged, they are considered unavoidable and remain essentially unchallenged (although the governments of China and Japan both invest heavily in comprehensive preventive health facilities). Adult Japanese women are to this day held responsible for the health and even for the occurrence of most illnesses of everyone living in their household. They are expected to live out their lives as nurturers of other family members, often to the sacrifice of their own health and well-being (Lock 1993a). It is also assumed that they should be stoic about any suffering they experience in order not to disrupt the household of which they are a part. This ideology, by no means limited to Japan, but manifest in an extreme form in that country,[4] was consolidated with the foundation of the modern Japanese state at the end of the last century. Despite the power and influence of biomedicine and an excellent public health care system for more than one hundred years, so that one might expect matters relating to health and illness to have been individualized, the ideology of female responsibility for family health remains pervasive in Japan.

Many women work hard to look after their own physical state, but it is usually for the sake of the family more than for individual well-being. This ideology is actively challenged today and dismissed outright by many women as discriminatory since the government foists responsibility for the health of many of its citizens directly onto the shoulders of individual women. Nevertheless, its influence is readily detected in the lives of millions of Japanese women as they care single-handedly for elderly relatives or for severely impaired family members (Lock 1993b).

We can gain some insight from these two examples into the somewhat different trajectory taken in recent Euro-American history when conceptualizing the relationship of the individual to society, and its resultant effect on allocation of responsibility for health and illness. The emergence in the nineteenth century of a reductionistic biology, in which nature is understood as the product of a set of laws entirely independent of both society and culture, permitted the hardening of certain ideas that had already been in the air for many years in Europe. The human body came to be understood as a universal entity, a product of nature, and subject to its laws. In contrast to bodies, individual persons, associated more with mind than matter, were thought of as unique (something about which Mr. Rogers repeatedly reminds young American children in his long-lived television program). On the basis of this dichotomous epistemology, inherent tensions emerged between the idea of the universal, invariant material body and individuals with their rich, culturally varied repertoires. Moreover, a second tension emerged between society and the aggregate of unique individuals out of which society was composed. Health and illness, subject to natural laws, were understood increasingly from the mid-nineteenth century on as falling largely within the domain of the rapidly expanding medical profession, members of which treated the bodies of individuals in their clinical practice as "cases" of specific diseases.

At the same time a counter vision of society and its mode of creation tempered the powerful drive of scientifically orientated clinical care. With the emergence of nation states in the nineteenth century and corresponding nationalist ideologies (and in much of the identity group politics that mark both national and international debates in the late twentieth century), the individual is understood as constituted primarily by and accruing worth through participation in a social collective or collectives, whether it be that of the nation, a culture, or the community. Thinkers as radically diverse as Hegel and Marx understood the individual as fundamentally a sociopolitical-economic entity, born into specific relationships and determined by them. Without society, which is prior, individual life could not exist, they argued. Many of the great social scientists of this century, most notably Emile Durkheim, followed this line of thinking, and its mark is evident in a large portion of social science research today. Such an approach is also present in much contemporary public health literature that focuses on the social determinants of health and illness. Despite these influences, however, a perspective in which the focus of attention in clinical practice is on individual minds and bodies remains dominant today. The point is not to argue that good clinical care of individual patients is not appropriate but rather to suggest that this is the approach that is overwhelmingly thought of today as the key to good health.

Although biomedicine is not a monolithic enterprise, and great variation exists among the practices of subspecialties and individual clinicians, it is probably safe to say that the majority of clinical practitioners equate illness with recognizable pathology and believe that health—that is, an absence of disease—can be measured through the application of various technologies to individual bodies; by extension, individuals can justifiably be made responsible for safeguarding, monitoring, and regulating their own physical condition.

Such an approach usually fails to appreciate, or else tries to circumvent, two important facts: first, that the subjective experience of illness does not stand in a one-to-one relationship with measurable pathology; individuals may feel and be unhealthy but have no manifest signs of disease. As is well known, the complaints of patients, notably women, are often not taken seriously unless they are can be readily classified as diseases. Second, a vast public health and social science literature shows a close association between inequities, in particular, poverty, and disease of all kinds. Despite this evidence, the allocation of responsibility to individuals for maintaining health is the dominant type of thinking, found not only among medical professionals but also in the public domain. This situation is in large part due to an unexamined acceptance of the idea that health and disease are just two sides of the same coin. Health means, quite simply, an absence of pathology. It is an ideology that is potentially reactionary, inherently competitive, and insensitive to issues of equity and justice.

The Seeds of Medicalization: The State and Health

As noted above, ideas about the relationship of the individual to society change through time and space and influence judgments about the allocation of responsibility for health and illness. Although the idea of the microcosm of the individual immersed in a social and environmental macrocosm was common in classical Europe (and was similar to thinking going on at the same time in China, with which there was probably some actual contact), this type of thinking was challenged early on from influential quarters. Elite Europeans living after the time of the physician Galen (A.D 200) saw doctors as "managers" of health and health as an inherently individual affair that had relatively little to do with communities, governing bodies, or the environment. Galen defined health three ways. He described it as the absence of dysfunction, gave a minimalist definition of physical health, and equated it with happiness and an abundance of energy. Instruction manuals for physicians and the literate minority spelled out correct regimen with respect to food and drink, sleep, wakefulness, sex, and the emotions.[5] In contrast to East Asia, where similar regimens were encouraged for the benefit of the social order, in Europe health became a value in itself—something to treasure as part of the good life (Von Staden 1992).

Only after the formation of the modern state following the French Revolution did the idea emerge that the burden of health care should not be left with individuals but that the state should take responsibility for the well-being of populations. This idea became the foundation for the development of state-managed health care plans, which were rapidly emulated throughout most of Europe and later in other parts of the world. Initially these moves focused largely on sanitation, an urgent requirement given the rapid expansion of crowded urban populations.

Since the early nineteenth century, a triangulation of interests among the state, the medical profession, and individuals has emerged with respect to health, at times in congruence with each other, but more frequently partially at odds. As we will see, a moral discourse in which location of responsibility for the preservation of health is a key issue is often a bone of contention among governments, the medical world, and individual citizens. Once government became implicated in health care, the way was opened up in the nineteenth century for promotion of the idea that health is a right—something owed to individuals by society. In post-Darwinian Europe and North America, under the banner of progress, a second idea, namely, that health can be *improved* and is not simply something finite and God-given, received enormous impetus. Individuals could actually contribute to society by improving their health and, reciprocally, society could ensure that only "healthy" individuals were permitted to reproduce. The idea of breeding better people is a very old one, but Francis Galton coined the term *eugenics* in the late nineteenth century to explicitly liken efforts to improve the quality of the human race to that of animal and plant breeding. In doing so, Galton made eugenics into a scientific endeavor in which the "biological roots of social degeneration" would be systematically investigated and eliminated by denying "unsuitable" individuals the chance to reproduce themselves (Kevles 1992).

In Pursuit of Health

The phrase *mens sana in corpore sano* (a healthy mind in a healthy body) has been attributed to Juvenal, writing in the first century. However, he originally wrote that one must *pray* for a healthy mind in a healthy body; stripped of context, the bon mot became a slogan for the self-help fitness movements that sprang up in nineteenth century Europe and North America.

Organizations such as the "crusaders for fitness" associated personal salvation and health with correct living, diet, and exercise (Whorton 1982). The doctrine of these "hygienic religions" was that, rather than simply praying for health, one worked for it. North American activists such as John Henry Kellogg and Horace Fletcher were explicit that changes in individual lifestyles would reinvigorate both body and spirit. In keeping with current theories of "social degeneration," the rhetoric of the day lamented the "social debility" evident everywhere (Green 1986) and claims were made that individuals who strove to increase their health could combat this shocking trend and recreate a healthy nation. Individual physical development was understood as an important step toward both human perfection and a prosperous social order (Fellman and Fellman 1981). Most of the activities of these organizations for fitness were directed at the emerging middle class, but the temperance movement preached the value of a "healthy" lifestyle to laborers and their families as a means of breaking free from the demon of alcohol. Thus deviant drinking was transformed from a sin into a moral weakness. Gilman (1988) has shown how syphilis, once it became recognized as a disease, was first associated with men, but by the eighteenth century the focus of attention had turned to women of "loose morals" who were its "source" (255).

Peter Conrad (1994) notes that the discourse about deviant drinking—renamed as alcoholism—has undergone a further transformation in recent times so that the dominant explanation today is usually that of a disease.[6] Medicalization has taken place, and moralistic judgments about alcohol use are, in theory, superseded. In practice, however, as is well known, a negative moral valence remains in connection with a whole range of medicalized conditions ranging from the use of alcohol and other stimulants, to sexually transmitted diseases and AIDS, fatigue, obesity, and bulimia.

Over the past twenty years a discourse countering excessive medicalization, particularly that of the female body, has become increasingly apparent. This "new health morality" (Becker 1986) has, Conrad (1994, 387) notes, transformed "health *into* the moral" (emphasis added). Wellness, the avoidance of disease and illness, and the "improvement of health" is widely considered as "virtue," and for some individuals takes on the aura of a secular path to salvation. Medicalization of distressed bodies proceeds apace, but at the same time a complementary move, that of "healthism" is something to strive for. Rather than a means to some other objective, one that may well contribute to society at large, the pursuit of health is now an end in itself.

Wellness, however, cannot always be separated out clearly from medicalization: The argument that women once past menopause should take hormone replacement therapy for the rest of their lives as a "preventive" measure against ill health is just one example of how the wellness as virtue movement becomes conflated with medicalization (see Chapter 8). Medical technologies become the means to individual control over the process of aging with its associated images of declining health. Once again the assumption is evidently at work that continued health can be equated simply with the absence of detectable disease.

Robert Crawford (1977), in writing about what he terms "a remarkable expansion of the health sector" over the past several decades, situates the pursuit of health in a framework of political economy. He notes that expansion of the medical sector in the 1950s and early 1960s went virtually unquestioned, the assumption being that increased medicalization would lead directly to improved health across all sectors of society. This expansion was first challenged in the United States in terms simply of equity and access. Later the women's movement provided a major critique of medicalization itself, pointing out the hegemony of medicine, and its role as an institution of social control. Self-help groups and alternative clinics were organized from this time specifically to promote the autonomy of women in connection with issues relating to health and illness (see also Chapter 5).

By the 1970s a perceived crisis created by the "aging society," as it has come to be known, contributed dramatically to an increasing sense of urgency that climbing health care expenditures deployed for the elderly must be curbed.[7] Political pressures were mobilized to cut health care costs at a time when citizens had come to think of health care not simply as a right but as an entitlement. Crawford (1977) cites Robert

Whalen, the commissioner of the New York Department of Health who asserted in the late 1970s that it was essential that people should assume "individual and moral responsibility" for their own health. John Knowles, past president of the Rockefeller Foundation, goes further.

> The idea of individual responsibility has been submerged in
> individual rights—rights or demands to be guaranteed by Big
> Brother and delivered by public and private institutions. The
> cost of sloth, gluttony, alcoholic intemperance, reckless
> driving, sexual frenzy and smoking have now become a
> national, not an individual responsibility, and all justified as
> individual freedom. But one man's or woman's freedom in
> health is now another man's shackle in taxes and insurance
> premiums. (Knowles cited in "Conference on the Future
> Direction of Health Care" 1995, 2–3)

Crawford argues that this victim-blaming ideology, established well before AIDS was recognized, was used to justify a retrenchment from rights and entitlements to health care. It also strongly reformulates health as an individual responsibility to which the collectivity need not contribute, for to do so would constrict the interests of society. Leon Kass (1975) went as far as to claim that it is inappropriate that "excessive preoccupations" about cancer lead to government regulations that unreasonably restrict industrial activity (42). Others took another tack and argued in the 1970s, in the face of striking evidence to the contrary, that poverty was on the decline, and that improved health would inevitably follow in good time (Somers 1971, 32).

These political moves, designed to foster a sense of responsibility by individuals for the occurrence of sickness, coincided with an increased awareness among large segments of the public that individuals have no control over the polluted environments in which they live, the quality of food they are sold, and the safety of medications they are prescribed. It was in this atmosphere that the wellness as virtue movement exploded, a movement actively encouraged by governments, since in theory it would contribute to a decrease in health care expenditures. The 1974 Lalonde report produced by the Ministry of National Health and Welfare of the Liberal Canadian government and entitled *A New Perspective on the Health of Canadians* is striking evidence of this trend. By 1978, 140,000 copies of this report had been distributed around the world. Eugene Vayda (1978) argues that its publication resulted directly from increasing anxiety on the part of governments, federal and provincial, about soaring health care costs, and a recognition that more medical services does not mean better health, a sentiment that was vigorously supported in a publication by the Canadian Institute of Advanced Research (Evans, Barer, and Marmor 1994; see also Burke and Stevenson 1993).

Controlling Health

On the basis of empirical research, Crawford (1984) produced what he termed a "cultural account of health" in contemporary middle-class North America. The results of open-ended interviews carried out in the Chicago area with sixty adults, female and male, from a variety of socioeconomic backgrounds, revealed two oft-repeated themes in respondent's accounts: one of self-control and a cluster of related concepts including self-discipline, self-denial, and will power. A second complementary set of themes were grouped around the idea of release and freedom. Informants repeatedly expressed the idea that exercising, eating well, giving up smoking and alcohol use, and so on are essential to good health, and moreover such activities were taken to be evidence of will power and self-control. Making time to be healthy was spontaneously ranked highly by the majority of informants who also noted that such behavior exhibited an active refusal to be coopted by the unhealthy society in which they found themselves.

Crawford (1984) argues:

> The practical activity of health promotion, whereby health is viewed as a goal to be achieved through instrumental behaviors aimed at maintaining or enhancing biological functioning, is integral to an encompassing symbolic order. It is an order in which the individual body, separated from mind and society, is "managed" according to criteria elaborated in the biomedical sciences. Medical knowledge, internalized and reproduced in our everyday discourse, represents a distinct, although by no means universal, way of experiencing our "selves," our bodies and our world. (73)

One of the master symbols of contemporary medicine and of North American society as a whole is that of control. Crawford (1984) suggests that by taking personal responsibility for health we are displaying, not only a desire for control, but an ability to seize it and enact it—we cooperate in the creation of correct citizens, thus validating the dominant moral order. He goes on to note that in this time of severe economic cutbacks individual bodies, "the ultimate metaphor," refract the general mood (80) as we attempt to control what is within our grasp. Although it is the economically deprived who are the most affected by budget constraints, Crawford argues that the middle class reaffirm their relatively protected status through personal discipline. Sandra Lee Bartky (1988) has pointed out that, for women, will power is often derived from an internalized self-surveillance associated with activities relating to beauty enhancement as well as activities that promote health (see also Morgan 1991, 1996a).

When interviewed by Crawford, many people expressed the idea that together with control must come release, usually through the fulfillment of instant desire and consumption. Crawford (1984) argues that it is not surprising that bulimia has emerged as one of the most common eating disorders, for the body is not only a symbolic field for the reproduction of dominant values and conceptions, "it is also a site for resistance to and transformation of those systems of meaning" (95; see also Lock 1990, 1993a). He concludes by considering what political implications can be associated with the fitness movement. Is it indeed a prior step to empowerment, or only part of the answer? Are individual lifestyle changes precisely what "power" requires of us at this historical moment? Is well-being as virtue being transformed into a dangerous fetish as Ivan Illich (1992) has suggested? After all, industry continues to pollute, corporations continue to grow while simultaneously making employees redundant as they maximize the use of technology, and increasing numbers of people, the majority of them women and children, live below the poverty line.

Some redress appears to be in order in connection with the inherent tension between the individual and society. Perhaps it is time to question the way in which in North America we tend to conceptualize individuals as inherently in opposition to the social. Together with a concern for individual health, rejuvenation of the idea of a healthy society may be a useful approach. Such a society is one that recognizes injustice, inequities, and an unequal distribution of resources and understands these problems as social in origin. Given the global economy of today, this includes a sensitivity to the exploitation of poor countries by the wealthy. A healthy society is one that has the courage to curtail greed, that questions the idea of endless consumption, built-in obsolescence, growth without end, and the idea that individuals can or should be in control of every aspect of their lives; it is a society that above all ensures that all its citizens have access to resources to avoid ill health. We appear at the moment to be moving in a different direction, one of fragmentation, extreme individualism, and widespread anomie, a condition that feminists must speak out against if we are to keep our sights on the politics of health and the responsibilities of society for the well being of individuals.

NOTES

Acknowledgments: I am grateful to Abby Lippman, Kathryn Morgan, and Susan Sherwin for thoughtful reading of and concrete contributions to this chapter.

1. Medicalization is the process whereby certain behaviors, problems, and events are conceptualized and treated as diseases; both the production of medical knowledge and its practices are implicated. See Chapter 5 for a full account of this concept.

2. "Geneticization" is a term coined by Lippman (1991). See p. 64 for a full definition.

3. I understand politics to be the way in which power is distributed and exercised among institutions and individuals.

4. The expectation that women will be profoundly involved in providing informal health care is found, with differing degrees of emphasis and in somewhat different forms, in many cultures. In analyzing the role of women as informal health care providers in the twentieth-century capitalist settings, Hilary Graham (1985) distinguishes three critical roles for women: providers of health with respect to the material, psychological, emotional dimensions of health with a strong emphasis on nurturing, healing, and caring; mediators of health with respect to the translation of cultural understandings of health and healthy practices into personal, private, and familial settings (think of the many child-rearing/health manuals directed at middle-class mothers; of the surveillance and diagnostic responsibilities with respect to identifying illness); and negotiators of health with respect to formal, public health care providers—whether they are physicians, nurse practitioners, or pediatric endocrinologists—and to the public institutions and structures that define a healthy community member. In cultures committed to the re-privatization of health care, these critical roles will, in all likelihood, become more prominent in the lives of women although, as Graham notes, the gendered nature of this labor and valuation may be camouflaged by communitarian language.

5. This regimen is not very different from the practices Belloc and Breslow (1972) identified as relevant to health and longevity seventeen hundred years later: seven to eight hours of sleep at night, eating breakfast, exercising, weight control, moderate (or no) alcohol, no smoking.

6. Commentators in the United States did, however, take the opportunity to label excessive alcohol use in the former Soviet Union as resulting from the communist regime under which people lived.

7. Much of the increased expenditure has been shown to be due to the extremely high use of tests and procedures made use of as surveillance of the well elderly.

4 The Politics of Health: Geneticization Versus Health Promotion

Abby Lippman

This chapter elaborates on many of the themes considered by Margaret Lock in Chapter 3. Her exploration of the politics of health and the limits of the biomedical conception of health as merely the absence of pathology/disease sets the context in which to examine the phenomenon of geneticization. Because it is fed by developments in molecular genetics, a discipline that is an integral part of biomedical practice and also tightly linked to financial markets (Cohen 1997), geneticization, like medicalization, not only is blind to issues of equity and justice with respect to health but erases them from the public mind.

This chapter considers geneticization as both an emerging ideology and as a set of practices, a combination that gives it enormous potential to divert attention from the structural changes necessary for true health promotion through its reinforcement of "healthism" (Crawford 1980), its assumptions of individual responsibility for the maintenance, if not the improvement, of a "disease-free" existence, and its enormous economic implications (profits for private biotechnology companies; alleged "savings" for governments).

Geneticization: An Ideology and a Practice

Geneticization is a term coined (Lippman 1992) to capture the ever-growing tendency to distinguish people one from another on the basis of genetics; to define most disorders, behaviors, and physiological variations as wholly or in part genetic in origin. It is both a way of thinking and a way of doing, with genetic technologies applied to diagnose, treat, and categorize conditions previously identified in other ways. The construction of a human gene map currently under way, a worldwide cooperative endeavor, is an expression of geneticization at the laboratory level. It has vast implications for the well-being of individuals, in particular because the concept of health is undergoing subtle reformulations as a result of this project and the applications of its associated technologies. The ideology of wellness as virtue, of health as an end, *the* end, perhaps, rather than a means or a resource, now takes on new meaning, one in which self-improvement and improvement of one's offspring—a neoeugenics—can potentially be put into effect.

The multiple international projects to map and sequence the one hundred thousand or so human genes permit the identification of an increasing number of molecular variations between people, thereby leading to the (unfounded) belief that differences among people can best be understood as primarily genetic in origin. With the completion of the map (scheduled for early in the next century, but perhaps sooner), the likelihood for an escalating process of geneticization is high.

The scientific investigation of molecular genetics is not inherently inappropriate, but the application of this knowledge in practice, as well as the fundamental changes it engenders in how we think about health matters, raise ethical and social issues of major importance. First, the categorization of people according to supposed differences attributed to their genes is primarily a political act with little or no biological basis (Lewontin 1991). Biological populations do not correspond in any straightforward way to ethnic or cultural groups (Lock 1993b). Second, not all "differences" or categories are understood as equal. And, third, we are already witnessing how information about "difference" is used to define new classes of illness, to predict future health problems of individuals in these classes, and to design preventive measures for them. Assumptions about the role of genetics in explaining these differences can only reinforce the view that they are somehow "natural" and that the stratifications in society they create are unavoidable (Nelkin and Lindee 1995; Hubbard and Wald 1993).

Both the substantial value loadings associated with differences[1] and the assumptions and expectations about genetic information create serious problems for women's health. Thus, while research, services, and policy networks that validate women's experiences as a way to promote their health are set in motion (for example, the five recently funded Centres of Excellence for Women's Health Research in Canada), parallel developments associated with geneticization are likely to present a formidable challenge to maintaining health issues as collective and political rather than individual and medical. The extent to which geneticization will lead to the further devaluation of specific groups of people is vast; it would be naive to think that developing genetic analyses in a society

that is already hierarchically gendered, racist, and classist and that systematically discriminates against those with disabilities can do other
than reflect and reinforce these attitudes (Wolf 1994). Thus, concerns involve more than discrimination; the alleged predictive ability of genetic
testing is also problematic, especially because it feeds into current notions of individual responsibility for health and health improvement.

Mapping of genes for susceptibility to complex and common conditions, the kind we will all probably some day experience in one form or
another (e.g., heart disease, cancer, osteoporosis) provides a tool to be
used in screening programs.[2] Such programs are currently under way
to identify those with a DNA pattern thought to be associated with specific selected conditions. These individuals can then be counseled about
behavior changes to make that are believed to lower their probability of
developing the condition for which they are alleged to be at risk. Thus,
if some future genetic test were to reveal that a woman is susceptible to
(predisposed to) heart disease, she might be counseled to alter her diet,
exercise, stop smoking, and transfer to a less "stressful" job, all alleged
to help her stay "healthy."

This predictive model takes for granted that awareness of one's personal risk status *as thus defined by genetic testing* is important to the individual (at best, a highly ethnocentric assumption: see Chapter 7) and
that awareness of it will encourage behavioral changes such as to prevent the future development of the predicted condition. This model
frames the individual as the agent of prevention. Not only is society's
obligation to remove the adverse social circumstances damaging to
health (including mutagenic damage to an individual's genes) left unexplored, but illness is transformed into a private event. The stage is
thus set for social control and "victim blaming" (Crawford 1977) of
those who do not follow what is allegedly "sensible" preventive advice.
Superficially seeming to give a woman "agency" then, the predictive
model actually is more likely to give others control over her.

Framing genetic testing for susceptibility as a way to educate individuals about their health "risks" may be particularly dangerous today
when cost containment is a primary criterion for governments considering health policies and practices.[3] As politicians seek to decrease financial contributions from the public purse for treating the sick, responsibility for becoming sick, for putting oneself at risk of becoming
sick or in need of medical care is increasingly shifting to the individual.[4]

A range of individuals and groups contribute to the popularity of
geneticization and the expanding use of genetic testing. Scientists above
all, but also government officials, funding agencies, biotechnology com-

panies, and the media all help spread an interpretation of disease in which distinctions are made between self and other, "us" and "them." The geneticization advanced by these many players creates whole new groups of disorders, "sufferers," and putative populations linked only by sharing the same statistical probability of developing some future condition.[5]

Groups are always socially constructed; real people overlap categories in many ways (Fee and Krieger 1993). The differences used to draw lines to create groups are merely one way to establish relationships between people. Neither difference nor sameness is fixed: both are contingent, expressed and understood in different ways in different times and places and for different purposes (Scott 1990). For example, equality of access to education, employment, and medical care, among other things, is often promoted these days through a deliberate inattention to certain commonly specified differences, particularly gender and ethnicity.

The mutability and constructed nature of difference demands careful attention. Attributing differences to genes obscures the politics of difference—as well as the indeterminate relation of genotype (DNA pattern) to phenotype (the actual individual).[6] To the extent that genes are (incorrectly) understood as blueprints for the inevitable, and phenotypes, therefore, are assumed to be "given," differences are naturalized and depoliticized.

Screening for DNA differences that are believed to influence how people behave, perform, resist (or succumb to) certain illnesses can only foster qualitative rankings of individuals: as women know only too well, not all characteristics and endowments are equally valued. Difference is rarely, if ever, neutral; the relationships it establishes inscribe values, with that which is different labeled as "abnormal" and often devalued. This means that gene mapping is not only about identifying a gene associated with, let us say, Alzheimer disease, but about showing how different those with it are from the normal "us" even before symptoms appear. By building upon processes already under way that set people apart from one another because of age differences (Robertson 1990), the DNA-Alzheimer associations further entrench an us versus them mentality. And although genetics is only one of the ways in which we look for and find differences, its links to medicine make it, perhaps, the most powerful discriminator today, for, as noted above, differences labeled as genetic in origin are (incorrectly) thought to be innate and "natural," fixed and unchangeable (see Strohman 1994 for an excellent discussion of the limits of genetic analysis).

We are now seeing humans, their strengths and their frailties, through what has been called a "genetic prism" (Duster 1990). This prism expands the surveillance capacities of biomedicine, yielding information that, combined with that from biological assays and other technologies, can be converted into numerical data for assessing the state of a body and identifying who is ill.[7] This focus reverses the order given priority in Osler's aphorism (cited in Herman 1991), so that attention goes first to "what sort of disease a patient has" rather than to "what sort of patient has a disease."

Throughout this volume, we emphasize how the idea of a (healthy) woman is mediated by her age, race, class, sexual orientation. To this array of mediating factors, then, another has now been added: genetics. And where medicalization has primarily been a diagnostic explanatory process carried out in a clinical setting, the entry of genes into an understanding of health/illness, means that prediction on a public scale takes on an important role.

Geneticization and (Who Is in) Control

In many ways, geneticization can be seen as a contemporary expression (expansion) of "lifestyle" medicine as practiced in North America. This apparent paradox, wherein internal biological factors become "managed" by behavioral adaptations, arises insofar as the reasons given for identifying DNA patterns are to counsel an individual about what she can do to avoid, or reduce the probability of, that to which she is said to be "at risk." Disease prevention, not health, is the issue and prevention becomes the responsibility of the individual. The objective is, therefore, to decode disease before its potential onset, not to understand health.

As a result, geneticization not only inappropriately makes some healthy women into patients, it compounds the problem by creating the possibility for them to be "bad"[8] patients if they do not follow advice, with further opportunity for social control. In addition, the "take charge" mentality of the genetic updating of lifestyle medicine is unlikely to encourage collective change, because individuals are fixed as both the loci and the agents of change. In addition, geneticization creates its own dynamic insofar as its existence influences health care delivery services and even law and social policies.[9]

The ongoing reform of the medical system in Canada and elsewhere impels close attention to geneticization. Conditions understood as genetic tend to be treated as individual matters. In fact, they are issues of public policy with "individual tragedies com[ing] out of public arrangements" (Karen Lebacqz, personal communication). For example, would the birth of a child with Down syndrome be seen as only a "burden" were policies in place that welcomed these children into society rather than shunting them aside?   ·

There seems to be a growing tendency to interpret the application of technologies in genetics and elsewhere as evidence of health professionals' "caring" for their patients.[10] Thus, the urge to do prenatal diagnosis because we "care" about the kind of children women have, to screen for DNA patterns allegedly linked to disease because we "care" about the health of women considered to be at an increased risk of cancer, and so on. This framing makes genetic medicine easy to sell. But perhaps we should start to consider these applications not simply as caring but also as potential threats to health. Offering prenatal testing to a woman does more than limit her choices about childbearing (can she really refuse?): it can diminish her well-being, a necessary component of health, during pregnancy.[11] On the collective level, too, it speaks loudly about the kinds of children we will welcome in society while more subtly transforming procreation from a process of giving life to one of giving genes.[12] Similarly, advertising tests for identifying genetic susceptibility to breast cancer does not prevent women from developing the disease, nor does it provide early diagnosis of a tumor itself. But it may limit their potential eligibility for employment or insurance coverage (Gostin 1991; Berner 1995).[13] Collectively, it highlights only a small proportion of breast cancers and privileges attention to breast cancer rather than some other serious threat to women's health (a threat that may require social, not individual, change). Moreover, women who are poor or vulnerable for other reasons, especially those who have disabilities, will hardly be cared for or have their health improved when they are likely to be the least able to resist the abuses of power attendant upon the application of genetic technologies, especially insofar as they are pushed into genetic testing in a further effort to control their behavior.[14]

Geneticization as Politics

Politics is about power: its distribution and its application by and through society. The process of geneticization is political because it redefines what we take to be significant differences between people and empowers new people and institutions to make these redefinitions. Regrettably, however, society is not considering sufficiently how it will respond to these differences—and our current responses are far from ideal despite instructive historical examples of the harms of arbitrary separations of the supposedly ill from the healthy (see Markel 1992). Thus, there might be potential for applied genetic technologies to have positive effects insofar as they truly provided new treatments and offered true choices about health and procreation for women. In the light of the past—and current—record, however, including the widespread discrimination faced by women, by people of color, by people with disabilities (indeed, by all persons seen as "different"), as well as an ever-increasing emphasis on "quality" as a defining element of people and things, there is danger real and immediate that these developments may be used in ways that restrict rights and choices rather than respect or enhance them.

Geneticization can be likened to a process of colonization as genetic technologies and approaches are applied to and take over areas not necessarily genetic. Attempts to find the gene "for" homosexuality or the gene "for" criminal behavior exemplify this process. In this respect, geneticization is similar to medicalization (see Chapter 5). To the extent that it rests on (genetic) stereotypes and prejudices that are deeply rooted in North American society (Wolf 1994), it is likely to be even more problematic than earlier forms of medicalization: who is to say what characteristic, trait, or behavior will be deemed abnormal or unnatural—or, more subtly, merely a source of suffering? The options are perhaps infinite (short stature, limited vision, addictions, homosexuality, learning disorders are but some variations that come to mind as already labeled and stigmatized for which a genetic basis is either alleged to be important or being sought), and in thinking about them, we must focus on more than persons already born. These—as all—observed variations have no intrinsic social meaning (Nelkin and Lindee 1995). The way we convert an observation into evidence of something is what matters (Longino 1990). And it is society—all of us—that imbues variations with social and political meaning and from which policies are then developed accordingly. Harm will come, not only because of discriminatory practices against individuals, something we might perhaps regulate, but also, as Susan Wolf notes (1994), because applying the rapidly developing technologies perpetuates the subordination of increasing numbers of groups, groups comprising people defined merely by notions about their genetic makeup. Moreover, although some things may seem innocuous case by case (predictive screening of an individual for some serious disease, prenatal testing of a pregnant woman, etc.), the cumulative and collective effects could be sufficiently offensive with respect to the kind of society we want to be(come) that they may do "genetic harm." Furthermore, because the gap between "diagnosis" (of a genetic disorder) and its "treatment" is growing, use of prenatal testing—followed by abortion if the fetus is found to have the condition sought—to "prevent" a problem from occurring may be increasingly encouraged.[15]

As several chapters in this volume repeatedly emphasize, health, however we define it, cannot be conceptualized without reference to politics and the power to name. There is no longer dispute that the primary determinants of health (status) include income, education, and employment; social arrangements, not DNA arrangements, determine women's health. This reveals that social factors under political control set the context for people's health. Furthermore, what we call health, and what is diagnosed as its absence, does not just come with a pre-fixed genetic—or other—label. Labeling itself is a form of social control by which some arbitrary dividing line is drawn between conditions that form a continuum to construct categories of convenience (e.g., tall/short, heavy/light).[16] One such category has traditionally separated health and illness.

Genetics is now refining these distinctions by drawing ever more lines to create novel categories. These lines delineate such people as the "not-yet" sick, the susceptible, the person "at risk."[17] Each of us will one day be fitted into one of these categories for something even if the "something" is not yet identified for all of us.[18] But in contrast to those who see this as a "democratizing" phenomenon, we suggest it may be a basis for oppression: true, we may all be at risk for something, but not all "somethings" are equal. Some states (of health) are already much more disvalued than others.

With susceptibility screening, as with prenatal screening, the mere availability of a test can change everything. This is made apparent when we consider one of the newest "hot" screening projects: testing women for the DNA pattern referred to as BrCa1.[19] For instance, will research to identify environmental conditions linked to breast cancer be valued if physicians can locate DNA variants and surgically remove the breasts of women with BrCa1 so that a cancer for which they may have a higher than average chance has a harder time developing?[20] Will new—and gentler—treatment possibilities be explored if one can detect these DNA variants in fetuses, even in fertilized eggs, and prevent those who might later be at risk from ever being born (Winston 1996)?[21]

Genetic susceptibility is *not* genetic disease, though the former too easily glosses into the latter. And in a context such as the Euro-American one of today where health is seen as the absence of disease, this "gloss" is made even easier as someone carrying a changed gene sequence—a demonstrable "pathology" to some—is necessarily, perhaps, seen as "not healthy." Susceptibility and illness are easily, if inappropriately, blended when things are seen as genetic, making health only the result of a biomedical failure to diagnose a (potential) problem. No matter that not all who are found to be susceptible for some condition will actually develop it.

Susceptibility screening that exhorts people to take responsibility for their later health, to change behavior and "live well," to do everything to avoid that for which they are said to be at risk (despite the fact that far more is unknown than known about these "everythings"), is likely to be more than just class- and gender-biased (we cannot all "live well") and short-sighted (poverty and violence are greater threats to health than genes). It may actually—and perversely—*protect* those institutions that themselves threaten health through discrimination, exploitation, pollution, and iatrogenesis (Tesh 1988). (The logic applied here appears to privilege cleaning out the victim rather than cleaning up the workplace.)

Increasingly, the idea of personal "genetic responsibility" is taking hold. At the minimum, it implies that an individual must learn that for which she may be susceptible and then do something to ward off the problem. This transfer of accountability from society to the individual potentially redefines "being ill" as "being guilty" (Gillick 1984) and makes illness private. It has the potential to shift the focus of concern from the outcome condition, the illness, to the individual's failure to follow advice. It sets the stage for social control and for "victim blaming" of those who do not follow what is supposedly "sensible advice" for their health. It creates a way to distinguish the "worthy" from the "unworthy" ill. Are governments that support screening programs going to want to pay for the costs of caring for those who actually do develop that for which they could have been screened but chose not to be, and for those who do not follow advice about what to do when given the results of testing? The debates over whether to provide intensive care at public expense for those injured while riding motorcycles without helmets or whether those with liver disease associated with excessive alcohol use should join the queue for liver transplants hint at what the answer by governments drastically reducing funding for health and social programs is likely to be.

Moreover, while it will be fairly straightforward to observe or document how "responsible" an individual is by seeing whether she does what is recommended for her in view of her supposed "genetic status," there may be no way to evaluate how sensible the advice actually is. Current knowledge makes it impossible to determine whether those who follow recommendations and do *not* become ill stay healthy because they are behaving well or because their genes are not really so "risky" after all. Yet these same current conditions mean that a woman's behavior can—and likely will be—judged.

The role of genes in influencing health and illness is far less determinative than the current publicity given to each new "discovery" would suggest. Media exaggerations have reached such intensity that gene searchers themselves now urge caution, but their subtleties are not yet being heard (eg., Epstein 1997). Even if the media hyperbole is toned down, however, seeing things "genetically," creating a genetic way of doing things as the routine (e.g., prenatal testing for all women thirty-five years and over), remains most troubling. It precludes asking the upstream questions about alternatives by boxing us into preset perspectives that focus on managerial matters such as finding ways to prevent "misuse" of some technology when we should be asking why this technology is being developed or used in the first place. It leads us to look for "genetic diseases" when we should be identifying and treating health problems of women.

Another Way of Seeing:
Health Promotion and Feminist Health

There is no clear separation of research, medical practice, politics, and health (see Zola 1978). Governments allocate funds for research and, in Canada, select what practices will or will not be supported by the public purse. Governments also protect the private sector and its investments in health research. They also set constraints on the support provided to maintain the economic, social, educational, and other structures and programs required for health. Consequently, what is decided on a societal level through public policies influences health and how we define it, irrespective of any clinical interventions applied to treat disease. This has made it reasonable to ask about biomedicine in general, genetic programs in particular, if the current application of resources in the domain of health and welfare diverts funds from areas that need development and sustenance if they are to provide what we and future generations will require to flourish. Despite the allure of genes, the "sex appeal" of fancy technology, and the quest for the "rescues" of biomedicine, are there ways other than medicalization and geneticization to approach matters of health? Will developing gene maps affect the funds put into social structures (schools, work sites, safe streets), the basics that are essential if the genes our offspring inherit are to make health possible for them. Does our understanding of ill-health and handicap as social constructs and not merely the presence of disease call more for "socialization" than "geneticization"? Does our understanding of a just society call for the elimination of diversity or, alternatively, the protection of human rights, dignity, and freedom for all of us who are, in one way or another, different from each other? (International League of Societies 1994). And if there are other ways of conceptualizing and working for health, what might these be? How might these be conceived?

Interestingly, many of the most exciting and insightful responses to the questions posed above that suggest there can be an alternative vision come from some key public health documents developed in Canada. These have provided frameworks internationally for considering health policies. (The fact that the promise in the more recent of these has yet to be fulfilled does not diminish the importance of these universally accepted statements.) Those I discuss here contain attempts to reappropriate power from biomedicine and biotechnology and to name and to respond to that which makes us ill.

In the 1974 document, "A New Perspective on the Health of Canadians" (familiarly called the Lalonde report after the federal health minister of the time), health is acknowledged to result not only from the medical care one receives but also from the interaction *at the level of the individual* (and the notion of the individual is stressed on purpose here) of four sets of factors: lifestyle, environment, individual biology, and the availability of health services. Although embracing these four factors represented a major change from earlier emphases on health services (i.e., medical care) as the sole factor of importance, attention really focused, however, on just two of these: lifestyle[22] and individual biology (see Chapter 3 for a possible economic rationale of this approach).

With respect to "individual biology" as a factor, there was growing attention at the time in Canada and elsewhere in North America and western Europe to seeking the genetic basis for individual susceptibility to disease.[23] In parallel, "lifestyle" was construed as those things people did that had an effect on their health: the allegedly controllable individual behaviors that if adopted would ward off disease. Thus, policy makers inferred from the Lalonde report that by getting people to change their (bad) habits and behaviors by having them adopt "healthism," one could prevent the onset of illness. More recently, some have come to believe the view, discussed above, that change would be most easily encouraged by identifying those whose genetic makeup makes them especially vulnerable to the ill-effects of their behaviors and habits.

In the decade following the Lalonde report, some attention began to be paid to environmental factors that might influence health, but the next major reworking of health politics in Canada as elsewhere is, perhaps, most clearly seen in the work done by the World Health Organization (WHO) through the Alma Alta declaration and the "Health for All Strategy" it announced, followed by the 1986 first international conference on health promotion. The latter was held in Canada, and a key document released at this time, the Ottawa Charter on Health Promotion, framed—and, for many, continues to frame—thinking about health matters (Charte d'Ottawa 1996). It also seems to have generated the current language used in Canada for discussing matters of health in the public arena through its definitions of health (generally, the ability of an individual or group to realize its ambitions, as well as a resource) and its focus on the "determinants" of this health.

As presented in the Ottawa Charter, "health determinants" are considered to be the prerequisites for health and include "peace, shelter, education, food, income, a stable ecosystem, sustainable resources, social justice and equity" (Hamilton and Bhatti 1996). As important as what was included, however, is what was not: medical care and a "healthy life style." In this regard, then, the document was quite revolutionary. In particular, and unlike the Lalonde approach, it appeared to move beyond the level of the individual to consider health and well-being in society, and the responsibility of social policy to enable citizens to improve and maintain health. This revolution is made apparent when one considers the five areas for action that were privileged in the Ottawa Charter. These include building healthy public policies, creating supportive environments, strengthening community action, developing personal skills, and reorienting health services to the needs of the "whole person" (Hamilton and Bhatti 1996). Clearly, these action areas privilege groups and communities, not individuals as separate beings. They emphasize structural (societal) change, not personal responsibility to achieve health.

Although Canada along with most countries participating at this conference adopted the Ottawa Charter and its goal of "Health for All by 2000," there is regrettably little evidence so far that the principles have been used to direct government activities related to health in Canada or elsewhere.[24] The document may have been revolutionary, but the revolution has not yet taken place (see Coburn and Eakin 1993 for a similar critique). Rather, the opposite seems to have occurred.[25]

Twenty years after Lalonde and a decade after the Ottawa charter, yet another reframing of matters of health is occurring in the Canadian public domain. This has been generated by widespread recognition that mortality and morbidity are linked to socioeconomic gradients and that people's behaviors and their biology, including their genes, *cannot* explain these associations. Yet, it, too, is in danger of being trapped in ways of thinking that will further delay movement from concern about disease and genes to an emphasis on health.

At present, there is general recognition of the complexity, multiplicity, and interdependence of the many factors that influence health (see, for example, Hancock 1993). But ways to address these remain controversial.[26] This controversy is captured in the contemporary Canadian debate mainly occurring between those who adopt a *health promotion* perspective and those who adopt a *population health* stance—along with a smaller but growing number of workers stressing the need to develop a research "paradigm" for health promotion based on overt recognition of the ideological and political nature of human knowledge (Eakin et al. 1996; Labonte and Robertson, 1996,)[27] or seeking to create some useful synthesis of the two approaches.[28]

The definitions of these "camps" as well as their implications for research and policy are still in flux and will not be detailed here. Suffice it to say that superficial similarities conceal fundamental differences between them, particularly with respect to conceptions of health and the importance of praxis.[29] Thus, health promotion conceives of health very broadly, recognizing the interdependence between states of health, education, work, prosperity, and the environment. In health promotion, well-being is primary, as are strategies to support individuals and communities seeking to build healthy public policy, emphasizing people's personal experiences and community actions, all the while acknowledging the importance of bottom-up approaches. A key concept in health promotion, therefore, is "empowerment."

By contrast, population health proponents, exemplified by the Canadian Institute for Advanced Research (Evans, Barer, and Marmor 1994) appear still to envision health mostly as the absence of disease and are focused primarily on macro-determinants. They explicitly link health to general economic prosperity and, in consequence, to social stability, economic well-being, and other population features. This "trickle-down" approach, as well as the emphasis given to studying health, mostly through epidemiology, is clearly more "conservative" politically than that envisioned in health promotion, which stresses action (praxis and practice).[30]

This contemporary view of health promotion could just as easily be the contemporary—even longstanding—feminist perspective on health, especially with respect to the emphasis on empowerment (see Ruzek 1978). Even before the Lalonde report, and certainly before the Ottawa charter, feminists in the 1960s and 1970s were taking political positions on health and became increasingly active. One defining event was the publication by the Boston Women's Health Book Collective (1976). Others, more local, include the report by De Koninck and Saillant (1981) on women's health and the creation of centers of and for women's health (Women's Counselling 1985). Not only did the feminist health movement focus on the demedicalization of women's lives, it also provided a means for women to work collectively, to determine their own needs, to develop their own responses, and to validate their own experiences and understandings of health with a view to promoting it rather than preventing disease. It provided a means for women to develop their own definitions of *well-being*. Generally such definitions have been—and are—defined for women, as they are for other subordinated groups, by those who claim to be their superiors. In the most politicized terms, then, the feminist health movement, as current health promotion theorists and activists, acknowledges that health arises from—and is based in—social arrangements at the household, community, national, and international levels. It further acknowledges that for women to be healthy, there must be an end to poverty, an increase in social justice (e.g., an end to racism) and eradication of cultural myths (e.g., an end to sexism). And, as do other social justice movements, it recognizes power relations as major factors in how life is experienced.

This movement continues, one hopes in more than theory, in the recent creation in Canada of feminist networks concerned either specifically with violence or, more generally, with women's health (e.g., the federally funded Centres of Excellence) (Cottrell et al. 1996). These groups have mobilized around what they define as matters of health in ways that emphasize the political dimensions of the major determinants of women's health, seeing them more as risk "conditions" that derive from power relationships in society than as risk "factors" that are identified either by individuals' genes or by their failures, for example, to eat, sleep, or exercise properly. Thus sexism becomes a determinant and risk condition that generates abuse of women; patterns of labor relations influence working conditions for women that generate health hazards (Messing 1995). Similarly, inequities in income, education, employment, working conditions, physical environments (inside and outside the home), social status, and social support are all health determinants and conditions of risk for the development of illness, determinants that must be addressed through health promotion activities.

These are not merely risk factors attached to individuals but conditions with a collective dynamic.

Public policies will be required to improve women's health. There are already policies recently developed and applied to improve biotechnological approaches to disease; they surely need now be harnessed for fostering health. This means, further, that public policies in multiple sectors must be examined specifically for their health impact, with questions asked, for example, about the potential effects on women's health of programs in education, housing, transportation, agriculture, labor, and so on. We do not argue that all policies are health policies but, rather, that their "health impact" needs assessment (not unlike current practices in Québec with respect to environmental impact assessments).

Many women in North America are now insisting that health matters cannot be disentangled from all else that matters in their lives; they recognize that many of the most important determinants of health (wealth distribution, housing arrangements, etc.) are beyond individual control, not because they are in any sense genetic, but because they reflect public policies to which women have had little input historically. To change, to improve women's health status, we need to change how women experience life.

NOTES

1. Genetic testing, whether before or after birth, allows for sorting people into categories that are already politically and socially ranked. These categories—sex and (dis)ability are perhaps the most obvious examples—come with historically conditioned identities. Consequently, as genetic information is increasingly used to impose a definition of normality, or acceptability, of health/illness on people, it can only reinforce the systemic and pervasive structural subordination of these groups. We live in a society where, in the words of the historian Mitchell G. Ash (1994), what we consider our ordinary social values are really "naturalized prejudices." And our "ordinary social values" clearly do not favor the ill, the different, the "other."

2. It is useful to distinguish *screening* from *testing*, especially in the genetics context. The first is a population-based activity to locate a subgroup of people likely to have that for which one is looking. The latter is individually based and seeks to determine if "a" actually has "b." In this regard, chronological age is a kind of screening "tool" for women at some increased risk of having a fetus with Down syndrome, while prenatal diagnosis by amniocentesis is a test to see whether the fetus actually does have an extra chromosome 21. For a general discussion of genetic screening and its problematic nature see Holtzman 1989.

3. For example, Hughes and Caskey (1991) praised the human genome initiative because it will allow "cost-effective customized presymptomatic care based on genetic predisposition" (3132). We are not aware of any studies that have compared the effectiveness of targeted versus generalized prevention strategies. The assumption that people will behave in "appropriate" ways only if they personally feel vulnerable is similarly untested. And see Burke and Stevenson 1993 for a critical discussion of the politics of cost containment.

4. Ironically, these economic savings may be more imagined than real. New technologies require more and more management and manipulation, not less, and these are often expensive. They also require more money and other resources and lead to reliance on professionals. One need only recall the sequelae of the "green revolution" for a cautionary example of this process (Shiva 1995).

5. For example, by privileging statistical probabilities of future events, otherwise heterogeneous women can get classified together as "women at risk of having a child with Down syndrome" or "women at risk of developing breast cancer" and then encouraged to follow the same biomedical regimen. All contextual factors in a woman's life are thereby erased with mathematically determined numbers alone creating homogeneity.

6. An instructive example is PKU (phenylketonuria), a biochemical disorder for which all newborns in Canada are screened. While those with classic PKU all have two changed copies of the gene that usually metabolizes a protein component in milk, successful treatment with a special diet allows these children to develop no less normally than their siblings who do not have these changed genes.

7. By contrast, questions about why this person is ill in this place and time are shunted aside.

8. It should be noted that that which may lead to a label of "bad" patient may be just that which is an example of a woman's resistance to medicalization, of her chipping away at biomedical power. For example, is a woman who does not take the hormones prescribed for her a noncompliant (i.e., "bad") patient, or a woman who has taken charge of her own life? Groups without power, whether they lack power because of gender, race, ability, age, or some other attribute, often use noncompliance, lack of cooperation, "misunderstanding," and similar strategies as active ways to challenge medical (and other power) dominance. In this light, it may be of interest to explore women's use of alternative medicine as much for its political as for its healing components.

9. For example, the presence of prenatal diagnosis means that ultrasound examinations must be available (to confirm a woman's reported week of pregnancy), that women see physicians at a particular time in early pregnancy (to be "eligible" to be tested), and that laws be in place to "allow" abortion well beyond the first trimester of pregnancy should a woman who is tested be told there is something "wrong" with the fetus. Geneticization also creates the potential for what is called "genetic discrimination" with respect to insurance, employment, adoption, and other facets of a woman's life (Billings et al., 1992; Lapham, Kozma, and Weiss 1996).

10. This framing is not limited to things genetic but may be seen to apply to other intensive biomedical/biotechnological interventions. For example, high-tech interventions among the dying elderly or very premature newborns may have their aggressive nature masked when presented as giving "care" to the person.

11. It perpetuates the dangerous assumption that birth with a disability is necessarily "suffering" and to be avoided at all costs (Silvers forthcoming). "We are trying to help people" (Epstein 1997).

12. I am grateful to Maria De Koninck for this point.

13. In the case of breast cancer, for example, the "options" for a woman who is tested and found to have a DNA variant associated in some families with an increased likelihood of later developing this disease (BrCa1, BrCa2, etc.) are particularly limited, with frequent mammograms and bilateral mastectomy the two most often suggested (see Kahn 1996). There is no prevention to be obtained by genetic testing (see Lippman forthcoming). Conversely, the real "risks" for a woman who is tested may be loss of health insurance or loss of a job promotion (Kolata 1997).

14. The parallel would be with such things as forced drug testing and interventions during pregnancy that are more frequent assaults on poor women of color than affluent white women, reflecting societal racism, assumptions about who can be a "good" mother, and the differences in sources of care (public vs. private) among women (Roberts 1996; Handwerker 1994).

15. Although it has long been recognized that prenatal testing followed by abortion is not primary prevention but merely a means to prevent the birth of someone with a detected condition, this term continues to be applied to these programs (Khoury et al. 1996).

16. Regarding tall/short: there is already a debate about those to whom pharmacologic treatment with growth hormone should be given and how short is "short enough"? Statistically, because of the variation and distribution of human heights, there will always be individuals in a lower 3 percent, no matter how the mean height may increase. This alone suggests that a permanent population for treatment will always exist; clearly, there is no firm line separating the "tall" from the "short."

17. It is also establishing new individuals and institutions with the power to name these groups or categories. As Lloyd (1994) notes: biotechnology has been given the power to "implement and enforce codes of normality." But, it has even more power, I think, to the extent that it also has the power to determine the legality of some acts (e.g., "selective" abortion is sanctioned after twenty-two weeks if a fetus has Down syndrome but it may not be legal if a fetus is "normal").

18. This concept was really captured by Jules Romain in his 1923 play *Knock; ou, Le triomphe de le medecin*: "les gens bien portant sont des malades qui ils ignorent" (Knock, on, the triumph of medicine: well people are merely those who don't know they are ill).

19. It should be emphasized that only about 5 percent of cases of breast cancer are currently thought to be associated with the inheritance of an altered BrCa1 gene (Kahn 1996).

20. Removal of the breasts does not mean that cancer cannot occur. There may be enough tissue remaining after surgery to allow the development of breast cancer. Furthermore, in the families at high risk for this disease, ovarian cancer is also far more prevalent than in the general population and mastectomy does nothing to change these odds.

21. Even more outrageous is the possibility medical professionals have informally discussed of using the well-established relationship between the risk of breast cancer and the length of the interval between menses and first pregnancy to argue for the hormonal treatment of young women so as to make them "artificially pregnant" to simulate a shortened interval! Where are the voices crying for changed work arrangements that would enable earlier childbearing for wage-earning women without threats to their later career advancement?

22. Fitzgerald (1994) notes wryly that we used to have lives, while now we have lifestyles.

23. Interestingly, while the focus on lifestyle has long been recognized as a consequence of the Lalonde report, the push to geneticization this document also provided has been generally overlooked.

24. This is not to deny the existence and growing strength in Canada of researchers, activists, and policy makers who do take the Charter principles and proposals seriously and who are working—against great odds, regrettably—to make them realities.

25. For example, disease-related issues are now seen with respect to their potential contribution to the gross domestic product of Canada (as well as the United States and several European countries). Here, as in the developing world, structural readjustment approaches being adopted (debt reduction, etc.) are premised on the view of health as important only insofar as those who are healthy can work and as the production of biomedical devices can contribute to the gross national product of a nation (at the same time as individuals must take all measures to avoid disease). Thus, this editorial from *Science:* "health research products and services and health care itself represent major sectors of the U.S. gross domestic product. Thus, a national commitment to emphasize health research and development will clearly stand to benefit physics, chemistry and engineering, as well as the life sciences; and US-based progress in a particular sector will also extend that sector's contributions to international trade" (Bloom 1995). Health, it would appear, is no longer even just the absence of disease but a barter item.

26. The "health" referred to here is clearly that of people living in the developed industrialized world where health concerns focus much more on chronic diseases of adult onset than on the infectious acute diseases (with AIDS and tuberculosis being two current major exceptions).

27. These authors call their approach "a critical social science perspective" and flesh out this model with the example of how smoking among young girls has been created as a health problem (Eakin et al 1996). Labonte and Robertson (1996) develop possible approaches for health promotion programs within this perspective.

28. A succinct presentation of one attempt at reconciliation between "health promotion" and "population health" appears in the "Declaration of Intent for Research in Health Promotion and Population Health" circulated at the 4th Canadian Congress on Health Promotion held in Montreal, June 1996.

29. Special thanks to Kate Frohlich for her input into my thinking on this matter.

30. To caricature or simplify their approaches in order to make their differences most apparent, health promotion gives priority to decreasing the (economic) differences between groups of people at different levels, to reducing income disparities, whereas population health gives priority to raising the level of the lowest group, to income per se. It is as if the former seeks to reduce the variation between groups, while the latter seeks merely to move the mean to a higher level without attending to between-group differences.

5 Contested Bodies, Contested Knowledges: Women, Health, and the Politics of Medicalization

Kathryn Pauly Morgan

During 1977–78, Leah Cohen, a social scientist, and Constance Backhouse, a lawyer, investigated women's health care practices in Canada in preparation to establish the Toronto Women's Health Clinic. Shocked by what they found, they wrote an article for publication in Canada's national newspaper, *The Globe and Mail.* In their article Cohen and Backhouse addressed such practices as:

- the overmedication of women, particularly with mood-altering drugs,
- high rates of unnecessary surgeries on the bodies of women in the form of hysterectomies, breast surgery, and cesarean section births,
- estrogen replacement therapy targeted to women pathologized simply by virtue of going through menopause,
- the frequency of crisis-oriented, technology-managed hospital births along with the absence of "legitimate" alternatives such as home births,
- suppressed information about the legality of abortion, hospital-introduced delays and quotas, and restricted access to abortion services, and
- negligence, avoidance, and trivialization of female rape victims by many physicians and health care professionals in emergency rooms.

Here's what happened to the article: "Although it was accepted by a senior editor, his superiors decided that the subject matter was not timely and that women readers would be unable to comprehend the statistical data" (Cohen and Backhouse 1979, 4). Not timely? Statistics such as the cesarean section rate "increased approximately 30% between 1968–1972" difficult to understand? I don't think so. Other explanations are called for. I interpret the Cohen-Backhouse experience as a political microcosm in relation to the larger politics of Western medicalization, a politics that involves women's bodies, women's health, and women's knowledges.

In their attempt to share their findings in a widely accessible, public journalistic forum, Cohen and Backhouse were not only engaged in publicizing their findings, they were also involved in the preliminary stages of what Jordan ([1978] 1993) calls the horizontal distribution of authoritative knowledge, a distribution pattern that she sharply distinguishes from carefully controlled hierarchical distribution patterns (152–54). By bringing into sharp public focus the ways in which the pathologization of women's bodies and women's psyches have been and continue to be translated into medically mediated harms, restricted choices, hostility, and negligence, Cohen and Backhouse explicitly challenged the ways in which dominant forms of medicalization often work in the lives of contemporary Canadian women. It is not surprising, then, that their work should be suppressed by a high status conservative publication.[1] It is not surprising that the very same sexist perception of women that can permeate the health care practices discussed by Cohen and Backhouse should be offered as a reason not to publish their article.

In order to see the Cohen-Backhouse experience as a political microcosm, it is necessary to understand the highly complex and dynamic sociopolitical structure of contemporary biomedical medicalization, to contextualize the exposition-suppression experience of Cohen and Backhouse in the larger setting of the North American and global Women's Health Movement,[2] and to address the epistemic politics of the Women's Health Care Movement.[3] In this chapter, I try to show how women's agency, women's health care practices, and women's political struggles around health care can be seen as a serious political drama involving contesting authoritative knowledge-seekers and providers. It is a drama in which medical authorities often believe that they alone are entitled to manage women's bodies, hearts, and minds and to prioritize women's health needs. It is also a drama in which some women, individually and collectively, contest that entitlement and struggle politically against the devaluing, the trivializing, the intimidating, and the silencing of women's voices, women's concerns, and women's health knowledge. Involving highly diverse modes of resistance, it is a drama of contestation over medicalization, over competing discourses, alternative paradigms, and diverging understandings, and over forms of consciousness. It is a global drama in which women have fought and continue to fight for authentic autonomy with respect to the politics of our health and our health care knowledge (see also Chapters 2, 7, and 8).[4] To paraphrase a classic text, it is a struggle for "Our Bodies, Ourselves, Our Communities, and Our World."

Medicalization: The Theoretical Model

In 1972, the social scientist Irving Kenneth Zola issued the following cautionary statement:

> Medicine is becoming a major institution of social control. . . . It is becoming the new repository of truth, the place where absolute and often final judgments are made by supposedly morally neutral and objective experts. And these judgments are made, not in the name of virtue or legitimacy, but in the name of health. Moreover, this is not occurring through the political power physicians hold or can influence, but is largely an insidious and often undramatic phenomenon accomplished by "medicalizing" much of daily living, by making medicine and the labels "healthy" and "ill" *relevant* to an ever increasing part of human existence. (Zola 1978, 487; emphasis in the original)

At its core "medicalization" refers to the unintentional or intentional expansion of the domain of medical jurisdiction (Conrad and Schneider 1980).[5] Incorporating a view of human beings as proper targets of medicalization, successful medicalization involves individuals, groups, and cultural institutions viewing (or coming to view) a domain or problem or condition or choice or life circumstance in medical terms.[6] Since this requires the continuous transformation of ordinary lifeworlds,[7] successful medicalization will involve shared cultural practices that support the legitimacy of using medical concepts, theories, and discourses to describe medicalized life phenomena and the acceptance of the use of medical interventions to "treat" them.[8] In short, successful medicalization must satisfy at least three crucial requirements.

1. The domain, process, or topic must be *definable and defined* in medical terms, that is, be assimilable and assimilated to dominant medical paradigms, theories, research, and methodologies and must be seen as only (or most) appropriately described through dominant medical discourse.
2. Medical authorities exercising the highest level of control over medical knowledge and treatments are seen as the only (or the most) legitimate authorities having the appropriate authoritative knowledge and control over the means and personnel to apply that knowledge to the medically defined "problem."

3. There must, ultimately, be widespread individual and group acceptance of the dominant conceptualizations of medicalization
and active participation in its diverse, interrelated macro- and
micro-institutions.

In his conclusion, Zola (1978) explicitly warns the reader that such
medicalization has the dangerous potential to lead to real evil because
the process is doubly camouflaged: first, as a technical, scientific one
that is purely objective in nature and, second, as a process done for the
loftiest of altruistic and benevolent reasons (502). As more and more
domains of ordinary life become medicalized, they become increasingly camouflaged as apolitical, and resistance comes to look increasingly irrational since health—an intrinsic good—cannot reasonably be
called into question. As a result, medicalization as a complex, allegedly benevolent process spreads, and the associated institutional
and personal disciplinary practices (Foucault 1973, 1979; Bartky 1988)
involve more and more pervasive aspects of social control justified by
the goals of preserving or restoring health and preventing disease (see
Chapters 3 and 4).[9] I am moved by Zola's original fears and I am impressed by his prescience regarding the pace and aggrandizing potential of medicalization (see Chapters 2, 3, 4, 7, and 9).[10]

Five Central Components

North American medicalization is extraordinarily complex (see Figure
1). I believe that unlike the relatively monolithic social control mechanism suggested by Zola's rhetoric—flowing like lava into more and
more areas of ordinary life—contemporary medicalization is better
characterized as a protean, dialectically shifting, social and political dynamic.[11] Contemporary medicalization has shown itself to be both responsive and powerfully supple when faced with challenges, resistance, appropriations, and political campaigns that have originated
with the Women's Health Movement and with other radical populist
health movements.[12] To understand this resiliency, I have generated a
theoretical model to clarify the multifaceted nature of medicalization. I
distinguish five dialectically related components in my Medicalization
Model, which I explain in turn by reference to Figure 1:[13]
1. Conceptualization through theories and paradigms
2. Macro-institutionalization through interacting social, economic,
political, and symbolic structures
3. Micro-institutionalization through direct and mediated doctor-
patient relations

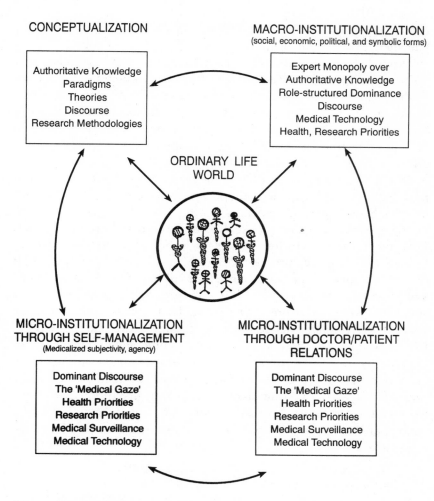

CONCEPTUALIZATION

Authoritative Knowledge
Paradigms
Theories
Discourse
Research Methodologies

MACRO-INSTITUTIONALIZATION
(social, economic, political, and symbolic forms)

Expert Monopoly over
Authoritative Knowledge
Role-structured Dominance
Discourse
Medical Technology
Health, Research Priorities

ORDINARY LIFE
WORLD

MICRO-INSTITUTIONALIZATION
THROUGH SELF-MANAGEMENT
(Medicalized subjectivity, agency)

Dominant Discourse
The 'Medical Gaze'
Health Priorities
Research Priorities
Medical Surveillance
Medical Technology

MICRO-INSTITUTIONALIZATION
THROUGH DOCTOR/PATIENT
RELATIONS

Dominant Discourse
The 'Medical Gaze'
Health Priorities
Research Priorities
Medical Surveillance
Medical Technology

Figure 1. Dialectical Structure of Medicalization

4. Micro-institutionalization through the lived subjective experience of personal medicalized self-management
5. Ordinary lifeworlds

Conceptualization

Successful medicalization is dependent upon medical knowledge having the status of authoritative knowledge, that is, upon acquiring the status of being the knowledge system that is seen as most relevant, most respectably based on evidence, and, hence, as most reasonable to acknowledge as authoritative (Jordan [1978] 1993; Davis-Floyd and Sargent 1996b; Foucault 1980a; Habermas 1981). Authoritative medical knowledge is dependent upon a community of knowledge gatherers and knowledge producers to define, develop, and employ the concepts, theories, central assumptions, and methodologies that are thereby accorded legitimacy by and through this process. Employing and reproducing the dominant forms of acknowledged medical discourse, medical theoreticians and researchers debate medical data, protocols, findings, and interpretations within a canonical set of theories, paradigms, and research methodologies.[14]

Those possessing authoritative medical knowledge become more powerful when they are able to appropriate or dismiss the dominant theories, paradigms, and practices of other discourses and other competing epistemic communities such as religious and moral authorities. This point is captured by the familiar "From Sin to Sickness" motto used to track the allegedly "progressive" and "enlightened" medicalization of various domains in North American culture such as alcohol consumption, high levels of activity in children, eating food, and homosexuality (Birke 1982; Conrad and Schneider 1980; Foucault 1980a; Fox 1977; Reissman 1983). Where other competing medical models may exist, the dominant model may label them "complementary medicine" or "alternative medicine" (if a pluralistic but potentially aggrandizing spirit prevails) or "quackery" or "hocus pocus" (if ridicule is politically most effective), or the dominant medicalizing institutions will have them eradicated or outlawed altogether. The powerful political implications of these epistemic maneuverings are underscored by Jordan, who remarks:

> Those who espouse alternative knowledge systems then tend
> to be seen as backward, ignorant, and naive, or worse, simply
> as troublemakers. Whatever they might think they have to say
> about the issues up for negotiation is judged irrelevant,
> unfounded, and not to the point. . . . Authoritative knowledge
> . . . also carries the possibility of powerful sanctions, ranging
> from exclusions from the social group to physical
> coerciveness. (Jordan [1978] 1993, quoted in Davis-Floyd and
> Sargent 1996b, 113)

As medical conceptualizations replace or are seen as superior forms of description and interpretation of ordinary lived experience, authoritative medical researchers, medical experts, medical knowledge, and medical discourse come to be seen by those living in medicalized cultures as the most legitimate expert conceptualizers of daily life (Code 1995a, 1995b; see also the discussion below). The medicalization authorities often come to have the power to control or exercise the implementation and material production of authoritative knowledge in specific research, funding, teaching, and clinical settings and in larger institutional structures such as courtrooms, schools, and prisons (see Chapters 9 and 10). In this way, authoritative medical knowledge is produced and then reproduced dialectically through the many and diverse macro- and micro-institutional sets of practices that constitute the variously positioned lives of those living in medicalized cultures.[15]

Macro-Institutionalization

Authoritative knowledge, theoretical paradigms, and abstract research methodologies lead a largely ethereal existence until they are realized in and through actual practice performed by real human beings in specific social, political, economic, and symbolic contexts. Just what medical conceptualizations actually take place and become dominant is a culturally grounded historical and material question (Foucault 1973, 1980a; Habermas 1981; E. Martin 1994; Oudshoorn 1994; Russet 1989; Schiebinger 1989, 1993; Tiefer 1995). Similarly, the direction of medical conceptualization is largely determined by health and research priorities arising out of the interests articulated in and by the medicalized culture. Often priorities are determined, within contexts of material and political constraint, by those in positions of cultural dominance, by the state, or by international regulatory agencies, but they may arise as well through political engagement of interested members and groups in the culture (Batt 1994; Browner and Leslie 1996; Gordon 1975, 1976; Kaufert 1996; Leavitt 1980; Sherwin 1992).

Many interlocking institutions are necessary in order for medical conceptualizers to attain and preserve their status as possessors of authoritative knowledge. In a high-medicalization culture medicalizing authorities create and expand a large variety of medical and medically related institutions in order to carry out medicalized research and to insure the (re-)production of medical authorities through specialized education, teaching, clinical practice, and therapeutic interventions. Correlatively, medicalized subjects often demand access to those institutions.

Consider, for example, the number of interlocking institutions surrounding the medicalization of conception, gestation, and birth in North American culture. If a woman (very likely white, privileged, apparently heterosexual, and apparently married) chooses in vitro fertilization as a route in which to conceive and bear a child, she may require access to a large variety of intersecting institutional and professional groups. Her choice involves networks of scientists and technicians whose fertility research in their laboratories is supported by multiple private and public funding institutions and the state, along with possible involvement with the following medical groups: geneticists, embryologists, fetologists, endocrinologists, neuroscientists, prenatal technicians, radiologists, genetic counselors, fetal-imaging technologists, fetal surgeons, anaesthetists, obstetricians, neonatal surgeons, neonatal pediatricians, intensive-care technicians, obstetrical nurses, laboratory technicians, hospitals, insurance companies, public health policies, autonomous professional organizations with professional codes, hospital administrators and boards, various kind of engineers engaged in developing genetic tests and technologies, medical computers and other monitoring and surveillance devices, the computer industry, the larger judicial system and juridical codes, the profit-oriented genetic and reproductive technology industries, the marketing industries, and the visual and print media (Basen, Eichler, and Lippman 1993; Corea 1985b; Morgan 1996a).

In principle, without complex forms of macro-institutionalization, medical conceptualization has no life, no lived authoritative status. It is instructive to observe and analyze the movement from conceptualization to macro-institutional realization. One striking feature of contemporary Western medicalization is the move to a culturally shared perception of the human body as a feared site of "virtual pathology" so that very real forms of medical control are taken up enthusiastically by members and specific groups in the medicalization culture in the name of "prevention" and "risk management" (Asch and Geller 1996; Crawford 1977, 1980; Lippman 1991, 1993; Lock 1996; Rapp 1989; see Chapters 3 and 4, this volume).

Two of the most recent examples of this in the lives of women in North America have been the conceptualizations of women's breasts and women's bones as such sites. Earlier conceptualizations of women's bodies were primarily directed to specific and real, actual instances of breast diseases and to bone fractures as evidence of loss of bone mass and strength. Catalyzed by the profit-oriented rise and widespread availability of the technologies of mammography and bone-scanning, these earlier conceptualizations were supplanted by much more broadly directed reconceptualizations of virtually all women's bodies as potential, presymptomatic, risk-laden sites (Coney 1994; Kaufert 1996; Love 1997).[16] This fear-laden perception that all women's bodies are sites of "virtual pathology" has resulted in much greater medicalization in the culture at large. (I return to this point below in my discussion of medical self-management.)

Politically, macro-institutionalization is most exclusionist when the authoritative medical knowledge embodied in the institutions is claimed to be—and is accepted as—the sole prerogative of particular individuals and groups who then use their expertise to provide "rational" justification for their position of hierarchical social, political, economic, and symbolic dominance in the culture (Habermas 1981; Smith 1990).[17] Where there is acceptance of the principle of expert monopoly over authoritative knowledge, social and political role-structured dominance follows as the experts exercise primary control over the medical discourse over the health and research priorities (within existing constraints), and over medical technology. In North America, medical experts, trained in medical schools and legally certified to practice by autonomous medical organizations, define, control access to, and exercise ultimate control over the legitimate use of the following: research investigations and protocols, screening devices and tests, expert-controlled interventionist procedures and treatments (such as surgery, vaccines, patches, implants, extrauterine fertilization, genetic manipulation, expensive hospital-based diagnostic and monitoring devices of all sorts), and prescription drugs and prostheses, and over other forms of technology and therapy deemed legitimate for preventative and rehabilitative purposes.[18] In Western industrialized countries, medical experts, medical practitioners, and medical institutions are thus positioned at the top of a health care–knowledge pyramid that pervades normal life. Formal legal and professional policy-driven monopolies guarantee the subordinate positioning of other health care researchers, workers, and providers in organizational and informal contexts.

As a consequence, health care institutions and practitioners who do not "fit" into this pyramidal structure are ignored, ridiculed, criminalized, or suppressed through a variety of institutional mechanisms. Similarly, given the epistemic dominance of a canonical set of research methodologies as the exclusive paths to knowledge, any claims to medical knowledge that arise from individual lived experience will likely be ignored, demeaned, or explicitly ruled out (Alcoff and Gray 1993; Code 1995b; Dalmiya and Alcoff 1993; Davis-Floyd and Davis 1996; Ehrenreich and English 1972; Jones 1988; Sargent and Bascope 1996). This is one of the reasons why the alleged authoritative knowledge claims of Cohen and Backhouse were not given expert standing in the press.

Micro-Institutionalization Through Doctor-Patient Relations
In Western industrialized medicalized culture, members of the culture are taught to see doctors as the benevolent holders of expert authoritative medical knowledge that doctors are believed to use for the therapeutic benefit of the community and individual patients. The

widescale cultural acceptance of this belief enables doctor-patient interactions and relations to function as powerful sites where the micro-institutionalization of medicalization can take place (Fisher and Todd 1983; Foucault 1973; Ruzek 1978; Sherwin 1992; Smith 1996; Todd 1989; see Chapter 7, this volume).

Individual doctors and patients are involved in complex, sometimes mutually reinforcing dynamics and negotiations. Often patients come to physicians, as David Schenck puts it, because of the "brokenness" of our bodies or of our hearts (quoted in Diprose 1995, 210). We often come in pain, uncertainty, dread, and terror, suffering from the loss of integrity. Although we may be healthy now (however that is defined by our culture or community), we may come to doctors for preventative reasons, to ward off pain, dread, and the loss of integrity later in our lives. Individual patients may want to be reassured by, and demand access to, precisely those medicalizing technologies the doctor controls as a way of trying to take control over uncertainty, over unpredictability, and over vulnerability.[19] This is a crucial aspect of relational autonomy where patients make choices from positions of oppression and personal vulnerability (see Chapters 2, 3, 4, and 9).

It is wise to remember, however, that doctor-patient interactions are highly political. The institutionalized power of the physician to diagnose, to discipline, to carry out surveillance, to expect confession and compliance to "doctor's orders" are particularly central to the exercise of authoritative knowledge built into hierarchical medicalized doctor-patient relationships (Code 1994, 1995b; Corea 1985a; Diprose 1995; Foucault 1973; Ruzek 1978; Smith 1996). This becomes clear when the expression of genuine patient disagreement is not seen as a real, respected option when weighed in the balance with the epistemic authority and institutional power of the physician. Resistance and refusal can be quickly labeled "lack of compliance" and can have frightening consequences, particularly for women and anyone vulnerably situated in oppressive circumstances (Morgan 1998; Weiss 1977).

When that happens, doctor-patient relationships function as micro-sites of oppression, of degradation—and of resistance.[20] It is also clear that doctor-patient interactions can, even in situations of power inequity, function as micro-sites of healing, as relations that are significant in restoring integrity, as providing liberating growth from abusive, repressive, or limiting constraints—in short, can function as relationships that empower the patient (Candib 1994; More and Milligan 1994; Pellegrino and Thomasma 1988; Smith 1996; see Chapter 9, this volume).[21]

Whether at the macro level or in day-to-day micro doctor-patient interactions, effective medicalization involves doctors seeing "the Other" through a professional, objectifying, clinical *"medical gaze,"* a complex perception in which the Other becomes "the vulnerable patient" simultaneous with the mutual acknowledgment of the medical doctor as the expert (Frankel 1983). Patients are expected to believe in the doctor's therapeutic competence and to trust in the doctor's good will because of the doctor's control over authoritative knowledge and over the dominant medicalizing discourse. Shifting any of these variables will significantly alter the politics of micro-institutionalization (Ruzek 1978).

Once constituted, from both a professional and a personal point of view, as a "patient," the patient comes into legitimate range for *medical surveillance.* While medical experts define the nature of the professional medical gaze and train medical students in its performance, often other mediating health care professionals and providers and individual members of the culture carry out "the doctor's orders." They are explicitly charged with exercising and translating the technological and therapeutic directives of the "medical gaze" through various forms of medical surveillance (Conrad 1992; Foucault 1973).

In high medicalization cultures medical surveillance is widespread as a differentially applied, culturally shared practice and can take on a complex variety of political forms. It can be exercised informally by family members and friends as well as by more likely role occupants such as teachers, administrators, members of the culturally identified "helping" professions such as social workers, nurses, and therapists, and by religious leaders charged with therapeutic responsibilities. The more pervasive the health-preventative and rehabilitative the medical practices are in a given culture, the more extensive the domains of surveillance can become (Crawford 1977, 1980; see Chapters 3 and 4, this volume).

Consider the following example. In the November 20, 1996, issue of *The Globe and Mail*, the subheadline read, "Smoking, poor diet, sloth lead to 70 per cent of [cancer] deaths" (A10). Reporting on a Harvard School of Public Health Report just published in the journal *Cancer, Causes & Control*, the five authors of the article attributed nearly 70 percent of all cancer deaths to a "sedentary lifestyle." The high institutional standing of the prestigious Harvard School of Public Health Report can be appealed to by health critics to provide justification for intensifying applications of medical surveillance to virtually all aspects of daily human life—movement, eating, and substance use (Crawford 1977, 1980; Graham 1990). Members of the culture may be encouraged to maintain medical surveillance in families, in supermarkets, in restaurants, at social gatherings—in virtually all public, social, and personal domains—in order to prevent the 70 percent of cancer deaths alleged to result exclusively from sloth-ridden lives marked by evil appetites involving potato chips and tobacco, and to explain and blame others' cancer on their failure to control such lifestyle factors. Studies have shown that often those patients who share economic and sociocultural affinities with their doctors and who report high levels of confidence in their doctors appear more motivated to participate in forms of medical surveillance (Davis-Floyd 1996; De Koninck 1990a, 1990b; Graham and Oakley 1981; Reissman 1983; Roberts 1996). Here it is wise to recall Kathleen Martindale's irate and sad comment (1996) in her posthumously published breast cancer narrative: "I already do all the alternative lifestyle stuff—I meditate, exercise, do yoga, eat health food, think positive thoughts and, yet I got cancer" (124).

Hard lessons learned from their patients' experience teach them that principled wariness is a more appropriate position to take than one of confidence.[22] It is clear that medical surveillance can take on sadistic and invasive forms with respect to particular populations of women such as incarcerated women (alongside enormous actual medical negligence) (Jose-Kampfner 1995). It can also occur in skewed and eclipsing forms in the lives of women who are open with their doctors about being lesbians or in the lives of women with known disabilities (Boston Women's Health Book Collective 1992; Martindale 1996; McClure 1994; Rockhill in Tremain 1996; Wendell 1996). As Susan Wendell (1996) remarks:

> Disability tends to be associated with tragic loss, weakness,
> passivity, dependency, helplessness, shame and global
> incompetence. In the societies where Western science and
> medicine are powerful culturally, and where their promise to
> control nature is still widely believed, people with disabilities
> are constant reminders of the failures of that promise, and of
> the inability of science and medicine to protect everyone from
> illness, disability, and death. They are "the Others" that science
> would like to forget. (63)

In other cases, necessary therapeutic medical surveillance can be withheld in the lives of high-risk women such as refugee women and homeless women.

Women are increasingly targeted for surveillance—largely as reproductively defined, instrumentally valuable "vessels and vectors" (Faden, Kass, and McGraw 1996; Greaves 1995). The medical surveillance of pregnant women occurs not simply in physician's offices but on the street, in restaurants, in public settings, and in the privacy of familial settings when medicalized norms of "the responsible pregnancy" are used judgmentally to evaluate and criticize the behavior of pregnant women, particularly with respect to alcohol and tobacco use.

For women who can afford it (either because of private insurance in the United States or because it is covered by public health plans in other industrialized countries) technologically mediated surveillance of pregnancy is becoming an increasingly normalized dimension of virtually every pregnancy and birth. As Browner and Press (1996) point out:

> Once a prenatal diagnostic technology becomes widely available it cannot be refused neutrally because refusal can be construed as a lack of responsibility on the part of the pregnant woman. Adherence to routines of scientifically based prenatal care, like AFP [alpha-fetoprotein] testing and ultrasound scans, is women's only culturally approved means of reassuring themselves, and others, that they are doing "all that can be done" to ensure a healthy pregnancy. (153)[23]

Increasingly, for many pregnant women who will ultimately have hospital births, a completely nontechnologized experience of maternity itself is becoming rare. Studies suggest that more and more women are demanding such surveillance in the name of choice and control—and their doctors are ordering the surveillance in the name of the responsible "technology-assisted" pregnancy (and as a way of avoiding possible litigation) (Browner and Press 1996; Davis-Floyd 1992, 1996; see Chapter 6, this volume).

In many cultures of the world, women occupy complicated positions in relation to medical surveillance and health care—as informal providers, negotiators, recipients, and mediators[24] as well as in their varied capacities as paid formal health care providers such as nurses, genetic counselors, midwives, and teachers.[25] Thus women are, generally, more likely to be involved in the complex dialectical process of engaging in the medical surveillance particularly of children and of their families and kin and of being prime targets for surveillance by themselves and others.

Summarizing the first three elements, I would say that the process of medicalization involves the creation and transmission of medical authoritative knowledge through mediating macro-structures and practices within which micro-institutionalizing doctor-patient relations are constituted through direct or mediated personal encounters. This is where the fourth element becomes important. Apart from situations of enormous political coercion, until there is active acceptance of this medicalization process by members of a culture in their ordinary lifeworlds, medicalization cannot function as a political form of social ordering and social control. This leads to a discussion of the fourth critical element.

Micro-Institutionalization Through Self-Management
In her powerful, insightful book *The Menopause Industry,* Sandra Coney (1994) claims:

> It is no longer possible for an individual to simply regard
> herself as a healthy woman in the prime of life. This can only
> be stated with authority if medicine has confirmed it by
> "screening" various parts of her body. She should submit to
> "monitoring" by periodic testing. For her breasts, there should
> be a "baseline mammogram," against which any changes in
> her tissues will be measured. She will develop a surrogate
> identity or alter ego—femina medica—in which she is defined
> by a series of computer printouts and x-ray films. . . . The
> woman who eschews protecting herself in this way is seen as
> inexplicably reckless and careless of herself. (26)

Clearly, a medicalized gaze and medical surveillance are most effectively produced and reproduced when individual members of the culture internalize, use, actively support, and demand the use of medicalizing concepts, discourse, and practices and when they not only comply with but seek out active involvement in medical technologies claiming medical discourse and vocabularies as their own. I refer to this as *medicalized subjectivity, or medicalized agency.* When this happens, not only does medicalization become a significant part of common cultural discourse, it becomes constitutive of the personal language of the individuals who experience themselves as active medicalizing subjects. As medicalized self-management develops, the rhetoric is often one of responsibility, control, self-interest, and self-determination (Boston Women's Health Book Collective 1992; De Koninck 1996; Kaufert 1996)—and the lived reality for a some people is a genuine increase of personal power and decision-making.[26]

For example, studies have shown that in North America, privileged pregnant women, who often bond socioeconomically with their middle-class professional obstetricians, are encouraged to feel apprehensive about the dangers of naive, unmonitored, technology unassisted childbirth. Pervasive technological monitoring and intervention throughout the birth are proposed to provide reassurance, to provide authoritative knowledge, as the remedy for such fears.[27] Just as "the healthy pregnancy" is medically defined and technologically mediated (Rothman

1986), so, too, the "ordinary healthy birth" is increasingly defined as "the medically monitored and technology-assisted birth." Women—particularly white, middle-class women—have been encouraged to adopt medicalizing discourse, to use mediating visually oriented medical technologies in the name of maternal-fetal surveillance, and to prize a technologically "assisted" birthing experience in a hospital setting. While some women report a sense of loss and alienation resulting from a technology-managed birth, others do report a sense of personal fulfillment as medicalizing maternal subjects who have chosen to appropriate the authoritative knowledge and technology of the experts and who claim to experience autonomy (Browner and Press 1996; Davis-Floyd 1994; Graham and Oakley 1981; Petchesky 1987; De Koninck 1988; see Chapters 2, 6, and 7, this volume).

Similarly, in North America, women's widespread demands for hormonal replacement therapy suggest that, in addition to associating particular experiences such as hot flashes with menopause, women are actively taking up the medicalization model of women's midlife as a potentially dangerous life stage involving a profoundly soul-altering Change (Coney 1994; Love 1997). Women are urged to combine this global pathologization of women's midlife with the more specific medical pathologization of menopause by researchers, endocrinologists, medical practitioners, and pharmaceutical advertisers as a "hormone-deficiency disorder" analogous to diabetes with a correlative need for lifelong medical intervention and control (Coney 1994; Sherwin 1992; Worcester and Whateley 1994; see Chapter 8, this volume).

The Ordinary Lifeworlds

Medicalization functions as a form of social control because it claims jurisdiction in the ordinary lifeworlds of individuals and groups in a given culture (Lindenbaum and Lock 1993). The degree and range of medicalization present in the ordinary lifeworlds of a given culture can be highly variable, as the central circle diagram in Figure 1 suggests. Various individuals (and, by extension, groups) in this diagram are represented as diversely medicalized and medicalizing subjects. For some, a particular area or zone or system of the body is a highly medicalized area, such as cosmetic appearance or fertility or the cardiovascular system, while the remainder may not be experienced through an internalized "medical Gaze" (Dyck 1995). Some members of the culture may not act or experience themselves as medicalized subjects at all—hence no surrounding serpentine symbol—while others may lead lives profoundly eclipsed as medicalized subjects. Similarly, the small circles representing heads are diversely characterized to indicate the highly varied responses that individuals and groups can have in relation to individual and collective medicalization.

Leaving aside contexts of involuntary medicalization and personal and political coercion, it is clear that a significant variety of personal and collective responses to medicalizing control do exist. Some individuals and groups *resist totalizing medicalization* and fight to shift the dominant discourse. For example, they may fight to shift totalizing discourses and replace them with phrases such as "people living with disabilities" or "people living with AIDS." Others may *fight for clear demedicalization or resist the dominant conceptualization* of medicalization in favor of some other model such as homeopathic medicine or the preservation of indigenous healing practices. Others may *fight for and demand access to medicalization* with respect to its macro- and micro-institutional forms demanding medical attention in such areas, for example, as the occupational health issues of migratory workers or more attention being directed to systemic environmental health issues concerning industrial pollutants (Messing 1991, 1995; Messing, Doniol-Shaw, and Haentjens 1994). Then, again, others may *argue for a shift in the basic conceptualization* element, for example, with respect to whether premenstrual experiences ought to be classified as a psychiatric disorder (Caplan 1993, 1995). Still others will *fight for a fundamental shift in health and research priorities* at both the macro- and micro-institutional level in such areas, for example, as AIDS and breast cancer.[28] While it is clear that medicalization can function as a powerful mechanism of social control, it is crucial to keep in mind its important political dialectical nature with respect to conceptualization and its macro- and micro-institutionalizations.

Two Cautionary Examples

Considered abstractly, as in Figure 1, medicalization might be thought of as a value-neutral, highly flexible social dynamic, the consequences of which may be good, bad, or neutral depending upon the content and contexts involved. Increased medicalization can promote important research and access to appropriate therapeutic interventions in the lives of human beings (Wendell 1996). Understanding communicable diseases as sicknesses that can be prevented, for example, through smallpox vaccinations and institutionalizing global preventative programs of inoculation that are widely accessible and effective at both the macro and micro levels can clearly be seen to be beneficial. Similarly, developing medical technologies such as fibre optic–based hysteroscopes so that organ-destroying fibroids can be removed vaginally from a woman's body without destroying her uterus is clearly an improvement over a bloody operation involving the use of a scalpel under general anesthesia (Gross and Ito 1991).

But medicalization is not always so benevolent. One of the most terrifying and instructive chapters for women in the history of Western medicalization involves the medical construction of lesbianism seen in the larger context of the medical control of any deviations from phallocentric institutionalized heterosexuality.[29] Following a general trend in the early twentieth century toward the secularization of forms of social control, the medicalization of lesbianism as a disease state began to dominate cultural discourse.

In the early twentieth century, determinist medical explanations of lesbianism alleged that lesbianism resulted in dangerous insane and "primitive" behaviors necessitating confinement in asylums to protect society from lesbian violence, perversity, and evil. These explanations lived side by side with the newer American psychoanalytic medical paradigms that viewed lesbianism as resulting from gravely pathologizing forms of regression, which caused lesbians to be more dangerous than homosexual men, consumed by aggressive hatred and hostility and dangerously psychopathic in their behavior. Stevens and Hall (1994) argue that because of the surrounding oppressive legal, political, and religious institutions, many lesbians and homosexual men in the late nineteenth century looked to the medical establishment as, potentially, more understanding and compassionate. As in some contemporary lesbian and gay circles, the hope was that, given the surrounding oppressive institutions, it was better to be viewed as sick rather than as evil or criminal. The hope was bitterly betrayed, however, as lesbians met institutionalized medical violence. Once medicalized, for most of the twentieth century lesbians (and gay men) suffered psychiatric confinements, medical and therapeutic ridicule and stigmatization, electroshock treatments, aversive therapy involving vomiting or dehydration, psychosurgery, hormonal interventions, and psychotropic chemotherapy (Birke 1982). This was accompanied by experimental degradation as medical researchers sought (and continue to search) for a biomedical cure (or, even "better," a preventative prenatal procedure).[30]

A second example involves the medicalization of maternal mortality. As Sohier Morsy (1995) notes, "the World Health Organization estimates that half a million deaths occur annually among women who are or have been pregnant during the previous forty-two days." Entitling her article "Deadly Reproduction Among Egyptian Women: Maternal Mortality and the Medicalization of Population Control," Morsy analyses how Egyptian women's fertility per se has been medically pathologized to satisfy the population control requirements attendant upon economic structural adjustment. Noting that a World Bank study identified "excess fertility" as "*a disease in developing countries* alongside malnutrition, anemia, tetanus, AIDS and sexually-transmitted diseases, diabetes, and others" (165, emphasis added), Morsy analyses how turning "excess fertility" into a disease and seeing the dying of Egyptian mothers as simply a medical problem medically pathologizes women's fertility. It also metamorphoses political population control itself into a medicalizing process allegedly devoid of any cultural or political agenda. (See Chapter 7 for an extended discussion of medicine's response to maternal mortality.)

What is the theoretical point of these examples? It is that it is imperative to locate any real life instantiation of the theoretical medicalization model in its historical and contemporary settings, to contextualize it with reference to larger material and ideological lenses and frameworks. Only in this way will we be able to understand the complex historical and contemporary contestations of medicalization by women and comprehend the radical epistemological politics of the Women's Health Movement.

Medical Conceptualizations in Context: Two Powerful Paradigms

As medicalization has developed in Western thought and practice, the conceptualization element involves two powerful paradigms: the biomedical model of the human body, and the "natural pathology" view of women.

Paradigm 1: The Biomedical Model of the Human Body
As we see elsewhere in this volume (especially Chapters 2, 3, and 9), in European and North American culture, medicalization often involves the entrenchment of a biomedical model as the exclusive "reasonable" paradigm in research and clinical settings as well as in macro- and micro-institutional settings (Rhodes 1990).[31] This model basically says that health (or the absence of health) is an internal property of a particular separate independent human organism. The individual living human organism is conceptualized as the proper subject of health and as the appropriate target for health care interventions. In its most atomistic form, this individualism is often carried out in principled, context-stripping ways so that differentiating systemic factors such as culture, race, historical location, class posi-

tion, gender, sociocultural age, sexual identity, political position, and disability status drop out of the picture altogether. If these factors are acknowledged in response to documented differences among particular groups of people, for example, with respect to mortality rates or hypertension, the differences are seen merely as naturalized biologically determined differences lacking any medical significance apart from their possible predictive value (Lock 1996; Scheman 1983). Health populations can then come to be understood simply as aggregates of such atomic individuals. Correlatively, health research, policy, and clinical and therapeutic practices and interventions are directed to specific individuals as individuals within populations.[32] Where it is manifestly impossible to treat people solely as detached separate subjects, such as in the case of genetically related persons or pregnant women, separate individualism can be sustained by denying the actual autonomous organic personhood of the women involved by reconceptualizing them, for example, simply as "vectors or vessels" (Faden, Kass, and McGraw 1996; Greaves 1995). This reclassification and shift of focus thereby eliminates them as separate subjects whose own health is a meaningful issue and directs attention to their sexual partners or to their (potential) offspring (see Chapters 3 and 4).

Biomedical individualism is often linked with a strong belief in naturalistic reductionism (Bem 1993; Birke 1986; Tiefer 1995), which maintains that the various biological factors, functions, and dimensions that constitute each of us at a given time really exist and function in ways that are fundamentally presocial or precultural. Belonging to human beings as biological organisms, they are seen as universalizable across the human species. Pneumonia is pneumonia regardless of where it occurs. AIDS is AIDS regardless of which human organism is the suffering carrier of the virus. In a reductionist model, decontextualized biological factors claim to be the only factors or the only significant factors that should be taken into account in generating and applying authoritative medical knowledge (see Chapter 10).[33]

While the biomedical paradigm has various limitations (Guttmacher 1997), it is difficult to see how it entails any oppressive consequences particularly for girls and women since such particularity is, by definition, ruled out by the paradigm. Further conceptual contextualization is necessary. We must move to a second important paradigm in Western biomedicine.

Paradigm 2: Essential Female "Natural Pathology"

One depressing and infuriatingly long legacy in Western European culture is the ideological and material multipathologization of women.[34] The ancient Greek philosopher Aristotle, in his biological treatise, "On the Generation of Animals" (1994), maintains that "a woman is as it were an infertile male; the female, in fact, is female on account of an inability of a sort; . . . *the female is as it were a deformed male*" (24–25, emphasis added). The alleged natural inferiority of "the female" is a dominant theme in Western religious and philosophical thought and continues to be the often sought after Holy Gender Grail. Although the pathology-conferring site or function has varied throughout Western history,[35] the conclusion has had a sickening monotony to it: women's bodies, women's minds, and women's natures are essentially and dangerously inferior to those of men.

In the nineteenth century rather than conceding any biological excellence to human females, Darwin asserted, in *The Descent of Man* (1874), the absolute inferiority of "the female" in *all humanly important domains*, an inferiority that, in a strikingly comprehensive process of racist racialization, he also assigned to virtually all non-European races in one fell swoop. Selective medicalization contributed to the new pathologization of menstruation, and technical scientific advances were used in support of crainiological demonstrations of women's inferiority and the inferiority of virtually all Black people (Gilman 1985; Haraway 1989). In the twentieth century, Western science often continues to "prove" women's natural inferiority by basing its arguments on the erroneous and often distorted medical conceptualizations of the role of "sex hormones" in women's bodies (Coney 1994; Fausto-Sterling 1985; Love 1997; Oudshoorn 1994) regardless of whether they are present or absent.

If hormones themselves are not sufficient, the multifaceted nature of women's fertility can serve as "justification" for the natural pathologization paradigm. In North America in the late twentieth century, a wide range of normal premenstrual changes in women are being classified as a mental disorder, "late luteal-phase dysphoria," which is potentially attributable to virtually all women who menstruate. Once so-labeled women become the appropriate medicalized subjects for pharmaceutical and psychiatric intervention (Caplan 1995; Fausto-Sterling 1985; Tuana, ed., 1989; Zita 1989). Analogously, in North America, in the dominant medicalization research, clinical literature, and popularly pharmaceutical advertisements, the ending of fertility is seen as requiring estrogen-replacement therapy to help women through the "withering" losses attendant upon menopause conceived as a universal disease state. (Clearly this is not universal. See Chapter 8.) Such losses are seen as involving the vulva shriveling so that it becomes "a dry narrow slit in some old women," the breasts becoming "pendulous, wrinkled and flabby," the skin of the breasts coarsening and becoming covered with scales, and the nipples losing their erective properties and erotic sensitivity (Coney 1994, 76).[36]

Psychologically, women are encouraged to pathologize themselves by volunteering to take tests such as the Moos Menstrual Distress Questionnaire, by describing their bodies through the often misogynistic rhetoric of medical and research texts (Caplan 1993, 1995; Fausto-Sterling 1985; Martin 1987), and by being assessed through personality testing instruments that structurally presuppose that only heterosexual submissiveness in women is normal and that female assertiveness signals a "dysfunctional gender identity" or abnormal phallic strivings (Fausto-Sterling 1985). Compulsory Western "normal" white, middle-class norms of subordinate, supportive nurturing become repathologized by medical therapists as the pathological state of "co-dependency" (Babcock and McKay 1995; Hagan 1993; Tavris 1992; Westlund 1997). Once again, and over and over, women are first medically conceptualized and then "diagnosed" as naturally sickly, blamed for being sick, treated as sick, and seen as irrationally pathogenic by nature. This carries important political consequences: women need to be and must be controlled by (preferably benevolent) men for women's and children's own good and for the collective social good. Patriarchal relations are necessary at both the macro- and micro-institutional level. More specifically, it is proposed that patriarchal medicalization must become normalized for the good and healthy society.

The prevalence of the "natural pathology" view of women leads to its inevitable corollary of (white, preferably healthy and able-bodied) males assuming pride of place as the most fully realized, reasonable research and clinical medical human paradigm available (and the principled oppressive dispensability of other males) (Bair and Cayleff 1993; Frankenberg 1993a; Frye 1975; Thomson 1997; Wendell 1996). A principled medical androcentric paradigm becomes the only conceivable norm with devastating health consequences for women (DeBruin 1994; Dresser 1992; Mastroianni, Faden, and Federman 1994; Morgan 1996b; see Chapter 10, this volume). Generalizing from this androcentrism, it is possible to read the history of Western medical research as reinforcing repeatedly the normativity of white male experience. This practice has proved dangerous and sometimes deadly to women.

Macro-Institutionalization in Context: 4 Frames

Consider the following:

> It is estimated that 75% of the 18 million refugees in the world
> are girls and women. Many of them experience repeated and
> brutal rapes at every stage of their escape. (Heise 1993b)

> In the urban Puerto Rican population in the United States one
> out of six babies has a low birth weight, childhood asthma is
> pervasive, and influenza and pneumonia are the third-ranked
> cause of death. In New York City women who are fortunate
> enough to work in the paid labor force in the textile industry
> experience health hazards such as brown lung or, if working as
> unregistered aliens, the oppressive conditions of the worst
> "sweat shops." (Zambrana and Hurst 1994)

> In Canada, because of northern health policy decisions and
> because of the selective use of health care resources which
> provides no community-based facilities for deliveries, almost
> all Inuit women have to be transported sometimes thousands
> of miles to urban hospitals for an average period of three
> weeks regardless of whether their pregnancies are deemed low
> or high risk. The federal government pays for this. (O'Neil and
> Kaufert 1995)

In each of these situations, women's experience of health and health
care is affected by the ways in which gender power politics are constituted by women's and men's defined reproductive and productive
roles, by the dominant domestic and global political economies involved, by multiple axes of oppression and domination based on such
factors as race, class position, sexual and gender identity, (dis)ability
status, by complex relationships to macro- and micro-medicalizing institutions and medical technology, and by varying relationships to
other dominant institutions in the culture. Women's health politics is always contextualized as women submit, accommodate, resist, sabotage,
negotiate, or appropriate medicalization from their own locations. This
is one of the important political insights about relational autonomy (see
Chapter 2).

   "Women's health is global"—this has become an important methodological postulate in women's health scholarship.[37] Reflecting far more
than simply an interest in aggregated or comparative geographical mo-
saics of women's health research, women's global health research seeks
out local, collective, and transnational intersections for a complex understanding of, for example, the role of poverty in the lives of women

and children (Jacobson 1993; Krieger 1994; Perales and Young 1988). One important dimension of this research is an interrogation of how Western biomedical medicalization has become a global form of (potential) social control, how its dominant forms of conceptualization become translated into contextualized powerful macro-institutions and culturally specific forms of micro-institutionalization. In contemporary medical macro-institutionalization, those experts and those macro-institutions that claim control over the authoritative knowledge central to Western biomedical medicalization and whose technocratic aspirations are closely linked to ideologies of control are often powerfully positioned by virtue of their critical alliances with other forms of social control in local and global economies and cultures (DeKoninck n.d.; Greenhalgh and Li 1996; Morsy 1995; see Chapters 3, 4, 7, and 9, this volume). Thus it is crucial to look at the social, economic, political and symbolic macro- institutional frames for contextualizing Western biomedicine. In carrying out global women's health research, at least four analytic methodological frames are necessary: (1) political economy, (2) dimensions of patriarchy, (3) relation to an ideology of technological control, and (4) structural alliances (see Figure 2).

Local and Global Political Economies
In Western industrialized countries the political economies are variants of welfare capitalism where the state assumes some responsibility for health care (and other social needs) on a large popular scale within a larger economic setting where control over material and economic resources is often dominated by a select number of individuals and powerful profit-oriented corporations. Oppressive ideologies and normalized ideological practices involving racism, class-bias, and ableism often result in differential access to actual health care (Krieger 1994; Silvers 1994, 1995). Highly variable access to wealth results in widespread poverty among women and children and among members of socially vulnerable groups in general. Major social resources are often directed to expensive, high-technology health research priorities that benefit relatively few, often privileged, members of the society (Basen, Eichler, and Lippman 1993; see Chapters 3 and 4, this volume).

On a global scale, neocolonial imperialism involving transnational control over local resources is likely to dominate. Often devastating destabilizing factors such as genocidal political practices, labor diaspora, war, and homelessness disrupt lives and place major strains on women for whom reproductive, familial, and community care-providing responsibilities are often central to their identities and roles in their nor-

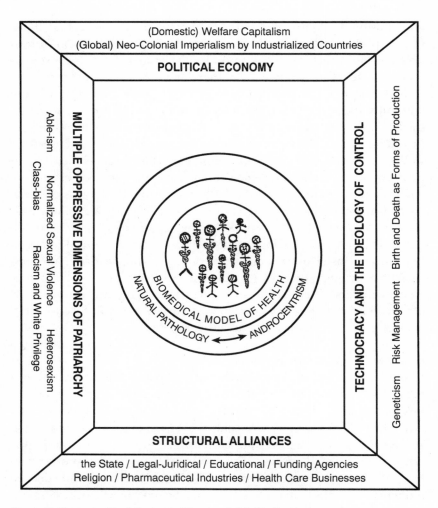

Figure 2. Contextualized Systemic Hegemonic Medicalization

mal lifeworlds (Ginsberg and Rapp 1991; Mullings 1995). International monetary agencies and policies, development agencies, international pharmaceutical industries, domestic markets, and local governments often promote Western biomedical medicalization as a form of "progress," as "enlightened medicine," thereby establishing its conceptualizations as authoritative knowledge and its experts as the dominant medical authorities (often in the absence of those support services that would realize the genuinely empowering potential of some forms of medicalization) (Ginsburg and Rapp 1995). Frequently, Western medicalization is tied to oppressive population control as a price to be paid for continuing foreign aid (Hartman 1987; Morsy 1995; Sundari 1994; see Chapter 7, this volume). Engaging critically with Western medicalization is a crucial part of many women's lives as they individually and collectively contest the political globalization of their lives.

Technocracy and Ideologies of Control

This frame refers to the cultural status accorded to Western technology—hence, "technocracy"—and to the ideological optimism and industrial profit to be made through the domestic lifeworld normalization of medical technology in Western countries and to the exportation of medicalizing technologies throughout the world. Given this mass exportation of Western medical technology and the presumption of the authoritative status of such technology over local technologies, each global realization of medicalization will involve some complex positioning in relation to Western technology and must be analyzed (Berer 1994; "The Human Laboratory" 1995).

One example in Western culture involves the medical conceptualization of the Human Genome Project, the growth of the macro-institutions based on the technologies for genetic testing and gene manipulation that appropriate the basic gene research, and the micro-institutionalization of genetic counselor–patient relations leading to the possible ascendancy of a cultural ideology of geneticism (Asch and Geller 1996; Hubbard and Wald 1993; Lippman 1991, 1993; Rapp 1989, 1990; P. Rock 1996; Wolf 1994; see Chapter 4, this volume). Once dominant, geneticization ideology and practices can create and reinforce power relationships in which some dominate by virtue of genetic superiority and others are subordinated because of medically defined genetic inferiority (Wolf 1994; P. Rock, 1996). Dominant geneticism would thereby involve a form of medical social control predicated on widespread technology-based geneticization throughout a culture (Lippman 1991, 1993; see Chapter 4, this volume).

Multiple Oppressive Dimensions of Patriarchy

Every woman has a complex relationship to patriarchy. Culturally specific patriarchal assumptions about women's nature, women's bodies, and women's health intersect with other potentially oppressive dimensions in women's lives, including the powerful forces of ableism, normalized sexual violence, heterosexism, class-bias, racism, and white privilege. Although, as "females," all women may be viewed through an androcentric "natural pathology" medical gaze as biomedical objects, often women experience a complicated double bind. This involves being simultaneously denied particularity and medically significant diversity through the context-stripping assumptions of the biomedical model while being treated differentially and, sometimes, in deadly ways if they are not women of privilege (see Chapters 7 and 9).[38]

This frame helps us to understand how, for example, the biological naturalizing of racialized categories in North America can intersect with context-stripped medicalized definitions of osteoporosis as a "white female disease" resulting in lack of attention to the prevention and treatment of osteoporosis in Black and Hispanic communities of women (Gamble and Blustein 1994). This frame helps us to understand why, as Carol Gill (1996) points out, most of the Western medical and social scientific research priorities on disability focus on men because being seen as passive, dependent, and incompetent is radically dissonant with masculine norms of activity, independence, and competence. Men with disabilities are expected to be seen as more devastated than women with disabilities, who are seen as simply more passive, dependent, and incompetent than usual. As a result, men are generally seen as more worthy subjects for medical research and as recipients for medical technology (R. Thomson 1994, 1997).[39]

Structural Alliances

It is clear that medicalization, as a complex social and political dynamic and set of institutions, does not ascend to a position of systemic hegemony or dominance in a given culture without powerful, mutually supportive alliances with other institutions. As it exists in North America, dominant medicalization is supported by and protected through powerful legal and juridical institutions that give preeminent status to medical experts and to medical knowledge. The state, health care industries, public and private funding agencies, insurance companies, and pharmaceutical industries provide financial support to medical schools and teaching hospitals. This practice underwrites the dominance of medical experts thereby further entrenching existing biomedical, misogynistic thinking. Especially in the United States, medicalization increasingly uses the power of the courts and the police to extend medical control in the lives of women by, for example, threatening and incarcerating pregnant women, by ordering court-enforced cesarean sections, by denying lesbians custody of their children because they have been deemed "psychologically unfit" by a court psychiatrist, and through involuntary competence hearings targeted at women (Jordan and Irwin 1989; Secker forthcoming; see Chapter 9, this volume).

On a global scale, multi-institutional neocolonial alliances have been formed that are committed to the globalization of Western biomedicine

and the concomitant appropriation or destruction of indigenous healing practices, nonmedicalized healers, and indigenous knowledges
(Mohanty 1991; see Chapter 7, this volume). These alliances thereby insure the continued multisystemic hegemonic positioning of medicalization politics throughout the world.

For a summary visual representation of the these remarks, refer once
again to Figure 2.

Contesting Medicalization Knowledge/Politics: The Critical Role of the Women's Health Movement

Contested bodies, contested knowledges—this is how I see the epistemic
politics between Western biomedical medicalization and the global
Women's Health Movement. From a feminist epistemological point of
view, I see this contestation as involving at least two complex, though related political projects. The first involves the (re)claiming of women's
subjectivity, women's agency. The second involves the (re)claiming of
epistemic power.

(Re)Claiming Subjectivity

From a hierarchical, expert-dominated medicalization point of view,
here is the ideal female patient: she is reasonably (but not too) intelligent, enthusiastic about but only sufficiently informed about medical
institutions, procedures, and technology to satisfy minimum legal consent conditions, cooperative with respect to the paternalistically motivated medically directed use of medical technology, convinced that institutionalized medicine and medical technology provide the best
health care in a larger macro-institutional setting where medicine enjoys pride of place, highly compliant with respect to following medical
orders, and cheerfully responsible with respect to medicalized self-
management (Morgan 1998; Sherwin 1992; Weiss 1977).

Women have not always been such "ideal patients." Nor are they
now. More particularly, women who identify with the Women's Health
Movement are extremely unlikely to demonstrate any potential to become such ideal patients. One of the earliest forms of political resistance
to misogynistic medicalization and to other violence in the lives of girls
and women has been the rejection of gender-specific norms of silence
(Doress et al. 1987). Stories of healing have always been told and publicly celebrated. More recently, women have told other stories. Women
have spoken out, telling of pain, of medical exploitation and coercion,
of fear in the face of powerful medicalizing macro-institutions, and of

degradation and violence directed at them by those entrusted with "the medical gaze" in micro-institutional settings and by those holding a monopoly over healing technologies.[40] Women have gone public with their stories of medical oppression, and women have gone public with their needs and their demands, sharing their aspirations for healthy bodies, healthy children, healthy families and communities, and a healthy planet. This movement toward the public and political, physically intimate narrative and the affirmation of the lived knowledge on which it is based—whether it is in villages or on prime time television, whether at quilting bees, at militant women's health rallies, or on the Internet—is a political act (Hannaford 1985; Klein 1992). Collectively, it contributes to a political movement in which women are empowered to challenge any medicalization model that promotes a picture of medical experts as universally committed to impartial benevolence.

In order for women to reclaim subjectivity, it is important for us to fight for recognition of the knowledge women have as healers, as knowledgeable informal and formal providers of health care, and as critical subjects who can take up a variety of political positions in relation to medicalization. In the context of the Women's Health Movement these positions often map onto those discussed above. Sometimes women's health advocates have *resisted totalizing medicalization* of various processes and states of women's bodies such as pregnancy, birthing, abortion, weight and body size, substance use, women's mood fluctuations and emotional lives, menopause in general, and experiences of violence. Similarly, many women's health activists have *fought for clear demedicalization* in areas such as women's sexuality and menstruation. Sometimes women and women's health advocates *have fought for and demanded access to medicalization* in such areas as access to anesthesia, and prevention and treatment of cardiovascular disease, vaginal cancer, toxic shock syndrome, as well as women-specific research into occupational health, environmental health, AIDS, systemic lupus, rheumatoid arthritis, and chronic fatigue immune dysfunction syndrome, linking them systematically to the pervasiveness of poverty and violence in the lives and health of many women (Sherwin 1992). In other contexts, women's health advocates have *fought for different medicalization* of areas of women's health such as personally distressing aspects of premenstrual stress (currently classified in the *Diagnostic and Statistical Manual of Mental Disorders* [*DSM-IV*] of the American Psychiatric Association as a psychiatric disorder, "Premenstrual Dysphonic Disorder," with all the medicalizing consequences attendant upon that "diagnosis"), and for different medicalization of personally distressing dimensions of menopause, osteoporosis, and breast cancer (Batt 1994; Caplan 1993, 1995; Coney 1994; Fausto-Sterling 1985; Kaufert 1996; Love 1997).

Women have also had the audacity to adopt a variety of critical positions in relation to medical research and medical technology (see Chapter 10).[41] In some cases women have fought to *change the technology* and technical procedures. For example, in the area of breast cancer, women have simultaneously pressed for more and better research, for the exercise of therapeutic choice in relation to a two-step surgical procedure should a biopsy demonstrate malignant tissue, and for the development of less invasive technical procedures with respect to the excision of malignant tissue. In other cases, women fought for access to medical technology such as early testing for cardio-vascular disease, woman-specific HIV tests, and chlamydia. In the struggle for access to better technology, women identified the limitations of mammograms for the prevention of breast cancer and for the early detection of lumps in women's breasts and argued for more sensitive technology. In the field of cardiovascular treatment, women identified not only the androcentric practices with respect to accepted techniques of treatment but pointed out that all the instruments that have been developed for heart surgery were intended for larger hearts of men of northern European descent. This is one of the main reasons why the outcome of bypass surgery is significantly worse for women, particularly for the many women of ethnic groups who are smaller than North American women of northern European descent (Ross and Sachs 1996).

There are other valuable epistemic strategies that the Women's Health Movement has deployed to promote women's subjectivity and agency in health matters. For example, women in the Women's Health Movement have turned their critical eye to ways in which authoritative knowledge was conveyed through the dominant paradigms, the curricula, and the ethos of the central medicalization training grounds, the medical schools and the teaching hospitals (Altekruse and Rosser 1992; Elston 1981; Ruzek 1978; Wear 1997; Weiss 1977). They have documented pervasive normalization of sexism, heterosexism, racism, and the pathologizing infantilization of women students and faculty. Medical school horror narratives now form a separate political genre in the critical archives of the Women's Health Movement.

In addition, there have always been women physicians who refuse to be completely loyal to male-dominated forms of medicalization (Theriot 1993). These women break ranks, they transgress, and sometimes they explicitly do so with the goal of empowering women. When they do this, they clearly contest the expert monopoly over authoritative medical knowledge and the hierarchical macro-institutionalization of Western biomedicine. They are an important part of the struggle to empower women, to transform and share authoritative knowledge, and to use their status to fight for the health of women on a global scale. For example:

- In 1976, women physicians pressured the Association of American Medical Colleges to establish the Office for Women in Medicine (Altekruse and Rosser 1992; Elston 1981).
- From 1986 to 1988, Nan Gartrell and her colleagues collected evidence and exposed the attitudes and practices among American psychiatrists involving the sexual exploitation of their patients thereby demythologizing the disinterested benevolence principle. She was refused funding for this research by the American Psychiatric Association and had to seek private funding. To its credit, the *American Journal of Psychiatry* published the results over a three-year period (Morgan 1998).
- In 1991, Bhooma Bhayana, a practicing family physician, published the important article "Healthshock" in *Healthsharing* in which she explained how Western health norms and practices produce insupportable healthshock for immigrant and refugee women in Canada. This undermines the universalistic, reductionist claims of the biomedical paradigm (Bhayana 1994).
- In 1995, listed as one of the top five hundred black health professionals in the United States, Diane Adams edits the important collection *Health Issues for Women of Color,* thereby emphasizing political contextualization as crucial in setting research and health priorities (Adams 1995).

These are just a few examples from a rich history. The point here is to acknowledge these and many other women physicians who align themselves with other courageous feminist health care workers in opposition to patriarchal medical practitioners, who put themselves at risk to transform the most sacred and entrenched aspects of Western medicalized social control, and who lead endangered lives on the front steps of abortion clinics.

What is important to emphasize in this section are the many ways in which women in the Women's Health Movement have fought and are continuing to fight for women's subjectivity, for women having a sense of entitlement to a self-determining voice in collectively and individually taking varied positions in relation to medicalization based on a reflective, critical assessment of women's own health needs and priorities.

Ideally this signals a move away from the constrained circumstances of oppression and toward greater relational autonomy (see Chapter 2).

(Re)Claiming Epistemic Power

Claiming subjectivity and agency is critically dependent on having access to relevant knowledge as the basis for one's choices in circumstances in which genuine choice is a real possibility. This is at the heart of epistemic politics, and it can involve a variety of moves. One important step is to demystify and democratize medical knowledge, thereby challenging the "credentialed expert" monopoly over such knowledge. In the 1970s the Boston Women's Health Book Collective, the Montreal Women's Health Book Collective, and other organizations published and distributed newsletters and journals even when it was illegal and in violation of standing obscenity laws, such as in Canada. Many diverse self-help groups selectively appropriated authoritative medical knowledge for their own purposes and generated their own knowledge from their collective lived experiences. Women who were not part of the community of medical experts demonstrated the power of women, collectively, to demystify and to share medical knowledge, to appropriate technical knowledge, and to translate it in empowering ways to large communities of women. Sometimes in the course of this political demystification, women challenged and changed dominant medical beliefs and research findings that held, for example, that cervical cancer was not a communicable disease (Boston Women's Health Book Collective 1992). They sought to empower women as knowledgeable health care subjects sometimes capable of bypassing medical control by testing new technologies themselves such as the cervical cap, by publicizing techniques for artificial insemination with turkey basters and other commonly available forms of "technology," and by learning the procedures for carrying out first trimester abortions and menstrual extractions without physicians present (Boston Women's Health Book Collective 1992; Jane [pseud.] 1990). Again, these strategies clearly contested medical expert monopolies over various forms of technology and knowledge.

Moreover, relying on new feminist theoretical classifications that emerged from systematic feminist theorizing and debates about human knowledge,[42] some women in the Women's Health Movement politically classified the lost and suppressed knowledge of women healers and the medically trivialized knowledge that women gained through lived experience as "subjugated knowledge" (Haraway 1991; Ruzek and Hill n.d.). From the beginning women health activists had argued that women were entitled to define their own experiences, to set their own health care agendas and priorities, to define what health and well-being meant in their own lived settings in their own communities. Now feminist epistemologists argued that not only was starting with women conducive to better health for women and politically crucial in the light of multifaced patriarchal medical oppression but that women's experiential knowledges should be seen as "privileged experiential epistemic standpoints."[43]

Increasingly, the Women's Health Movement has sought to destroy the psuedo-universality of the biomedical model and biomedical medicalization by redefining the knowledge base for women's health in a way that is woman-centered, culturally and politically contextualized, and committed in principle to addressing the cultural diversity, the oppressive differences, and the global systemic interconnectedness of women's lives.[44] This involves an important principle of grounded particularity.

But it is possible and important to go further. Dorothy Roberts, in her bold and persuasive article "Reconstructing the Patient: Starting with Women of Color" (1996), rejects any anemic "perspectival-inclusion" approach to standpoint theorizing. Roberts argues that "because women of color experience the intersection of gender and racial oppression, they may have unique critical insights to offer" (117). Roberts states as her purpose:

> to identify how the perspective of poor women of color—their
> particular relationship to the institution of medicine—can
> uncover the way in which the practice of medicine, particularly
> the doctor-patient relationship, perpetuates hierarchies of
> power, can highlight women's forms of resistance to medical
> control, and propose a vision for transforming medical ethics
> and the health care system. (116–17)

In privileging the experiences and the critical insights of those most oppressed by racialized, class-biased, ableist medicalizing discourse, research, and clinical practices, Roberts explicitly decenters the privileged status of white, middle-class males and those women affiliated with them. She not only identifies and argues for the existence of legitimate knowledge within communities of women oppressed through medicalization; she privileges that knowledge, thereby inverting the dominant epistemic pyramid.

The epistemic politics of medicalization provides a way to think about women's struggles to contest dominant discourses, to propose alternative paradigms, to produce diverse understandings and forms of consciousness, and to unify highly diverse modes of resistance to harmful medicalizing forms of social control. At the heart of this contestation is the clear perception of the political and epistemic necessity and urgency of collectively breaking the monopoly of expert knowledge, democratizing that knowledge, and starting medical conceptualization, research, priorities, and therapeutic practice "from the lives of women" (Harding 1991).

As girls and women struggle to claim full subjectivity, full personhood, our bodies and our choices are often the embodied site for powerful forms of resistance as well as domination. For such a politics of resistance to be meaningful, we must experience lived, principled respect, freedom from poverty, freedom from the fear of personal and political violence, and freedom from other systemic forms of oppression (Edemikpong 1992; Young 1990). For our struggle to result in autonomy and authentic agency it must be waged in a context of social justice that guarantees various rights: rights to privacy, rights to bodily forms of self-determination and fertility control, rights to literacy and to the relevant knowledge needed to maintain health, to make genuinely informed decisions, and to use medicalization for genuine empowerment (Sherwin 1992; Chapter 2, this volume).

As Madeline Boscoe, an advocacy coordinator at the Women's Health Clinic in Winnipeg acerbically points out, "Women aren't just asking for pink walls, a warm speculum and kinder doctors" (quoted in Williams 1996, 49). In fact, we're not asking, at all. We are engaged in a political fight for shared knowledge, for collective power, for health, for bodily integrity—for ourselves, our communities, and our world. This is a far better politics than a politics of fear, compliance, morbidity, and death. It is a fight we dare not lose.

NOTES

Acknowledgments: I wish to thank Marilynne Bell, Robbie Davis-Floyd, Susan Sherwin, and an anonymous reviewer for their helpful comments on this chapter.

1. Cohen and Backhouse's experience is politically aligned with other efforts to expose harms in relation to women's health. See the article by Anonymous (1993) detailing the censorship and manipulation of her research in the context of the Canadian Royal Commission on New Reproductive Technologies. See also the narratives of danger and suppression in the controversial video "The Human Laboratory: Experimenting on Women in the Third World—Good Science or Gross Exploitation?" (1995). For other extended publicly documented examples, see Paula Caplan's struggles (1993, 1995) with the American Psychiatric Association.

2. I am using the singular form of the noun "the Women's Health Care Movement" for purposes of abstract referential simplification. I do not intend it to signify that there is only one women's health movement, or that there is, in reality,

a monolithic global health movement. It is important to recognize the enormously diverse, culturally specific, often pluralistic movements for women's health.

3. In this chapter, while I position myself critically in relation to already existing theoretical models of medicalization, I see myself constructing my own theoretical model that I contextualize and frame. In addressing the "epistemic politics of the Women's Health Movement," I am engaged in a synoptic reconstruction using this theoretical model for interpretative purposes. I am not committed to an overall intentionalist analysis of what particular individuals intended to do as activists in a political movement (although sometimes their epistemological intentions are explicit). Clearly, there are many complex and valid ways to interpret the politics of women's health. This is but one way.

4. See, for example, Boston Women's Health Book Collective 1992; Browner and Leslie 1996; Davis-Floyd and Sargent 1996a, 1996b; Driedger and Gray 1992; Ginsburg and Rapp 1995; Koblinsky, Timyan, and Gay 1993; Petchesky and Weiner 1990; Sargent and Brettell 1996.

5. Correlatively "demedicalization" refers to the relatively rare shrinking of or the explicit de-institutionalization of medical jurisdictional control in a particular domain. It is important to note that this is possible both empirically and politically given proof of harmful medicalization or in political struggles for normalization or revalorization of such aspects of identity as sexual identity or disability (Balsamo 1997; Hausman 1995).

6. Obviously not all attempts at medicalization are successful. Some fail altogether. Others are diversely taken up by particular individuals and members of a culture or group. For an example of an extraordinarily successful, and theoretically illuminating, model of medicalization see Leonore Tiefer's analysis (1995) of the phallocentric medicalization of male sexuality (involving definitions of the "perfect penis" and the medicalization of impotence) seen in relation to the institutional expansion of the urology and sexology professions.

7. I am using the term *Lifeworld* in the somewhat technical meaning it has acquired in the phenomenological and critical theory traditions (Habermas 1981; Merleau-Ponty 1962; Smith 1990; Smith 1996). It refers to the world of (often precritical) lived experience involving a familiar and easy acquaintance with and lived experience of customs, interpretive patterns, and world views by those individuals living within a culture or subcultures. Often aspects of and frames of one's own lifeworld(s) are seen unproblematically as "given," as "obvious," as "natural." As a consequence, challenges to individual and group dominant lifeworld paradigms can have a profoundly disorienting effect because of their constitutive roles in identity and in their collective way of "being in the world." When one lives in multiple potentially totalizing lifeworlds, for example, as an aboriginal lesbian with AIDS in a white urban setting, multiple lifeworlds exist that must be negotiated.

8. Main theorists of medicalization include: Conrad 1992; Conrad and Schneider 1980; Fox 1977; Foucault 1965, 1973, 1979, 1980; Illich 1976; Irvine 1990; Reissman 1983; Tiefer 1995; and Zola 1978.

9. When prevention is defined in terms of expert-mediated access to diagnostic and monitoring technologies coupled with extensive "life-style" conceptualization models, medicalization can become increasingly pervasive in a culture.

10. See the following for more specific analyses: Conrad 1992; Crawford 1980; Foucault 1980; Illich 1976; Irvine 1990; Lippman 1993; Morgan 1991, 1996a; Reissman 1983; Tiefer 1995.

11. I want to stress the dialectical, interactive nature of my medicalization model for both theoretical and political reasons. It commits me to looking for patterns of interaction, challenges, transformations, and resistances, and to principled openness to change. I believe it is important to avoid any a priori monolithic "top down" picture of medicalization politics at the level of theory. On the other hand, when medicalization becomes powerfully institutionalized in the context of a militarized neocolonial economy where profit-oriented transnational pharmaceutical companies play a major role, it clearly involves "top down" politics of domination and subordination. This is a separate, empirical issue that I do not want to minimize. This is why I have built principled framing into the model.

12. See Adams 1995; Batt 1994; Caplan 1993, 1995; Coney 1994; Corea 1985a; Dreifus 1977; Moss 1996; and Oakley 1984.

13. Unlike other medicalization theorists, I distinguish four elements in my model. Although other theorists refer to self-management as an aspect of medicalization, they do not cite it as a major component. I believe that is a mistake that results in an undertheorization of "medicalized subjectivity" lived phenomenologically in the context of an increasingly "medicalized life" in the context of one's daily lifeworld. I have given this element distinct standing so that empirical and normative investigations of lived medicalized subjectivity are methodologically called for by the model.

14. Where radical innovation enters in involving theoretical changes and genuine paradigm shifts, more emphasis is likely to be placed on those canonical research methodologies that have authoritative status, thereby strengthening the methodologies.

15. It is important to keep in mind that the term *medicalized culture* does not refer to a single kind of culture. It is possible to categorize cultures as "high" or "low" medicalization cultures. Similarly, it is possible to categorize them as "homogeneously" or "heterogeneously" medicalized according to whether a single model or varied medicalization models are present in the culture. Similarly, a culture may be characterized as "unmedicalized" from the point of view of Western biomedical medicalization but "high medicalized" from the point of view of a medicalization dialectic operating with respect to, for example, indigenous medicalization. Analogous remarks can be made about individuals in those cultures.

16. Analogous medicalization dynamics are at work in Europe and North America in the lives of white men with respect to the alleged "disease" of testosterone deficiency, and the very real disease of prostate cancer.

17. For a classical study of the extraordinarily clever North American rise and stabilization of Wyeth-Ayerst's hegemonic dominance of the "replacement hormone" market with Premarin, as women's drug of choice—for menopause, for osteoporosis, and for heart disease—see Love 1997, particularly the chapter "The Medicalization of Menopause." See also Coney 1994, chaps. 1, 3.

18. Available studies in ethno-medicalization suggest that access to authoritative knowledge and control over medicalized technology are critical in assessing the politics of medicalization in a variety of cultural contexts. Bair and Cayleff 1993; Browner and Press 1996; Davis-Floyd 1992, 1996; Davis-Floyd and Sargent 1996a; Feidler 1996; Graham and Oakley 1981; Rapp 1989; Ratcliff et al. 1989; Tremain 1996; Wendell 1996.

19. Ironically, deeper and deeper involvement in medicalization technologies may prove more likely in cultures committed to liberal ideologies involving rhetorics of self-determination and choice. This is separate from the issue of whether, in fact, a particular choice does involve self-determination. For examples of diverse ways of appropriating (and thinking about appropriating) medicalizing technologies, see Browner and Press 1996; Davis 1993, 1995; Davis-Floyd 1992; Jordan (1978) 1993; Love 1990; Kaufert 1996; Morgan 1991, 1996a; Rapp 1989, 1990; Rothman 1984, 1986; Shanner 1996.

20. For empirical examples and further discussion, see Arms 1975; Code 1994, 1995b; Komesaroff 1995; McPhedran et al. 1991; Morgan 1998; Rich 1985; Shanner 1996; Sherwin 1992; Stark, Flitcraft, and Frazier 1994; Smith 1996.

21. For a wry, politically poignant summary of these points, listen to Barbara Ruth in her poem "Lament to the Medical-Industrial Division of the Capitalist Patriarchal Complex" (1996).

> I like some docs.
> The ones I like
> Do what I ask them to
> At least most of the time
> Realize I'm both brilliant and brain-damaged
> Have the good taste
> To answer my questions
> In my vocabulary
> Like anyone would
> As a common courtesy
> Act like it's no big thing,
> . . . .
> Neither deny or abuse
> Their power.
> . . . .
> They tend to have a hard time
> Keeping their privileges. (97)

22. For extended particular studies see Bair and Cayleff 1993; Batt 1994; Bhayana 1994; Corea 1985a; Fee 1983; Fee and Krieger 1994; McClure 1994; McPhedran et al. 1991; Saxton and Howe 1987; Scully 1980; Sherwin 1992; Todd 1989.

23. Like other feminist social scientists, Browner and Press document women's highly diverse responses such as acceptance, dismissal, modification, and scepticism in relation to other prenatal advice coming from the official medical experts.

24. See Davis-Floyd and Sargent 1996a; Ginsburg and Rapp 1995; Graham 1985; Jordan (1978) 1993; Koblinsky, Campbell, and Harlow 1993; Mahowald 1993.

25. For an extended critical discussion of why and how women are "suited" to be genetic counselors and how gender considerations play very complex roles in the politics of genetic counseling see Rapp 1989, 1990. Analogous roles and expectations were directed to female field workers in the early eugenics movements (Carlson 1998).

26. Compare Coney 1994; Davis 1993, 1995; Davis-Floyd 1996; Lorde 1980; Love 1990, 1997; Martindale 1996; Morgan 1991, 1996a.

27. See Arms 1975; Boston Women's Health Book Collective 1992; Basen, Eichler, and Lippman 1993; Browner and Press 1996; Corea 1985b; Morgan 1996a; Reissman 1983; Rich 1985; Rothman 1986.

28. Asch and Geller 1996; Batt 1994; Bassett and Mhloyi 1994; Bell 1989; Carovano 1994; Corea 1992; Faden, Kass, and McGraw 1996; Hoangmai, Freeman, and Kohn 1992; Overall and Zion 1991; Sherwin 1992, 1996a; Triechler 1988.

29. For documentation and discussion of the pathologization of lesbianism see Birke 1982; Foucault 1980a; Gilman 1985; Irvine 1990; Jackson 1987; Raymond 1979; Rich 1980; Sherwin 1992; Stevens and Hall 1994.

30. Stevens and Hall (1994) document how demedicalization in one form (removing homosexuality from the high status diagnostic manuals) is often accompanied by renamed medicalization (as in the case, for example, of "gender identity dysphoria," which may be applied to many of the same individuals if, for example, a lesbian reports depression) or by new forms of pathologizing medicalization with the baptizing of a new syndrome called "homophobia" for which analogously invasive forms of treatment may be prescribed by progressive expert psychiatrists and therapists, thereby keeping the macro- and micro-institutions in place.

31. Here it is important to recall that it is possible to work with a different medicalizing model of human nature and still engage in medicalizing politics. Medical anthropologists have demonstrated how Western biomedicine is but one of a large range of powerful health theories of human nature with established cultural traditions (see Chapter 3).

32. In the Western context of healthism and self-help ideology, often the medicalizing recommendations to lifestyle practices and changes are directed to (invisibly privileged) self-determining, individual rational human organisms romantically conceived as purely autonomous individuals fully capable of voluntarily, easily, intentionally making whatever health-related changes are needed. This is, of course, a completely mythic construct that can function in

highly punitive ways in oppressive contexts. See Crawford 1977, 1979, 1980; Fee and Krieger 1994; Martindale 1996; Perales and Young 1988; Sherwin 1992; Wendell 1996; and Young 1990 for more extended discussions. See also Chapter 3.

33. Analogous decontextualizing can also take place in the area of assessing competence. When *competence* is understood as a universally standardized purely cognitive capacity, competency standards, testing instruments, and clinical protocols for assessment will, on principle, omit crucial gender, class, and other sociocultural factors. If a person is deemed to be incompetent by a biomedically trained expert assessor because this assessment is based on an inadequate model of competence, it can have harmful and unjust powerful legal and judicial implications. Here decontextualizing this form of medical surveillance has the potential for extensive social control. See Secker forthcoming.

34. This remark is not meant to imply that women are "naturally pathologized" only in Western European cultures. This is clearly not the case, although where colonial and neocolonial domination has taken place, there will be at least a conceptual overlay (if not dominance) of European pathology assumptions.

35. For extensive historical documentation of this variability, see Easlea 1981; Jacobus, Keller, and Shuttleworth 1990; Jordonova 1989; Lowe 1982; Martin 1987, 1990, 1991; Russet 1989; Schiebinger 1989, 1993; and Tuana 1993. A recent variation on this theme has been the description of subhuman features of women's bodies, such as hormones and microcellular structures in ways that naturalize female passivity and rapine models of male-female interaction as normal. For sources see the Biology and Gender Study Group 1989; Hubbard 1990; Martin 1991; Spanier 1995.

36. Coney (1994) documents in detail how the early misogynistic descriptions have been taken up by medical experts in medical texts and have been given technical status. See also Kaufert and McKinlay 1985; Love 1997; Martin 1987; Morgan 1979; Worcester and Whatley 1994; Zita 1993.

37. For a sample of women's health research where this is an explicit methodological principle see, e.g., Davis-Floyd and Sargent 1996a; Ginsburg and Rapp 1995; Jordan (1978) 1993; Paltiel 1993; and Whiteford 1996.

38. For examples of how this double-bind operates along different axes of oppression such as race, class, (dis)ability status, sexual orientation, and "Third World" status, see Gajerski-Cauley 1989; Giachello 1995; Perales and Young 1988; Roberts 1996; Silvers 1994, 1995; Tremain 1996; Wendell 1996; and White 1990.

39. For example, androcentric assumptions also permeate much of North American occupational health research with the consequence that often women's occupational health concerns are left unconceptualized and invisible, skewed, trivialized, or eclipsed by androcentric explanatory and clinical models. See Karen Messing's highly original, paradigm-shifting research in this area (Messing 1991, 1995; Messing and Mergler 1995; Messing, Doniol-Shaw, and Haentjens 1994).

40. For a range of sources incorporating political health narratives see the Boston Women's Health Book Collective 1992; Butler and Rosenblum 1991; Campling 1981; Corea 1985b; Davis 1995; Dreifus 1977; Laurence and Weinhouse 1994; Martindale 1996; Matthews 1983; McPhedran et al. 1991; Morgan 1998; Rich 1985; Ruzek 1978; Shanner 1996; Tremain 1996.

41. See, for example, Dresser 1992, 1996; Mastroianni, Faden, and Federman 1994; Love 1990; Ratcliff et al. 1989; Rock 1996; Rosser 1994; Sherwin 1994.

42. For a sample of this feminist scholarship see Alcoff and Potter 1993, incl. Bibliography; Antony and Witt 1993; Bannerji 1995; Bar On 1993; Braidotti 1994; Code 1991, 1994, 1995a, 1995b; Collins 1990; Dalmiya and Alcoff 1993; Davis-Floyd and Davis 1996; Duran 1991; Haraway 1991; Harding 1991, 1993; Harding, ed., 1993; Hawkesworth 1996; hooks 1989; Jones 1988; Longino 1990, 1993; Mohanty 1991; Morgan 1995; Nelson 1993; Scheman 1993; Smith 1990.

43. Advocates of what might loosely be called "standpoint theory" include Bannerji 1995; Code 1991, 1994, 1995a, 1995b; Collins 1990; Dalmiya and Alcoff 1993; Davis-Floyd and Davis 1996; Haraway 1991; Harding 1991, 1993; hooks 1989; Mohanty 1991; Morgan 1995; Scheman 1993. See Bar On 1993 for major reservations about marginality and standpoint theory. For an extensive critical review of this literature, see Longino 1993. (Clearly there are some classical Marxist roots to standpoint epistemologies.)

44. See, for example, Adams 1995; Boston Women's Health Book Collective 1976; Davis-Floyd and Sargent 1996a; Ehrenreich and Fuentes 1981; Fee and Krieger 1994; Ginsburg and Rapp 1995; Koblinsky, Timyan, and Gay 1993; Lindenbaum and Lock 1993; Malterud 1992; Mastroianni, Faden, and Federman 1994; McClure 1994; Ruzek and Hill n.d.; Sherwin 1992; White 1990.

6

Agency, Diversity, and Constraints: Women and Their Physicians, Canada, 1850–1950

Wendy Mitchinson

Historians' interpretations of the past are very much influenced by the period in which they write. Until the late 1960s, historians of medicine (many of whom were physicians) tended to see the medical profession and the care it provided in a very positive light. They saw the story of medicine as one of advancing progress, each generation of physicians building on the advances of the previous one, with doctors as altruistic people whose only goal was to help their patients.[1] By the 1960s, however, more critical voices were being heard as the medical establishment was challenged by those who felt that medicine had become too bureaucratized, that many physicians were more interested in making money than in helping patients, that medicine had become so specialized that physicians no longer saw their patients as people but as specific body parts, and that the medical profession had established hegemony over health care. At the same time, the self-help movement, as epitomized by the antismoking and physical fitness campaigns, focused on the ability and need for people to take health care out of the hands of physicians and place it in their own to offset what many saw as the medicalization of society.[2] Feminists who were part of this critical groundswell argued that if patients in general had not been served well by the medical profession, women patients in particular had been especially ill served. Feminist historians in turn often emphasized the way in which women in the past had been victimized by the medical establishment.[3] Such an interpretation has proved valuable in stimulating research and calling into question the "objectivity" of medicine.

In recent years, the medical profession in North America has been considerably weakened and many practitioners feel under siege. Perhaps for this reason, historians of medicine are recasting the previous interpretations of the female patient-doctor dynamic and while not abandoning the critical feminist stance are building on the work that has already been done and probing the complexity of the interaction.[4] Within this context I argue three points. First, women were not passive. Rather they participated in building their relationship with physicians through various demands, negotiation, and renegotiation when they were patients themselves and when they were acting in defense of other women as patients. Such participation does not mean, however, that what resulted corresponded to women's expectations. Unintended consequences often occurred, some of which led to increasing medicalization of women's lives with which many were not happy. Nor does the recognition of limited patient agency mean that the relationship between women and doctors became equalized. It did not. Second, in examining the physician–female patient relationship, it is important not to see a generic patient and a generic physician. Patients varied according to race, class, age, ethnicity, ability, and so on, and the intersection of one or more of these categories with gender shaped how they reacted to and how the physicians reacted to them. While physicians tended not to be as diverse in characteristics as their patients, they certainly did not speak with one voice. Physicians in general had more power than patients but how that was played out varied with the individual physician and patient. Third, physicians experienced constraints that limited their ability to act as so-called free agents. Just as women were never "totally passive," neither were physicians ever "all powerful." Just as women were, physicians were products of the society and period in which they lived. While I argue that women did have agency and physicians experienced constraints, I do not suggest that the pendulum of historical interpretation is shifting back to a prefeminist position. To the contrary, the feminist awareness of the difference in power between woman patient and physician has not disappeared but has been nuanced to suggest the complexity of human interaction. Linda Gordon in her book on family violence (1988) points out the difference in the power relationship between women living in poverty and the social workers who were attempting to help them. She argues that this power differential did not mean that we can predict what would happen in any given situation; rather, individual women could negotiate and shape their own lives even if women as a group could not. Gordon is differentiating here between individual and collective resistance. Similarly in the medical world, women often had the power to resist as individuals but lacked power as a group to change the system (18). But I suggest that a similar differentiation can be made between the individual practitioner and the medical profession of which he or she is a part, and that in this instance it is the practitioner that may have less power of action than the collective profession. In addition, medical practice is the result of a complex dynamic involving not only the patient and physician but culture as well. What is being suggested, then, is that historians need to be careful not to overly dichotomize the relationship between female patient and physician.

While my arguments can apply to much of western European and North American society in the late nineteenth century and the first half of the twentieth century, the specific context is Canada. In many respects, the situation in Canada was very representative of what was occurring elsewhere. Canadian medical schools taught from, and Canadian medical journals reprinted, international medical literature. New medical technologies or skills developed by practitioners in other countries were quickly taken up Canadian practitioners and vice versa. Many Canadian physicians took medical training in Great Britain or on the continent. Nonetheless, by focusing on a specific place, we can better take into account any local nuances that a more broad-ranging overview would overlook.[5]

The Historical Context

It is easy to understand why feminist historians found problematic the traditional concept of medicine and physicians as benevolent. Time and time again, the pronouncements on women by physicians in the past reveal a belief that women's bodies were socially deterministic and flawed.[6] H. B. Atlee, head of gynecology at the Dalhousie Medical College, Halifax, in a 1931 article he wrote for the *Canadian Home Journal* reminded his largely female readers that "a woman's physical upbringing from her earliest years must have childbearing as its aim and end. . . . It means that woman must carve out a feminine way of life, a way that differs from the male as her destiny differs from his."[7] Percy Ryberg in his popular advice manual *Health, Sex and Birth Control* (1942) made it clear to his readers that "the goal of every girl was to marry and to procreate" (35). And Marion Hilliard, one of North America's leading obstetricians, more than twenty years after Atlee's pronouncement, argued in her best-selling *A Woman Doctor Looks at Love and Life* (1957) that pregnant women were very much dominated by their physiology, that hormonal changes could result in their being "out of control," and that pregnancy could introduce "split personality effects" even in the most docile of women (23–24). Similarly, she felt that menopause led to "emotional upheaval" as a result of "hormones and certain glands behav[ing] eccentrically" (152). What these views and others reveal is that many (even most) physicians believed that the reproductive system was the defining characteristic of a woman, that it determined her social role in society, and that it was problematic. Such views cannot be dismissed as antiquated musings with little repercussion. As Margaret Lock and Kathryn Morgan argue (see Chapters 3, 5, and 8) medicine was and is one of the dominant institutions of twentieth-century society and was part of the reordering of that society.

Various historians of Western medicine have accounted for this physician perspective in three ways. First, in the latter decades of the nineteenth and first half of the twentieth centuries, doctors tended to see the male body as the norm of how an adult body should work. As seen from the above examples, physicians saw women as different from men and those differences seemed to be based on their physiological distinctiveness. This had not always been true. Until the eighteenth century, physicians viewed the female body as a "lesser" version of the male. At that point it began increasingly to be seen as different from man's. Anatomy books, for example, began to make distinctions between the way men's and women's skeletons were depicted (Duden 1993; and Fee 1979; Gallagher and Laqueur 1987; Laqueur 1990). By the mid-nineteenth century, medical literature deemed the differences between female and male bodies more significant than the similarities. But despite the emphasis on difference, the male body continued to be viewed as the norm and physiological "events" in women, such as puberty, menstruation, and menopause, were often viewed as sources of weakness.[8] Some critics have also suggested that in Western society self-control and self-mastery have been "cultural preoccupations" and experiences such as menstruation and menopause appeared "outside" mastery (Pirie 1988, 640).[9] Evidence abounds that physicians accepted a form of biological determinism with respect to women. As the medical argument went, women's bodies, especially their reproductive systems, were much more complex than men's and thus more could go wrong with them. In addition, the complicating factors of menstruation, pregnancy, childbirth, and menopause were stresses that male bodies simply did not experience. It was not women's fault, but they did pay the price in ill-heath because of "natural" weakness.

Historians have also pointed to the tendency within medical culture to generalize women patients to the wider community of women.[10] Doctors endowed healthy women with the problems of ill women; the real problems of some became the potential problems of all.[11] As Janice M. Irvine (1990) has argued, any strategy built on the differences between men and women "is closely allied to either a biologically or a culturally based essentialism, falsely universalizing a set of historical and social relations" (22). In medicine, the phrase *women's diseases* or the phrase *women's bodies* reflects that essentialism. The conclusion that emerges from the medical literature using such phrases is that women's bodies are all the same and prone to all the same ailments. The conflation of potential and actual is made. This was particularly true in the area of childbirth where the reductionist view of women as solely reproductive "machines" became dominant. What feminist critics, as part of the Women's Health Movement discussed by Kathryn Morgan in Chapter 5, have tried to do is to raise awareness of this essentialism and the degree to which it is socially constructed (Lowe 1982). The female body is a biological body but it is also a gendered body and as such has a history. Certainly the perspective on women's bodies has changed over time. For example, as noted, until the eighteenth century, physicians conceptualized the female and male bodies as essentially similar—indeed the reproductive system of women was a reflection of the male but manifested internally and not externally.

A third factor that helped explain past medical perceptions of women was the power differential between patients and physicians, especially when the former were women and the latter were men. Until recently, the concept of patient rights has not been strong in medical ethics or in law. Emphasis was more on physician obligation to do what he or she considered best for the patient, sometimes even despite patient wishes.[12] In the first half of the twentieth century, the status of the medical profession in Canada was very high. Most physicians, because of their practice and status in the community, were middle class and, given the social expectations of the time, most were white men, and, outside the province of Quebec, of British heritage. Within this general context of patient-physician inequality, all women were doubly disadvantaged in that they were patients and they were women, individuals in society who were felt unable to measure up to the male norm.[13] This meant then that women, who as a group were considered weaker and different from men and consequently inferior to men, were faced as patients most often by a man who was part of an increasingly powerful profession and a member of a gender that represented public power in the country. The result was that because of their position, physicians were not as likely to listen to their women patients as they were to their men and to see in women's bodies the concrete expression of female inferiority and subordination.[14] Within the context of the late nineteenth and early twentieth centuries, changes within the medical institution accentuated this disadvantage. Gynecology was becoming a major surgical specialty predicated on women's bodies' being problematic, and childbirth was increasingly becoming medicalized. The pressure was on women to seek medical help when their bodies seemed to give them difficulties. A dependent relationship thus developed.

Interaction Between Women and Physicians

In recent years, feminist historians have been modifying the traditional view. Although the above interpretation has advanced our understanding of the woman patient–physician relationship and was a needed corrective to the traditional approach to medical history that preceded it, it simplifies both women as patients and the physicians treating them. For one, it tends to downplay the existence of a patient-physician dynamic, a give and take within the relationship, even though that relationship was unequal in terms of power. An examination of history reminds us that the patient-physician dynamic was composed of both sites of resistance and sites of compliance, that women as individual patients did have some agency.[15] Some groups of women also had a strong collective voice. Thus agency could be both individual and collective. As Susan Sherwin points out in Chapter 2, however, agency does not negate oppression. The latter places limits on choice, and while choices may be made by women (either individually or collectively), the range of choices are circumscribed by class, race, ability, and so on, especially gender, and attitudes toward them in any particular period. When a woman entered a physician's office, she had made the decision to go. Such a decision was influenced by many factors: the ability of the woman to pay for medical assistance, the social context that encouraged her to see medicine as a "science" that could respond to her needs, and her own feeling of comfort with the individual physician, affected as it was by the age, gender, race, religion, and so on of both. Whatever the influences, she was the one who decided to seek medical aid and we have to acknowledge that decision even at the same time we recognize the limitations of choice certain individuals or groups experience. When the focus remains medicine, the limits on women seem and are significant. If we broaden our perspective to include the issue of health as suggested by Margaret Lock in Chapter 3, then the situation shifts in an important way. Too often, historians lose sight of the fact that going to a physician was only one of many choices that women had before them to insure their health. Women sought to maintain and improve their health through midwives, through public-health nurses, through self-help networks, and through the experience of living with their bodies; they read advice in popular health manuals and women's magazines; they took patent medicines; they learned from the experience of older women,[16] and they could resort to alternative medicine. Each of these options needs examination in order to understand the degree to which individual women and women as a group could be or could not be empowered.[17] For example, in 1931, Jenny Pincock of St. Catharines, Ontario, was instrumental in forming the Radiant Healing Centre, which used "radiant rays" and "psychic healing" to help those who were ill. Sometimes used as an alternative to orthodox medicine and sometimes as a supplement, the Centre was part of a wider Spiritualist community that was particularly attractive to women.[18] The Radiant Healing Centre did not survive the depression, nor did it cater to a large number of people, but it is an example of the ways in which individual women could act to meet their own needs. What the existence of the Radiant Healing Centre suggests is that there were various sources of "medical" authority and that women could seek multiple sources, not just one. It also suggests a way in which women's voices could be heard.

Although the recognition that alternatives to orthodox medical care were available is important, the historical emphasis on the female patient–physician dynamic is not unwarranted. It is a response to the increasing medicalization of our lives and an attempt to explain how this occurred (see Chapter 5). The area of main concern for feminist historians has been reproduction and I want to examine four aspects of this: the decline in midwives, the increasing medicalization of childbirth, and the control of reproduction through birth control and abortion. North American critics have been particularly concerned about the decline of midwives and the emergence of childbirth as a medicalized event. They have envisioned a profession in opposition to midwives because of vested self-interest and using its power to drive out midwives and establish a medical monopoly over childbirth. Midwives are seen as the preservers of "natural" childbirth and somehow the representative of the woman and her agency.[19] There are many problems with such a view but three are worth mentioning. One is that the image of childbirth as "natural" is problematic. Birthing is socially constructed and controlled in *all* societies and seldom did the parturient woman act alone in determining how her child would be born even when midwives were present (see MacIntyre 1977). Thus the birthing woman, unless alone, did not have control over the birthing process and the switch to doctor-"managed" birth from midwife-"managed" birth may not be as significant a change as has been suggested. Certainly there needs to be a great deal more research on midwives in Canada before we can make an assessment about the amount of control a birthing woman had when attended by a midwife compared to the amount when attended by a physician. Maria De Koninck's discussion of midwives in western Africa (Chapter 7) suggests that we cannot assume that midwives are necessarily going to be sympathetic to women in labor. Did more negotiation occur between a parturient woman and a midwife than between the woman and her physician because in the former case, until fairly recently, both were female? In believing so, are historians in danger of essentializing women?

Was the degree of negotiation dependent on training? In nineteenth-century Canada, few midwives had formal educational training. Nor did many have "apprenticeship" training. For most of the nineteenth century, many women lived isolated lives where they were fortunate to have any woman, let alone a midwife, with them in childbirth. Was the degree of negotiation dependent on time spent with the patient? The historical consensus is that midwives came and spent time with the woman during most of her labor and stayed afterward to help care for the family and give the woman some respite. The physician, on the other hand, is usually portrayed arriving after labor has started and, assuming he arrives on time, delivers the child, then leaves. The midwife's presence is certainly more pervasive at one level. At this point, we cannot say with certainty how women in mid-nineteenth-century Canada viewed midwife-assisted birth compared with physician-assisted birth. We know very little about *how* midwives helped women or *how* interventionist physicians were. After this period, the question becomes somewhat ahistorical since by the end of the century few midwives existed and the nature of physician's involvement had altered with the emergence of "scientific" childbirth.

The traditional historiography has blamed the decline of midwifery and thus the decline of woman's control over childbirth on the opposition by doctors. But the story is not quite so straightforward. Not all physicians were hostile to midwives. Many were quite willing to work with them and were respectful of their talents. Others distinguished between trained and untrained midwives and confined their hostility to the latter (Mitchinson 1991, 162–75; Connor 1989, 128–87). Nonetheless, even those respectful of "trained" midwives did not support or encourage that training, with the result that by the end of the nineteenth century, physicians in Canada were in control of childbirth. From that position of power, they publicly opposed the introduction of midwives when it was put forward as part of the original mandate of the Victorian Order of Nurses (VON) as envisioned by the National Council of Women of Canada (NCWC). But they were not alone in their opposition. Nurses, too, were not supportive of the midwife tradition, seeing in it a threat to their own efforts to professionalize. In the early twentieth century, most nurses and physicians continued their opposition (Buckley 1979). Nonetheless, many physicians recognized the need for midwives in isolated communities where there were few or no medical personnel. In the first half of the twentieth century, for example, a fairly cooperative relationship between midwives and physicians in Newfoundland existed (McNaughton 1989). What this has suggested is the danger of generalizing groups. The members of the NCWC who endorsed the creation of the VON wanted midwives. Nurses in Canada, however, did not. Yet nurses were potentially future childbearers; they were familiar with the issues of midwife-assisted versus physician-assisted births. Their decision not to support midwives had elements of vested interest just as that of many physician-opponents. Thus the decline in midwives was not the result of a gender conflict, that is, male opponents versus female supporters but was rather more complex.

The irony of the traditional view of midwife decline and its emphasis on the "woman-centered" nature of a nonphysician birth is the absence of the patient, the woman who should be center stage.[20] It would appear that the patient did not exist or if she did, had so little power as to be invisible. But power is not a "thing" held by one group over another. "It is continuously enacted and re-enacted, constituted and reconstituted" (Felstiner and Sarat 1992, 1452, 1454.) Doctors could have held sway only if women themselves had preferred to go to them rather than to midwives. There is little evidence that Canadian women opposed in any significant way the decline of midwifery. Indeed, evidence abounds that many women *wanted* physicians involved in childbirth. In nineteenth-century Canada, childbirth was the second greatest killer (next to tuberculosis) of women in their middle years. Women wanted a way to lessen the risk to themselves and the children they lost at birth and saw the practitioners of medicine as possibly providing that insurance. In midwife-assisted births, when problems arose that the midwife could not handle, both the midwife and the family of the woman often called in a physician. As early as the 1820s in York (Toronto), the Society for the Relief of Women, in an effort to aid women in childbirth, provided a midwife or, "if required," a physician (Mitchinson 1991, 164–65). There was a sense of doctors' having additional expertise based on the perception of the value of their "scientific" training. Thus a midwife was deemed fine—up to a point.

The switch from midwife- to doctor-managed birth is part of what many have seen as the medicalization of childbirth. The process cannot be denied but it was partially in response to many women's demands. This does not mean that the outcome was what they wanted; outcomes are never predictable. By the end of the nineteenth century, childbirth had become medicalized in that physicians attended most births, even though those births still occurred at home. In 1899, only 16 percent of Ontario births were unattended by physicians and only 3 percent were attended by women considered to be midwives or calling themselves that (Mitchinson 1991, 167). More doctors were available and women were having fewer children and preferring to have doctors attend them in the hope that physicians could deliver them safely. Birthing at home, however, meant doctors had to respond to the domestic situation where family and friends were present (Leavitt 1995, 26). Physicians were not immune to the demands of their patients and patients learned very quickly what medical care was available. An early example of this was the patient of one physician who, six months after anesthesia was introduced into childbirth practice, "begged" him to give her chloroform to ease her pain. Doctors also reported their patients' wanting their husbands present at birth and agreeing to it. This shift to physician-assisted birth was not without its political aspects. In 1897, for example, the Act to Regulate Maternity Boarding-Houses and for the Protection of Infant Children passed in Ontario made it mandatory that only a "legally qualified medical practitioner" could attend births in hospitals or maternity homes (Mitchinson 1991, 168, 178, 197). This was in response to the incredibly high infant mortality rates of such homes. When it is remembered that hospitals and such homes catered to unwed women and very poor women, its significance becomes clear. The state could not yet tell middle-class women who they should have to assist them in birth but they could tell poorer women. The alliance between the state and medicine was being forged.

By the 1940s the next step in medicalization of birth had been achieved as the majority of children were being born in hospitals. The real push for this began in the 1920s because of the concern about high maternal mortality rates and physicians' consequent commitment to extensive prenatal and postnatal care. Demands for increased care meant that it was much easier for patients to go and see physicians than for physicians to travel from patient to patient. Add to this increased technology surrounding childbirth, and the hospitalization of childbearing women, from the medical point of view, seemed necessary. Hospitalization also increased the power of the medical institution since it was an environment controlled by doctors not patients.[21]

But this shift to the hospital did not occur in a vacuum. The concern about maternal mortality rates was part of a pronatalist push that received added reinforcement with the loss of life in World War I. The pressure to increase Canada's population by lowering infant and maternal mortality rates became an especial focus of middle-class women and their organizations. Such women were behind the creation of many maternity hospitals and the introduction of maternity wards within general hospitals. They believed that such facilities would provide women living in isolated areas, with few medical practitioners, a place to go for childbirth. Many women believed that hospital birth represented safety for them and their babies. For poorer women, hospital births provided a much needed rest before going back to the demands of their families. Hospitals, however, were environments controlled not by women but by physicians and because of the relative social position of women to doctors (most of whom were men), hospital births had the result of increasing women's dependency and in a sense altered what choices they could make. The hospital accentuated the use of medical discourse, which many women adopted to describe their experience of birthing, thus medicalizing it and perhaps alienating them from it.[22] But the interaction of the woman and her physician or the physicians and hospital was not unmediated. As a result of the baby boom of the war years and immediately after, the time a woman stayed in a hospital for childbirth decreased from approximately two weeks to ten days. Partially a result of the actions of some physicians who had been advocating it for years, the real impetus for the change was economic. Obstetrical wards were so crowded because of the baby boom, they simply could not afford to keep women on their floors for the extended period. In this instance the arguments of some physicians for the benefits of early rising and shorter stay after childbirth combined with economic exigencies to lessen somewhat one aspect of the medicalization of childbirth.[23]

One of the criticisms of the shift from midwife- to doctor-managed and from home to hospital births has been the increase in intervention that followed both. But intervention is not necessarily an imposition by physician on patient. As already seen, in the late nineteenth century, patients often demanded the intervention of the physician through anesthesia. Intervention is not bad in and of itself. Rather, it is the nature and circumstances of the intervention that need to be explored. One of the more interesting stories in the history of childbirth is the introduction of twilight sleep. It, too, reveals unintended consequences. Viewed by many as painless childbirth, twilight sleep in the early decades of the twentieth century was especially popular in the United States, compared with Canada. It involved the use of scopolamine during labor because of its tendency to cause amnesia. Thus a woman in labor experienced pain but she did not remember it afterward. Some American women had been exposed to twilight sleep in Europe and returned to their own country insisting that American doctors offer women this alternative. Partially as a result of this collective pressure, which they exerted through the popular women's magazines, and the individual pressure middle- and upper-middle-class women exerted on their doctors, many physicians in the United States and elsewhere adopted the procedure. But it was a complicated and delicate one and in some respects a very interventionist and doctor-dominated one, best performed in a hospital (Sandelowski 1984, 3–26). The women who demanded twilight sleep certainly wanted their voices heard with respect to shaping their childbirth experiences and were quite successful in doing so. But the result was in some respects a diminishment of their involvement in childbirth.

If childbirth itself has revealed the complexity of patient-physician interaction and the existence of and problematic nature of patient agency, the effort to prevent reproduction did so as well. Historians have discovered that long before a birth control movement began, couples had been controlling their fertility and, as evidenced by the decline in the birth rate in Canada and the rest of Western society by the end of the nineteenth century, had been successful. The irony of the twentieth-century public movement for birth control in Canada, and the United States as well, was that many of the birth control clinics run by predominantly Protestant women were insistent that physicians be involved. This may have been a result of these women being predominantly middle-class and able to afford physician care, which they considered superior and safer to nonphysician care. They also supported the use of the diaphragm, which they and physicians believed necessitated medical involvement to insure a proper "fit." In setting up their clinics, these women wanted to offer poorer women the best care available and also win the support of the medical community. Doctor-run clinics would, they hoped, do both.[24] Prompting middle-class women to become involved in birth control as a public issue was their belief that women had the right to control their fertility and also the specter of parents not being able to support their families and those children becoming a charge on the state or worse. Such concerns were reflected in a handbill entitled *Birth Control; or, The Prevention of Conception*, written by Georgina Sackville and available in western Canada. In it, Sackville asks women, "Are you the mother who either through 'ignorance' or because of some 'religious belief' with half a dozen 'accidental children' shoddily clothed, under-nourished, dragging to her skirt, refuses to take any precautions which would prevent the birth of another weakling?" (Trott, 1984, 105). Such attitudes were especially popular in the 1930s as a result of the Great Depression and reflect a strong eugenic overtone.

An alternative to medical control emerged at the same time as the women-run clinics. The Parents Information Bureau, which was established by A. R. Kaufman, a Kitchener, Ontario, industrialist, discouraged medical involvement, believing that it would be difficult to convince poorer women to come to clinics and see a physician. Instead, Kaufman had his "nurses" distribute free samples of birth control (condoms plus jelly) in poor neighborhoods. Although perhaps not always as effective as the diaphragm, such means were easier to use and cheaper to purchase and did not require physician input (McLaren and McLaren, 1986, chap. 5). They did, however, unlike the diaphragm, necessitate male cooperation. Within the Canadian context, then, middle-class women were aligned with the medical profession to make physicians the gate-keepers of birth control. Once obtained, birth control was in the hands of women. A. R. Kaufman, on the other hand, tried to put birth control directly into the hands of many more women. Kaufman's motives, however, were hardly feminist. His birth control method necessitated male involvement and his concern, like that of many middle-class women reformers, was to limit the procreation of "undesirables" by the working class.

Abortion provides one last example of an area of interaction between women and physicians. Historians are discovering the frequency with which women resorted to abortion in the past. Abortion was once thought of as the desperate act of young unmarried women, but what has become clear is that married women, too, were equally desperate. Some women sought a way out of an unwanted pregnancy on their own. Others turned to physicians, even at a time when abortion was illegal except for medical reasons. A careful reading of patient records allows a woman's voice to emerge even though distorted through the various people writing the record. For example, Martha McNamara, a single twenty-two-year-old waitress from Newfoundland, entered the Victoria General Hospital, Halifax, on January 9, 1931. In September 1930 she had missed her period and so in early October had taken some pills to encourage menstruation. She began to bleed in mid-October and assumed that this was her regular period since the timing was right. She stopped bleeding and then began again two days later. On Monday, January 5, she obtained more pills from her physician and took a large dose (7–8) for the next three days. She began to bleed again and entered the hospital, whose record notes, "Patient admits having had opportunity to become pregnant." Part of a fetus was found in the vagina and removed.[25] The fact that her physician gave her the pills without testing her for pregnancy is suggestive of complicity on his part. This is quite amazing considering that abortion was illegal except in the most exceptional circumstances. The narrative also reveals the agency of Martha. She went to a physician for a problem that she diagnosed in a way that would allow him to help and her to accept that help. When she first took the pills she was very early in her pregnancy. When she returned for more pills, however, she was approximately four and one half months pregnant and it is unlikely that there was doubt about her condition; still there was no suggestion that the physician was suspicious. Perhaps he did not have to be; he knew very well what the pills were for and the legal situation was such that if he wanted to help her he had to be complicit. It may also have been that he, like many other Canadians, had concerns about a single woman having a child, especially in a period of economic downturn. Whatever his reasons, the case reveals a physician willing to acquiesce in a lay diagnosis; he acknowledged the power of the patient or connived with her in the fiction of missed periods and gave her something to bring about an abortion. The patient-physician relationship, as this example illustrates, is somewhat analogous to a series of storytellings, both patient and physician participating until they agree on a version even if it represented quite differing agendas for each (Felstiner and Sarat 1992, 1454–55).

From the above examples of interaction between women and physicians, it is clear that women exerted some agency. As patients, they often chose to call in physicians rather than midwives. They put pressure on physicians to respond to their needs in the birthing room as is evidenced in some women's demands for anesthesia, for the presence of their husbands, and for twilight sleep. Even those most vulnerable, those seeking illegal ways out of a pregnancy, could negotiate with some physicians. Through group pressure, women also exhibited the ability to act in their own behalf or on the behalf of other women. Women's groups often saw physician care as better than midwife care and provided for it through their charitable societies. When doctors were not available, midwives were the next-best-thing as evidenced in the NCWC's support of the VON. Women's groups were behind the setting up of many of the maternity wards in hospitals, and those middle-class women who supported woman's rights to birth control felt this was best done through a medically controlled environment. The demands placed on physicians by their women patients and women's groups did not establish a relationship of equality between doctors and women. It was a negotiated relationship and the consequences of the negotiations could be unexpected, even unwanted, and varied from situation to situation.

Diversity of Women and Physicians

If the ability of the woman patient to negotiate depends on the specifics of the situation or issue, it also depends on who the woman and who the physician is. Historians have emphasized the diversity of women in the past, making it clear that women as a group cannot be generalized. Jane Roland Martin (1994) has pointed out, however, the dangers of stressing diversity to the point of being unable or unwilling to generalize and thus advance our understanding of the past. Nonetheless, within medical history, the tendency has been to juxtapose "women" in opposition to "doctors." But we need to ask which women and which doctors. As many of the examples have indicated, women were not of one mind. Middle-class women often aligned themselves with physicians with respect to childbirth. Only when doctors were unavailable did they endorse midwives, as in their support of the VON. Nurses, on the other hand, aligned themselves with physicians in this battle, not wanting to alienate physicians and fearful that midwifery with its inclusion of home care would taint their efforts to professionalize. Not all women endorsed birth control—certainly Roman Catholic women restrained by their religion did not, nor did many others, believing it would open the floodgates of sexuality.

At an individual level, women decided whether to seek out medical assistance and whether to accept the medical aid proffered. As seen in the example of abortion, they could negotiate with the physician about what they wanted done and fashion a story of what was wrong with them in an attempt to achieve the results they wanted. While this seldom equalized the power relationship between patient and doctor, it did suggest a degree of choice and agency on the part of individual women that helped offset the power of any individual physician. The ability to do this was dependent on many factors. For example, the class of the woman patient could dictate how the physician responded to her. For all of the period under review, there were few medical insurance schemes and those going to a physician were expected to pay. Hospitals, which had their origins as charitable institutions, maintained a sliding scale to ensure that those people without funds would be cared for, and private practitioners as well tended to carry their own complement of charity patients. What this meant, however, was that for many working-class women, physicians were consulted rarely. When such women did seek out medical advice, cost would be an issue and if they did receive the advice free because they could not pay, they became the objects of charity. In either situation, the dynamics between patient and physician would have been much different from that between a middle-class woman and her physician. In the latter situation, the woman was paying for a service and could expect to receive it. The class of the patient also colored attitudes toward her and treatment given to her. Many nineteenth-century physicians, for example, believed that working-class women gave birth more easily than did middle-class women and could endure pain better (Mitchinson 1991, 37). This appears to be very similar to what Margaret Lock in Chapter 8 refers to as "local biologies"; that different cultures and different eras see bodies differently. In the same period, ovariotomies became a fad among many gynecologists to relieve nervous complaints and other physical problems of women. Some physicians advised their colleagues that working women might require the operation more than middle-class women. The latter could be offered less invasive treatment because they had the time and money to afford a leisurely therapy. Working women, however, could not; they needed something quick and effective such as surgery—a response to the reality of their lives.[26] Marital status and age, too, influenced treatment. Physicians were very hesitant about operating on young, unmarried women if it meant it would remove what chances they had to bear children. Married women who already had children or older women nearing menopause did not elicit the same concern (Mitchinson 1991, 263–77). Thus who the patient was helped determine the outcome of her meeting with a physician. Depending on who she was she could expect certain attitudes and be faced with different choices.

If historians have been less than sensitive about the diversity of women and how various class, age, and even religious factors (among others) limited or expanded their agency in relation to physicians, they have been even more so concerning physicians. Medicine is a dynamic profession that is constantly evolving. Certain procedures are introduced, accepted, challenged, dismissed, with new ones taking their place. In most periods, several of these stages occurred at the same time, inspiring healthy debate among groups of physicians. Doctors seldom spoke in one voice. While this lack of unanimity can be seen in many areas centered on the treatment of women, I discuss three: general intervention in childbirth, cesarean sections, and estrogen therapy.

Critics of medicine have focused on the degree of intervention in childbirth that has occurred. No one would deny that this has happened but it is important to note that many physicians questioned that intervention and the nature and need for it. Dr. Tye, a Chatham, Ontario, physician, in 1882 observed that "after seeing all the forceps and scoops and other iron instruments, he really congratulated himself that he was not a woman" and noted that in his own practice he seldom felt the need to resort to them but trusted in nature.[27] Not all followed his practice, as evidenced in the complaints made by some physicians and patients alike that the ill health of many women stemmed from the poor childbed customs of physicians.[28] Gynecologists, in particular, saw the medical practices surrounding birth as the cause of much ill health in women, and contributory to fertility problems.[29] Gynecologists, in expressing their concerns, were, of course, trying to insure the well-being of their patients and other women but also to raise their own status in relation to general practitioners.

In recent years, concern about intervention has focused on the frequency of cesarean sections. Yet not all physicians followed this trend or liked that many of their colleagues seemed particularly eager to do so.[30] Nevertheless, the reasons for the surgery help explain the eagerness. It was originally devised for those women who, for health reasons, could not survive "natural" childbirth. In the nineteenth century, this group included not only women with ailments such as heart disease but also those women who, because of poverty, had been malnourished and, consequently, because of rickets, suffered from deformed pelvises. For such women, the birth canal was such that birth could not occur by vagina. To save these women, doctors had to sacrifice the child through mutilating operations. It was no wonder that many physicians welcomed a procedure that would help them avoid such a decision. With better nutrition, however, some of the reasons for C-section disappeared; but, instead of declining in frequency, it increased. Three factors may have accounted for this. One was the increased size of the babies being born and another was the shift from concern about saving the mother's life (which was perhaps not in danger) to saving the baby's. The latter became of particular concern given the declining birth rate for most of the first half of the twentieth century. A third factor was that its safety had improved. By the late 1920s and after, references abound to how "simple" and "easy" the operation was and how "dramatic" and "spectacular" its results. Indeed, critics made the argument that it was the combination of the two that accounted for the increase in the use of the procedure. Practitioners were attracted by the status that performing such a procedure conferred—through increased patient fees and the apparent complexity of the procedure compared to vaginal birth—without having to cope with the risk normally attached to such serious intervention. But as critics reminded their colleagues, the increasing safety of the operation had not eliminated all risk.[31] What the C-section example reminds us is that intervention in childbirth has long existed but its nature changes, in this instance from mutilating operations to C-sections. It is also noteworthy that not all physicians supported the adoption of C-sections and that the reasons for them change over time. Nor should we forget that such intervention could and did save lives. The issue then is not that all intervention is bad but rather what kind of intervention was involved, when, for what reasons, on what women, and performed by whom.

If physicians were not of one voice with respect to C-sections, neither were they unanimous in endorsing hormone therapy, especially estrogen therapy for menopause in the late 1930s and 1940s. Critics have argued that such therapy has medicalized a process that for most women is an unproblematic experience. As Margaret Lock points out in Chapter 8, many physicians in Japan would agree with this. In the mid-twentieth century, many physicians would have agreed as well. When the use of hormonal extracts for menopause began to be introduced, some expressed concern. Beckwith Whithouse, professor of gynecology and obstetrics at the University of Birmingham, in the 1933 *Canadian Medical Association Journal* argued that ovarian extract treatment and the "oestrin they contain" could lead to uterine hemorrhage and could act as adrenaline and accentuate the hot flushes.[32] A leading Canadian gynecologist, H. B. Atlee, complained about the rise of all the hormonal preparations and the proliferation of trade names, which led to much confusion about what they actually were.[33] Evan Shute of the University of Western Ontario in 1939, too, stressed the proliferation of therapies for menopause, especially the "indiscriminate use of estrogens."[34] In a significant article published in the 1945 *Canadian Medical Journal*, J. S. Henry, a physician from Montreal, discussed the negative affects of estrogen therapy and its links to cancer.[35] Others echoed his concerns, although perhaps not with his intensity, some feeling they could overcome the negative repercussions through more judicious prescriptions.[36]

As the above examples indicate, doctors often did not speak with one voice. Sometimes this diversity of voices was connected to the situation of the individual physician. In the late nineteenth century, a study of obstetrical care in Canadian hospitals revealed that such care was fairly conservative. Hospitals at that time had few paying patients and the doctors associated with them were often attached to university medical faculties. When a comparison of use of forceps was made between hospital patients, usually poor women, and those of private patients at home, the incidence was much higher for private patients. Obstetrical intervention in general seemed less in hospitals than in private practice. While ability to pay was certainly one factor, the rhetoric of hospital- and university-affiliated physicians did tend to be less interventionist than that of others in the profession (Mitchinson 1991, 219). Area of specialty also divided physicians. As noted, some gynecologists were willing to blame the poor childbirth practices of their nonspecialist colleagues for the gynecological problems that some women experienced. General practitioners in the late 1920s and 1930s criticized surgeons for resorting to C-sections more than was needed. What this stresses is the danger of generalizing physicians, not distinguishing individuals from the collective group and its culture, or distinguishing one group of physicians from another. We cannot equate physicians with the institution of medicine in a straightforward manner. This does not mean we cannot make generalizations about groups, indeed we must to make research comprehensible and meaningful. But we need to be aware of the tension that will always be there between the general and the specific.

We also need to understand that the same physician could hold somewhat conflicting views of women. For example, a reading of the medical literature suggests a strong belief in biological determinism as it pertained to women's bodies. At the same time, the belief was offset by a recognition that social factors, too, could account for women's health problems. For example, in the nineteenth century, the idea existed that "civilization" caused female problems, that civilization had refined modern women to such an extent that the experiences that "primitive" women supposedly found unproblematic, such as childbearing, were now posing difficulties. Of course, no commentator wanted to return to the past. Women had gained as well as lost with the advance of civilization. Women it was felt simply had to bear the consequences of change and some physicians saw their role as helping women to cope with those consequences. Early in this century, J. A. MacKenzie, the assistant medical superintendent of the Nova Scotia Hospital (for the Insane), in Halifax, quoted authorities to substantiate the idea that hysterical symptoms in pubescent girls were not unusual. In his view, however, this was not because of the "femaleness" of girls but because of the limitations of girls' lives; they did not have the same outlets that men did to release nervous tension; thus it was the social context, not the body that led to hysteria.[37] Although many physicians did give recognition to the gendered nature of women's lives and their bodies, there was very little that they could do about it. They, as most people did, accepted society as they found it and simply tried to alleviate the problems of living in it. They tended to accept the "naturalness" of gender but then so did most Canadians. At times they focused on certain aspects that they found problematic and it is important for historians to analyze the issues on which they did make a stand when they did so and the reasons for it.

Constraints on Physicians

In the feminist literature on doctors' treatment of women, the constraints experienced by women patients are given pride of place. This is as it should be since the patient is the individual who is most vulnerable. But it is difficult to understand the physician response to women patients without appreciating the constraints experienced by physicians as well, that is, the way in which patients, societal norms, and medical culture placed limits on and shaped their response. As already suggested, any evidence of women acting on their own behalf placed limits on what an individual physician could and could not do. Each meeting between patient and physician is situated within the context of their individual lives, experiences, and training. For example, patients do not see their bodies in the same way that physicians do. The patient's knowledge is an embodied knowledge, one that is experienced. At times this results in physicians and patients talking at cross purposes.[38] Physicians, envisioning medicine as "scientific," want precision and this is something that is not always forthcoming. In a study of women's medical records in the first half of the twentieth century, it was clear that women did not remember their medical histories with the degree of specificity physicians expected of them, suggesting that their priorities about their bodies did not "fit" the medical model.[39] Their perception was situated within a social and cultural context. Similarly, the power of physicians as a group was part of the broader social-cultural context of the past (Felstiner and Sarat 1992, 1458).

Historians have been interested in how physicians became so powerful. Early historians of medicine used to argue that it was a result of progress, the consequence of physicians, through the advances of medical science, being able to offer their patients treatment that worked. Most historians of medicine today have rejected the link between medical efficacy and medical power, arguing that the latter preceded the former. Rather, the rise of medicine was linked to other trends in modern society. The main one was the emergence of science as a counter to and substitute for religion as the source for understanding the natural world (which included the body). If at one time people had looked to the Bible for guidance in understanding the world about them, by the end of the nineteenth century, they increasingly looked to science and comforted themselves that, since science was "objective," it truly reflected the divine purpose. At the same time that this alignment was occurring, allopathic medicine was gaining an apparent monopoly. In mid-nineteenth century Canada, physicians had numerous competitors—midwives, purveyors of patent medicine, and a broad spectrum of groups whose members also called themselves doctors—homeopaths, Thomsonians, and eclectics. By the end of the century, however, most of these groups had been eliminated, absorbed, or marginalized. Medical education had been standardized and there was only one route to medical practice—a university education. The alignment of medicine with science and the narrowing of "medical" expertise to one group raised the status of physicians and gave them, in the eyes of many, the aura of experts on a wide variety of issues.

One of those issues was the nature of women's bodies and women themselves. But doctors' views on women did not exist in a cultural vacuum; they were shaped by the wider culture of which they were a part. For example, as we have seen, the overtones of biological determinism with respect to women were evident. Furthermore, such determinism was not confined to the medical profession. It permeated much of Western society in the nineteenth century and the early decades of the twentieth century. Doctors were not unique in believing that women differed in "kind" from men, that their reproductive systems determined their physiological responses as well as their place in the society of the time. Most commentators reflected this view (Mitchinson 1991, 30–41 and chap. 2; Houlihan 1984; Klein-Mathews 1979; Mawhood 1989; Nash 1982; Wilson 1977). The culture influenced physicians to see women in a particular way and physicians provided the culture with the scientific legitimacy for doing so. The relationship was a dynamic and symbiotic one and it is that symbiosis that feminist scholars have pointed to as evidence of the socially constructed nature of medicine.

The moral values of society limit what a physician can or cannot do or what particular physicians can or cannot do. Historians have often focused on the male gender of most physicians as an explanation for physicians' treatment of women. Underlying the criticisms concerning male physicians is the belief that women physicians would treat women differently. Few historical analyses of this issue have been done. One U.S. study that compared a woman-run hospital with that of a man-run hospital concluded that few significant differences existed (Morantz-Sanchez 1985).[40] This does not mean that gender is not a factor but suggests that it is not a "deterministic" one, which of course it cannot be since it is socially constructed. Gender could at times limit physicians' options. This was particularly true in the early and middle decades of the nineteenth century when a "male" midwife was viewed by many as immoral and when an internal examination was seen as equivalent to moral rape.[41] However, the wider status and power of men in society coupled with the rising prestige of medical "science," eventually overcame such concerns. If gender could limit, other factors as well intervened and complicated physician agency. Attention has been paid to doctors' opposition to birth control. This opposition was made clear in most public pronouncements in the nineteenth and early twentieth centuries. But birth control was illegal. The Criminal Code of Canada stated:

> Everyone is guilty of an indictable offense and liable to two
> years' imprisonment who knowingly, without lawful excuse of
> justification, offers to sell, advertises, publishes an advertise-
> ment of or has for sale or disposal any medicine, drug or article
> intended or represented as a means of preventing conception
> or causing abortion. (McLaren and McLaren 1986, 19)

This remained the law in Canada until 1969. To speak out on a subject that was both illegal and, given the mores of the time, highly suspect morally by many would have been difficult. It would also have alienated significant groups in society, such as Catholics (including many Catholic women), from whom many physicians' patients came. Nonetheless, interviews with women who reached sexual maturity during the 1930s and 1940s suggest that many women who could afford access to private physicians had little difficulty in accessing birth control from them before marriage.[42] Public pronouncements and individual actions did not necessarily coincide. Protestant physicians may have been concerned about the illegality of birth control (except for medical purposes) but they had little difficulty morally, since many of the Protestant churches had publicly removed their prohibition from the use of birth control by married couples for the purpose of spacing births. Catholic physicians, however, continued to be restricted by both law and Church doctrine.

The nature of medicine itself was a limitation. It is a truism to say that medicine was a combination of art and science but it is one that holds. Much of a physician's skill came from experience and an intuitive sense of what might ail a patient or what might work for a patient. Each individual had his or her own responses to illness, to medication. Physicians consequently worked in a context of uncertainty much of the time. Medication might work but the reasons for it could be unclear. What should work might not. It is difficult for any person to deal with uncertainty, especially when people's lives may be at stake. Medical technology has played an important role in helping offset this uncertainty. Within medical culture and the wider culture generally, technology represented the "science" of medicine and as such was supported as a way of legitimizing what physicians did. Measuring through technology offered a "certainty" that was comforting. It became a part of medical culture and as such difficult to question. Similarly, doctors acted according to the prevailing treatment within the medical culture at any particular time. Certain physicians innovate and discover that new procedures can offer patients relief from their pain. When ovariotomies were first introduced, the mortality rate was such that few were willing to perform them. As they became safer to perform, largely because of the acceptance of antiseptic practices, the mortality rate declined. More physicians adopted the surgery and expanded the indicators for it. Whereas once ovariotomies were to be performed only when other therapies had failed and double-ovariotomies only when menopause would be guaranteed to cure the problem, they became an alternative therapy to cure a wider range of physical ailments as well as sexual and emotional ones.[43] At that point, the efficacy of the procedure was questioned, most often by those within the profession, alternatives suggested, and newer and "better" procedures took over and the cycle of innovation, adoption, expansion, and questioning began once again.

The nature of medical culture in the past can and needs to be questioned. But for those who practiced medicine, it was difficult, though not impossible, to escape. Some physicians were able to challenge the norms and assumptions of that culture. While the power exerted by any individual patient placed constraints on physicians, those constraints paled in comparison to those faced by the patient. Furthermore, whereas the wider social context of which medicine was a part could limit the power of medicine through laws and mores, that context has at the same time generally expanded the power of medicine through, for example, the alignment between medicine and science.

My argument is that we need to be sensitive to the broader context of society when we attempt to change one aspect of it, in this case, medicine. Scientific "knowledge" is culturally and historically produced and as such is difficult to change by a concentration on the knowledge only. Feminist scholars have been raising important questions about the nature of science and whether what passes as science today and in the past is science (Haraway 1989; Harding 1991; Hubbard 1990; Schiebinger 1993). The application of science has real repercussions on our lives. Nowhere is this seen more than in the "science" of medicine. Perhaps for that reason, it has become a major focus of feminist scholarship. The relationship between women and their physicians has not been a simple one, nor has it been a one-dimensional one of the physician "acting" on the woman patient. This view does a disservice to the women and physicians of the past and ignores the dynamic, albeit unequal, relationship between them. It essentializes both groups and ignores the constraints that have limited the ways in which physicians can respond and undervalues the determination of women to resist. Nor is it productive for understanding the past or creating opportunities for change in the present.

Contemporary feminist critics argue that medicine ignores the *experience* of women. They point out that the medical profession has had an overly narrow view of health and have called for a widening of that definition to include issues related to poverty, abuse, disabilities, and so on (Canadian Advisory Council on the Status of Women 1995, 6, 18, 22). The expansion of the definition of health is necessary if health is not to remain exclusively a biomedical concept. But this expansion of definition cannot occur outside a social and historical context. One problem with a more encompassing definition of health is that it is being proposed in a society that still connects medicine and health. That connection needs to be altered if we are not to expand the medicalization of society even more. Challenging that connection is the goal of feminist health ethics.

NOTES

Acknowledgments: Research for this chapter has been funded by the Social Sciences and Humanities Research Council of Canada (SSHRC) and by the Hannah Institute for the History of Medicine. The Program for Scholars and Artists in Residence funded by the Rockefeller Foundation in 1994 also provided me with an opportunity to develop many of the ideas in this essay.

1. The traditional interpretation to medical history can be seen in the numerous biographies of physicians, the histories of medical institutions, and the histories of medical "advances," and in general histories of the profession.

Many of these were written by practitioners who also wrote medical history. In recent years, this interpretation has declined in part because of the entry of trained historians into the field of medical history. For an overview of medical history in Canada see Mitchinson 1982, 1990; Mitchinson and McGinnis 1988, introduction; Shortt 1981.

2. See the Chapters 3, 5, and 8 for a more detailed examination and definition of medicalization.

3. See Arnup, Lévesque, and Pierson 1990; Atkinson 1985; Barker-Benfield 1977; Delaney, Lupton, and Toth 1976; Ehrenreich 1973; Ehrenreich and English 1979; Haller 1971; Haller and Haller 1974; Kern 1975; Litoff 1978; Mort 1987; Rothman 1982; Showalter 1985; Strong-Boag and McPherson 1986; Tew 1990; Vertinsky 1990. This interpretation is also reflected in studies of modern maternity and medical care. See Abramson 1990; Arms 1975; Bleier 1984; Coney 1988; Corea 1995a, 1985b, 1992; Currie and Raoul 1991; Dreifus 1978; Grant 1992; Haire 1972; Martin 1991; Mendelsohn 1981; Nechas and Foley 1994; Oakley 1980; Raymond 1982, 1993; Rowland 1992; Scully 1980; Shaw 1974; Todd 1989. See also De Koninck 1981, 1988; Quéniart 1988; Saillant and O'Neill 1987. One of the few works that examines the historical treatment of men is Parsons 1977.

4. For past views of women's bodies see Duden 1993; Fee 1979; Gallagher and Laqueur 1987; Laqueur 1990; and particularly the article by Schiebinger (1987). For an excellent study of birth in the modern period see Davis-Floyd 1992.

5. This chapter focuses predominantly on English Canada. The tradition of French Canada was very closely aligned with that of France and also was very much influenced by the predominantly Roman Catholic faith, which did influence medical approaches to issues such as birth control and abortion.

6. One of the few works that does not see the physician view as problematic is Shorter 1982. Shorter sees doctors as the rescuers of women from the flaws of their own bodies.

7. *Canadian Home Journal*, November 1931, 83.

8. Margaret Lock, Chapter 8, reveals that not all cultures have viewed menopause as problematic. For a discussion of how the physical body and intelligence is constructed by culture and the environment see Lowe 1982, 91–116.

9. Such a view, while perhaps applicable to the late nineteenth and twentieth centuries, may not be as applicable to other eras and be a reading back into the past preoccupations of the present. It is also very much culturally specific to the West.

10. For an excellent study of the problems of essentializing see Spelman 1988.

11. For example, at the end of the nineteenth century many physicians questioned the wisdom of encouraging pubescent girls to continue their education. Because physicians saw that some young women had problems with menstruation, they felt that young women in general would be better advised to concentrate their bodies' energy on developing a healthy reproductive system rather

than dissipate it by trying to educate themselves. Such a view makes sense only when it is remembered that late nineteenth-century physicians believed that energy was finite and once lost was not regained. Because the male body was not as complex as the female, it did not need the same amount of energy for development and so boys could be encouraged to further their education.

12. This was particularly seen in the area of consent. The idea of consent being informed did not really exist as we know it until the late 1950s. Doctors were required to tell patients what was going to occur, but there was little emphasis placed on making sure that they understood or that they were aware of all the options available to them. Even if patients had been, they still were dependent on the physician who was part of the system that constructed the knowledge and the language used to explain that knowledge.

13. For an example of how women's bodies put them more at risk with respect to physicians see McLaren 1986. Although sterilization was in theory not gender specific, the reality was that many more women were sterilized than men.

14. Other factors such as race, age, and ability play into this as well. Some women would have more power than other women and indeed some women would have more power than some men patients.

15. In recent years, historians have been seeing agency as positive and heroic but there is no necessary reason why it should be. Agency is limited, confined, influenced, and shaped by so many different factors that it is impossible for any person to have total agency. What historians need to discuss is degree of agency or types of agency.

16. For an example of women dealing with their own bodies see Davis 1983.

17. For example, women's magazines were often a source of information but they were more often than not owned and run by men. The articles written by women on health matters often used physicians as sources of authority.

18. Jeff Warner, "'A Most Un-Christian Affair': The Maines, the Pincocks, and Spiritualism" (paper, Department of History, University of Waterloo, 1995), 36–39.

19. Many works exist that promote a fairly uncritical view of midwifery and that see the medical profession and its hostility as the explanation for the decline of midwifery. See Benoit 1989; Biggs 1983; Burtch 1994; Corea 1985a, 14; Donnison 1977; Laforce 1990; Leavitt and Walton 1984; Litoff 1978; Mason 1988; Oakley 1976, esp., 18; Oppenheimer 1983. Shorter (1982, 58–62) takes quite an opposing view of midwives.

20. For a discussion of the ability to read women's voices from medical texts see Theriot 1993.

21. For an excellent study of the prenatal and postnatal concern see Arnup 1994 and Comacchio 1993. For a description of the medicalization of childhood see Dodd 1991 and Raymond 1991.

22. For a discussion of the difficulties of patient-physician discourse see West 1984.

23. The irony is that in Canada today economics is forcing women out of the hospital after only a one- or two-day stay. This is proving to be problematic for nursing mothers.

24. Annau 1992; Dodd 1982, 1983, 1985; McLaren and McLaren 1986, ch. 5. Margaret Sanger in the United States also wanted physicians involved in birth control. See Gordon 1976; Kennedy 1970; Reed 1978.

25. The names of patients have been altered. Victoria General Hospital, Halifax, patient no. 1205, register no. 1087, Surgical Dept., Martha McNamara, admitted January 9, 1931, discharged January 20, 1931.

26. Class was not a constant variable. In the case of C-sections, middle-class women were more at risk because they could afford to pay for them.

27. Public Archives of Ontario, William Canniff Papers, MU 490 Package 3, Canada Medical Association, 1882, reports from newspapers.

28. *Practical Home Physician*, 1884, 974; *Canada Medical Record* 26 (January 1898): 4. See also Mitchinson 1991, 256–57.

29. *Canadian Medical Association Journal* (hereafter *CMAJ*) 10, no. 10 (October, 1920), 901; *The Public Health Journal* 14, no. 6 (June, 1923), 243; *CMAJ* 19, no. 2 (August 1928), 228; *Canadian Journal of Medicine and Surgery* 66, no. 3 (September 1929), 71; J. M. Monroe Kerr, J. Haig Ferguson, James Young, and James Hendry, *Combined Text-Book of Obstetrics and Gynaecology for Students and Practitioners* (Edinburgh: E. and S. Livingstone, 1993), 360; *Maclean's* 63 (July 15, 1950): 49.

30. For examples of patients demanding C-sections see *Canadian Public Health Journal* 25, no. 3 (March 1934): 142; *CMAJ* 37, no. 1 (July 1937): 37; *CMAJ* 39, no. 6 (December 1938): 531.

31. For examples of C-section being seen as easy and dramatic see *CMAJ* 5, no. 11 (November 1915): 968; *CMAJ* 14, no. 10 (October 1924): 907; *Canadian Practitioner and Review* 49, no. 4 (April 1924): 210; *CMAJ* 21, no. 6 (December 1929): 656; *CMAJ* 24, no. 4 (April 1936:) 473. For the medical belief that C-sections were still dangerous see *CMAJ* 20, no. 6 (June 1929): 647–48; *Canadian Journal of Medicine and Surgery* 75, no. 2 (February 1934): 46.

32. *CMAJ* 29, no. 6 (December, 1933): 590.

33. Public Archives of Nova Scotia, Medical Archives Collection, file 318, "Medical Society of Nova Scotia, Executive Meeting, 1936," 5–6.

34. *CMAJ* 40, no. 1 (January 1939): 40.

35. *CMAJ* 53, no. 1 (July 1945): 311-37

36. *University of Toronto Medical Journal* 24, no. 3 (December 1946): 72; *CMAJ* 58, no. 3 (March 1948): 252; *Alberta Medical Bulletin* 13, no. 1 (January 1948): 67; *CMAJ* 60, no. 3 (March 1949): 309; *Alberta Medical Bulletin* 15, no. 1 (January 1950): 15. Hormones are controlled substances and it is doctors who control them.

37. *Maritime Medical News* 14, no. 12 (December 1902): 437. MacKenzie, however, did feel that menstruation added to the build-up of this tension. Other physicians worried about the consequences of other social stresses such as education, social restraint, and better hygiene. Dudley 1902, 26–27; Hall 1917, 184; *Woman's Century*, April 1920, 10; Graves 1929, 159; Ryberg 1942, 3.

38. For an investigation of difficulties in discourse between patients and physicians see West 1984. See also Fisher 1986.

39. See *Montreal Medical Journal* 29, no. 9 (September 1900): 652, for women not knowing their dates of menstruation. Also, Jane Granger when she entered the Montreal General Hospital in 1902 recalled having had "some" operation but was not clear what it was. In 1930 when Mavis Denton entered the Victoria General Hospital, Halifax, she could not recall whether instruments had been used in a previous birth. McGill University Archives, Montreal General Hospital, RG 96 vol. 163 Patients Casebooks Gynaecology, 1902–4, patient no. 2, Jane Granger admitted January 6, 1902, discharged February 19, 1902; Victoria General Hospital, patient no. 1924, register no. 957, Surgical Dept., Mrs. Mavis Denton, admitted December 30, 1930, discharged January 4, 1931.

40. That women are not necessarily more sympathetic to other women than are men are to women is evidenced by the work of Helene Deutsch (1984).

41. The irony is that today many male physicians feel under siege because women patients often prefer to see a woman gynecologist rather than a man.

42. These interviews were taken for a new project on which I am working that examines medical treatment of women in Canada from 1900 to 1950.

43. For a detailed examination of ovariotomies see Mitchinson 1991, 258–77.

7

Reflections on the Transfer of "Progress": The Case of Reproduction

Maria De Koninck

Over the past several years, while studying various aspects of women's health, I have focused on pregnancy and childbirth. There are two main reasons for my interest in these events: they represent meaningful experiences for women, and the conditions under which they take place are closely related to women's place in society.

Childbirth has special status because it is an essentially female act, women's "visible" contribution to reproduction. How childbirth and pregnancy are treated in a particular culture often reveals interesting and significant aspects of social relations in that culture (Handwerker 1990). For example, here in North America, as in other so-called developed countries, pregnancy and childbirth are under the responsibility of medicine and medical experts.

Recently, my involvement in international health led me to deal with an issue that specifically concerns developing countries: maternal mortality.[1] While mortality associated with pregnancy or childbirth has become relatively rare in North America and in Western Europe, it remains very frequent in developing countries. It has become a reproductive health priority for many feminist organizations and appears more and more as a favored field of action in the discourse of multilateral organizations such as WHO (World Health Organization), UNFPA (United Nations Population Fund) and UNICEF (United Nations International Children's Emergency Fund) (UNICEF 1996). The main motivation for this interest lies, without a doubt, in the striking disparity in maternal mortality rates that persists in different countries around the world. The international community's political attention was also focused on the issue when the importance of women's contribution to Third World economies and the loss that their early deaths represents was brought to light (World Bank 1993).

In the following pages, I present some thoughts on the dilemmas, paradoxes, and contradictions that seem inherent in any policy aiming to reduce maternal mortality. My thoughts are based on my field experience in West Africa and are structured around three dimensions: (1) the foundation of the modern approach developed in the perinatal field, which is part of what we want to "transfer," that is, the notion of risk; (2) the current understanding we in our society have about Third World women's experiences; and (3) the actual transfer of our obstetrical technology. An ethical reflection on women's health care, such as the one we present in this book, cannot evade concerns about what becomes of this care when exported in other contexts.

Before dealing with maternal mortality in the specific context of my field experience, I wish to place the issue within the broader context of women's health.

Women's Health in the West: The Standards

Several health indicators point to a notable improvement in women's health in industrialized countries over the past few decades. This improvement is most evident in women's longer life expectancy, and this is partly attributable to a marked reduction in reproductive mortality. In fact, once mortality among women of child-bearing age declines, women's biological advantage becomes apparent and they have a longer life expectancy than men (Santow 1995).

This overall improvement in women's health must be placed in context. The context is one of socioeconomic and cultural changes in the conditions of women's lives, including greater access to education and the job market, and greater recognition of women's legal and economic rights. There have also been considerable changes in health resources, such as accessibility to birth control methods and to abortion, as well as stricter monitoring of pregnancy and birth with the development of specialized services.

Generally, in industrialized countries, women's life expectancy is no longer as closely tied to their reproductive functions as it once was and still is elsewhere in the world.[2] Overall rates of maternal and perinatal mortality and morbidity have dropped considerably in the West.

This observation is not, however, unilateral. Debate concerning the causes and consequences of the observed evolution persists. Indeed, there are many different interdependent factors that can be used to explain the improvement in life expectancy and the decline of certain pathologies. For example, education acts by enabling women to gain knowledge, by delaying the age they begin having children, and by providing the possibility of playing other roles than that of mother. Access to income gives women a certain independence in the area of reproduction and facilitates the use of health resources. Beyond simply identifying factors, it remains difficult, if not impossible, to analyze the specific role of each of these factors in isolation, be it biological, economic, social, cultural, or environmental.

Moreover, once certain problems have been resolved or reduced, new ones can appear that make any attempt at a definitive assessment even more problematic. For example, an increase in life expectancy implies aging, a phenomenon that is not simply a benefit since it involves the appearance of new problems or the accentuation of existing ones such as the prevalence of cancers and of pathologies more frequent in the elderly.

Progress also comes with some unforeseen and adverse effects. These are generally associated with the global phenomenon of the medicalization of women's bodies and experiences. The term refers to a greater medical control over women and the sanctioning of medicine as the legitimate expert in these experiences. The women's health movement has developed a critical analysis of the medicalization of pregnancy and childbirth, faulting medicine for having transformed normal and natural events into illnesses. Reproaches focus on dehumanizing aspects of this medical trend (more recently described as technicization) and the problems generated by medical interventionism: the chain of interventions, iatrogenic complications, and so on (Arms 1975; Rothman 1982; De Koninck 1990a; see also Chapter 5).

Recent studies on the subject indicate, however, that the medical institution cannot be considered the sole culprit in the situation; as indicated in Chapter 6, women have been active players in the increased availability of medical interventions during pregnancy and childbirth. An analysis of the interactions between women and experts and the history of women's struggles for better birthing conditions, particularly regarding pain control, reveals that women themselves have contributed to the entry of medicine in this area of their lives (Leavitt 1986; Mitchinson, Chapter 6, this book). Furthermore, women's endorsement of a mentality in which planning is a central value and of a technocratic culture leads to their support for the use of technology in the field of reproduction (De Koninck 1990b; Davis-Floyd 1994).

Even if we acknowledge that the adverse effects of medicalization are the result of a social dynamic and not the unilateral action of experts, it nonetheless remains that the events surrounding pregnancy and childbirth have become highly medicalized. This medicalization is far-reaching and is evident in the approach taken, the resources utilized, the places where pregnancy and childbirth can legitimately take place, their supervision, and the rate of intervention, including surgery.

The consequences of the medicalization go beyond observable phenomena such as high cesarean section rates, for example. They concern the broader issues of social relations, they affect women's images of themselves and of their potential, and they justify the control to which women are subjected as reproducers, which raises the issue of women's autonomy regarding their reproductive experiences. One of the most significant impacts of medical control over the experience of childbirth is, without a doubt, the feeling of incompetence it tends to generate in women. At the heart of the phenomenon of medicalization is the notion of risk; many women have internalized the discourse on risk that dominates the perinatal field (Quéniart 1988). An increasingly strict monitoring of pregnancy, according to constantly evolving medical criteria, which goes as far as the supervision of pregnant women's habits, places women in a position of responsibility for the health and normality of their infants. A series of dictates defines both what a pregnant woman can and must do and what she cannot and must not do. This phenomenon is neither new nor is it specifically Western. Everywhere rules have existed and continue to exist, whether they be beliefs, food taboos, or the like. The difference lies in the nature of the expertise (medical), its scope, how it is exercised (most notably through technology), and how it is applied (sometimes including legal decisions), and since this expertise goes hand in hand with the growing preoccupation with the fetus, one may add the arguments invoked (De Koninck and Parizeau 1991).

Obstetrical practices are permeated with technological developments and technological logic currently determines how events unfold. Women's experiences all too often involve feelings of solitude, apprehension, fear, and disappointment (De Koninck 1988).

The evolution in women's health in industrialized countries is filled with paradoxes. While considerable gains have indeed been achieved, some of the consequences, such as the high rates in surgery, the control of women's behaviors in the name of prevention, and the deskilling of women's knowledge and practices (Beauregard and De Koninck 1991), are viewed as negative by the women's movement. It is also difficult to assess the factors responsible for such gains because the factors are complex and they interact with one another. It must also be remembered that "women" as a social category covers a highly diverse group of people. Belonging to a social minority (aboriginal people, immigrants, etc.)

or to a disadvantaged social class can substantially modify the quality of women's experiences and thus have an effect both on life expectancy and on the frequency and seriousness of morbidities.

Despite these reservations, women's health in industrialized countries, from a transcultural perspective, is highly enviable, especially with regard to the specific issues of pregnancy and birth. This remains true even if greater life expectancy is accompanied by new problems. When measured by several health indicators, it is markedly better than that of women in less privileged countries where morbidity and mortality rates remain very high. This explains why the practices developed in industrialized countries become the standard. From this perspective, the criticisms concerning the adverse effects of the increase in medical interventions can sometimes seem secondary.[3]

Maternal Mortality: The Issue

In 1995, when I took my sabbatical leave, I had many questions in my mind about the acceptability of transferring our health practices related to childbirth, and these questions became all the more acute during the time I was away. I spent the year in the field, first at WHO's Family Health Division in Geneva and more specifically within the Maternal Health and Safe Motherhood Unit, where knowledge is brought together before being standardized. Then I went to West Africa, hoping to gain some insight into women's experiences.

The issue I focused on throughout that year was maternal mortality. According to available data, the human development indicator that reveals the greatest disparity between industrialized and developing countries is the risk of death among pregnant women. The ratio is 200 maternal deaths in the Third World to 1 death in the West (Tinker and Koblinsky 1993). The number of women who annually die of pregnancy or birth-related causes is currently estimated at 585,000, and 99 percent of the cases occur in the Third World (UNICEF 1996). The most frequent direct causes of death are the same throughout the world: hemorrhages, infections, hypertension, labor obstruction, and abortion (WHO 1995a). There is a broad consensus that the majority of these deaths could be avoided. Moreover, maternal morbidity is also very frequent. It has been estimated that at least 20 million women annually suffer from severe, long-term disabilities associated with pregnancy and childbirth (Türmen 1994).

Such a noticeable disparity cries out for a remedy. Indeed, concerted efforts at the international level began when information on the number of deaths became general knowledge (Rosenfield and Maine 1985). The first international conference on the subject was held in Nairobi, Kenya, in 1987 (organized by WHO, the World Bank, and UNFPA). The Safe Motherhood Initiative was launched at this conference and attention was focused on the extent of the phenomenon of women who "die in silence" during childbirth. Through the use of statistics emphasizing disparities, a rapid and energetic response was put into motion. The consequence of this strategy was that maternal morbidity, which was also very high but viewed as less dramatic, did not attract as much attention and was not as well documented as mortality. Efforts were mobilized around mortality and aimed to save lives rather than prevent or treat the pathological consequences of a difficult pregnancy or birth (Graham and Campbell 1992).

The goal of reducing maternal mortality from that time on appeared to many international health workers as a priority in the movement to improve the health of women in developing countries. However laudable, the actions necessary to achieve this goal have far-reaching implications that may not be obvious at first sight. First, the goal was established on the basis of the evolution observed in industrialized countries. This situated evolution contrasted markedly, however, with the situation in developing countries. When strategies for action are being determined, they most often appear as a transfer of knowledge or practices, and any transfer raises a number of issues, some of which I illustrate further on. As anthropologists and sociologists have clearly demonstrated, dispensing Western biomedical services in non-Western contexts can be a double-edged sword (Ginsburg and Rapp 1991).

The issue of transfer becomes all the more pertinent in the case of women's health and reproduction. Reproduction is at the heart of gender relations and is closely connected to the perception of women's role that dominates in society. The many debates surrounding "reproductive rights" during the last two world conferences (Population and Development, in Cairo in 1994, and Women, in Beijing in 1995) remind us of this. Reproduction cannot be reduced solely to its biomedical dimensions; sociocultural and political components can prove decisive for any action in the field. Even the definition of reproductive health adopted by multilateral organizations implicitly acknowledges that social, cultural, and political dimensions play a part in its construction (Nations-Unies 1994). Any action aimed at one aspect of reproductive health must take this into account and cannot be limited to the transfer of specific medical practices.

A consensus is emerging among international experts that the best approach for reducing maternal mortality is to organize emergency obstetrical services. This view is based on an assessment of the successes and failures of the various strategies attempted to date (Prevention of Maternal Mortality Network 1995). Since the first international conference on maternal mortality, a variety of programs have been created and projects have been set up in many countries, but little progress has been made. One of the arguments used to explain the fact that maternal mortality rates remain high is that too much has been invested in antenatal care. It seems that the approaches that were tried did not give the expected results and the effectiveness of these approaches in reducing mortality has partly come into question. These criticisms lend support to the advocates of curative-type interventions such as emergency obstetrical services.[4]

While I was in WHO, the debates around this issue were very animated. Some actors in this field preferred giving priority to emergency obstetrical services, while others were more inclined to favor an "essential" services approach that would promote a balance between preventive and curative care in the organization of health services. For my part, throughout my time at WHO, I insisted that we take a close and careful look at the role of social factors, and more specifically, of gender relations and women's status in maternal mortality. I also wanted to emphasize the potential of creating adverse effects in transferring technology-oriented interventions without considering these aspects. I expressed fears that the medicalization process could take place very rapidly in settings where women are not in a social position to offer some resistance because of their lack of information and legal rights. Supporting the organization of health services including emergency services is definitely a valuable option, but the context in which it takes place must be taken into account. Issues such as access to care, expert/lay relations, information given to users, the right to accept or refuse medical decisions, and so on, are not incidental but determinant components of health services and might require social measures.

Promoting biomedical solutions is not sufficient. It is my conviction that Third World women are victims, not of their reproductive potential, but of social conditions and gender relations that transform their reproductive experiences, including the lack of access to adequate care, into pathologies and death. Even though we cannot decide what is best for them, we know, based on our own experience and on theirs, that status enhancement (defined as access to education, better economic conditions, and greater possibilities for deciding their own future), leads to greater longevity and better health. We also know that these conditions constitute empowerment (Karl 1995).

Not everyone agrees with an approach that promotes social actions as much as biomedical interventions. Although almost everyone believes that educating girls, raising the age of marriage, and making birth planning more widely available are key factors in reducing maternal mortality and morbidity, they are considered medium- and long-term changes. When weighed against more technical means that target the organization of services and most notably of emergency services, they lose their attraction, partly because it is allegedly more difficult to measure their effects. Moreover, these different dimensions may even be considered as distinct from one another instead of interacting, as if the value of women's lives in a society did not participate in the definition of the type of care that is put into place and in women's potential access to it.

To have an impact on social factors, one must necessarily move beyond the field of health because the measures one may want to adopt call gender relations into question, involve several sectors, and, what is more, require a political will that is not always forthcoming. The need to enhance women's status is not denied in development agencies, but the means of doing so, when not completely out of reach, seem too complex or politically threatening.

My preoccupation with the adverse effects of "progress" in the perinatal field, most notably the medicalization of pregnancy and birth, found few echoes in a context concerned with identifying the best means for saving lives. Nevertheless, my concerns did concur with the warnings of some midwives involved in international health and working for WHO who fear both an increase in interventions and a decline in the organization of prenatal services to the benefit of curative obstetrical acts (Thompson 1995).

A Field Experience in Africa

After leaving WHO, I spent six months in Benin (previously called Dahomey), in West Africa. Although I was more skeptical than ever about the judiciousness of transferring obstetrical technology to developing countries and preoccupied by the consensus that was building in favor of the emergency care solution, I remained convinced that the inequality between the situation of women in industrialized and developing countries as regards perinatal care was totally unacceptable and required action. My intention in going to Benin was twofold: to spend

time with women there in an effort to better understand how they experience their situation, and to assess whether, based on their remarks,
it would be possible to identify the most strategic means of having an
impact on the situation, taking their specific situations into consideration. I carried out empirical research aimed at fulfilling these objectives.

Benin, which had a population of 5 million in 1992, is considered to
be one of the poorest countries in the world. It gained its independence
from France in 1960 and, after being under a marxist-oriented military
regime for seventeen years, became a democratic country with the national conference held in 1990. The most important city is Cotonou, with
over 400,000 inhabitants. This city was the site of the Francophone sum-
mit in December 1995.

In 1992, 80.1 percent of Beninese women were illiterate. The overall
fertility rate was 202 per 1,000 and the synthetic rate was 6.1 children
per woman.[5] One-third of married men are polygamous. Officially, the
maternal mortality rate is 473 per 100,000 live births, but this is considered an underestimate; in 1996 UNICEF estimated it to be 990 (UNICEF
1996). In 1993, only 3.42 percent of the national budget was allocated to
health. There is one national hospital in Cotonou, one hospital in each
province, and health centers in the communities. Half of the women
giving birth are attended by a professionally trained person (Commission nationale pour l'intégration de la femme au développement 1994;
Ministère de la santé 1993, 1994; Ministère du plan et de la restructuration économique 1994).

The study I did was exploratory.[6] I carried out interviews with nineteen women, thirteen of whom had had obstetrical complications and
eleven of whom had had a cesarean section. I had access to survey questionnaires each had already completed on the events related to their
pregnancy and childbirth. They had all given birth in a hospital. Their
sociodemographic characteristics were varied, particularly age, religion, occupation, place of birth, ethnic origin, marital status, level of
schooling, and number of previous births. I met with thirteen women
living in the city (eleven in Cotonou and two in Ouidah) and six living
in villages in the countryside. Eight of them were illiterate, three had
been to school for less than four years and three for less than nine years,
and five had studied for over ten years. This high level of education can
be explained by the fact that the selection was carried out from hospitals, even though the majority of women interviewed had not planned
to give birth there. It can also be explained by the fact that many lived
in Cotonou or in Ouidah, where literacy is higher than in rural settings.
Five of the women were in polygamous marriages and fourteen in

monogamous marriages; of these nineteen, eleven lived with their husbands. Their ethnic origins were: nine Fons, three Adjas, two Sahoués, two Gouns, one Mina, one Dodoméghé, and one unknown. Fifteen of them stated they were Roman Catholic, including four of the five women in polygamous marriages, who thereby indicated that their adhesion to the religion was not necessarily orthodox. This absence of orthodoxy must be interpreted in regard to the transformation taking place in Benin, as elsewhere in West Africa, with marked social changes associated with urbanization. Urbanization is generally accompanied by a mixture of representations and practices. Three of my informants said they belonged to a traditional religion and one stated she had no religion. Four were primipara (first pregnancy), eleven had had between two and five pregnancies, and four had had more than five.

No statistical generalizations can be based on a sample so small and so diverse and constituted from hospital records, because hospital births are not at all the experience of the majority of women.[7] But despite the absence of statistical representativeness in the study population, the nature of information gathered confirms the relevance of speaking to women in order to better grasp their personal experiences and their perceptions of pregnancy, childbirth, and health services if one hopes to reduce maternal mortality.[8] Individual interviews proved effective as a source of strategic information for defining solutions. They elucidated the factors that, depending on the interviewee, influenced the course of events: available information, understanding, decision making, obstacles to receiving care, and so on. Women's comments also confirm the scope of the issues raised by the current practice of transferring a different way of doing things to developing countries at three different levels. The first is the framework within which actions are developed, through the prism of risk. The second is women's status and gender relations, and the third, which is related to the first two, is women's relationship to health services. I explore each of these issues in more detail now.

Risk Approach: An "Exportable" Concept?

Based on the remarks of the women interviewed in Benin, their perceptions of the dangers associated with pregnancy and birth appear completely foreign to the notion of risk that prevails in Western medical culture. When asked to describe their experiences, several talked about childbirth and referred to death as being an integral part of it. In Benin, there is a saying that when a woman is pregnant, she has one foot in the

grave: "The day of delivery, you are between death and life and when
you do that, you can die as you can survive" (October 30, 1995; hereafter
10/30/95). The respondents' comments confirmed this view. One interviewee, an illiterate Catholic woman who lives in the countryside and
who was taken to a hospital during her labor and subsequently lost her
child, leaving her with two living children after six pregnancies, said:

> Birth is an experience between life and death. You don't know
> whether you will survive or not. You no longer have any control
> over anything. That's what giving birth is about. You see that
> giving birth is a mortal act. God forbid, but there are children
> who are born only to be taken directly to the land of the dead or
> else others who survive with their mother; others prefer to die
> alone and leave their mother alive. That's how it goes. Life and
> death exist side-by-side during childbirth. (9/11/95)

Another woman, the mother of five living children after seven pregnancies who lives in the countryside and practices a traditional religion,
is married to a man with three wives. She explained her attitude toward
events: "Once you're pregnant, especially from the beginning of the
pregnancy, you have already accepted everything: you have accepted
death, illness, and so on." She continued by describing her feelings during her last birth.

> What came to mind was: Will I survive? Will I go home alive?
> Will I die? Birth is the land of the dead, because you're no
> longer alive when the baby comes out. What if the baby comes
> out and you find yourself where you're not supposed to be?
> That's why you have such thoughts." (10/3/95)

Medical interventions can be perceived in the same manner, as revealed by comments from a street merchant about having her first child:
"They operated on me. . . . I understood because they shaved my "road
to the spirit" [pubic hair] and I told them it did not matter, that if I survive, it would be better, otherwise too bad" (10/18/95). Interpretations
associating death and childbirth were generally communicated to us in
religious terms. Such a prospect is accepted as God's will. A young
monogamous Catholic Fon merchant told us that after her second cesarean section: "I felt that God had done something great for me. He was
merciful. I didn't think I would still be here after all the bleeding. I felt
a great joy when I realized this" (10/10/95).

Among Beninese women the loss of a child can also be described as
part of the order of things. An illiterate woman living in a monogamous
marriage in Ouidah told us of the deaths of two of the seven children

she gave birth to: "They went away. One boy and one girl. They will be up there preparing the way for me" (9/26/95).

Another woman spoke to us of her experience. She is a salesperson in Cotonou living in a polygamous marriage and had undergone a cesarean section. She already had three children, and the fourth one died several months after the birth: "Lots of people have died that way. I continue thanking God. And the child only lived a few months before going back. However, I don't complain too much, everything God does is good" (9/29/96).

These accounts demonstrate how the approach dominant in industrialized countries is part of an essentially different cultural model. In the West, the approach is based on risk assessment and the object is to exert greater control over events. Women's reproductive experiences are scrutinized in an effort to identify the risks they might present. In prenatal clinics, pregnant women are classified according to their degree of risk: high, low, or "no risk" groups. Risk assessment is based on their characteristics (age, number of previous births), medical antecedents, and, increasingly, their habits (smoking). Although the notion of risk has long existed in the area of pregnancy and childbirth, it has been used as a basis for classification and differential treatment only since the 1960s (Alexander and Keirse 1989). Control may be exerted over women's habits, and in certain cases, interventions such as cesarean sections can be imposed in the name of the fetus (Davis-Floyd 1994). The use of coercion (extension of social pressure) appears to ensue from the risk assessment approach, as defined by medical experts. Once one or several risk factors have been identified, physicians attempt to make pregnant and birthing women abide by their instructions. The risks are viewed as a threat to the woman or to the child in utero or to both, a threat with which the physicians are acquainted and that they believe they can remove.

The medically managed risk assessment approach in the perinatal field is now accepted as the international standard (WHO 1995a). This explains why health workers in developing countries are increasingly trained and encouraged to identify high-risk women. This process is taking place in societies where risk as a concept may not have the same social meaning and function because of the cultural backgrounds. A question may be asked here: When local Western-trained medical personnel adopt the risk assessment approach, what type of interaction may we expect them to have with women who consult them and whose references remain those of their own cultures?

The concept of risk as understood in the West today is indeed the result of profound social and cultural changes. It has not always meant the presence of a threat or danger. Instead, it used to refer to the probability of any event occurring. The modern sense of the term reflects the spread of rationalism coupled with a growing preoccupation with safety and the need to prevent any possible complications. It is rooted in an ideology of controlling environmental conditions through the use of knowledge developed on the basis of scientific criteria. Its use in the social field conveys a distancing from interpretations based on spiritual beliefs or religion.

> A theology of catastrophe is slowly yielding to a secular view
> putting into perspective a series of potentially predictable, and
> therefore avoidable, if certain precautions are taken, harmful
> causalities. . . . The philosophy of the Enlightenment invented
> the accident. Risk was established at the human level in
> relation to an environment posited as indifferent to God's
> designs. (Le Breton 1995, 28; my translation)

Furthermore, the discourse on risk corresponds to our modern way of controlling behavior and practices. "The calculation of risk is deeply entrenched in science and manufacturing and as a theoretical base for decision making. . . . The concept of risk emerges as a key idea from modern times because of its use as a forensic resource" (Douglas 1990, 2, 3). Other concepts such as "taboos" and "sins" have played a role (or continue to do so) in moralizing or politicizing dangers, but not necessarily in the same way, according to Mary Douglas. Risk is a modern norm for managing social life.

"For most epidemiologists, risk exists as a statistical construct, a product of analyzing aggregate data in a particular way (Imber 1988). Clinicians abstract the vocabulary of the epidemiologist, the epidemiological language of risk, from its place in scientific discourse and insert it into their own argument about childbirth" (Kaufert and O'Neil 1993; reference to Imber 1988). Risk can refer to different factors: biological demographic characteristics, social conditions (poverty), or habits (alcoholism). Medical personnel recognize the cause-effect relationship to illness, even though it has not always been explicitly demonstrated; the same is true of the relationships between factors (Goldberg 1982).

Proposing this approach for use in the perinatal field in developing countries raises a dual issue. On one hand, the notion of risk does not have the same meaning in other cultures, so transferring practices based on this approach requires a change in mentality.[9] On the other hand, the new expertise emphasizing medical personnel's involvement may reduce women's role in reproduction, challenging the quality of their experiences. Yet one must not, as statistics indicate, idealize the experiences of women living in contexts that have not been medicalized (MacIntyre 1977).

Thus, the women interviewed in Benin said that they are aware that pregnancy and birth entail "risks" (which in general they refer to as the possibility of dying, with only one of our participants mentioning that she had feared giving birth to a child with a handicap), but many describe these "risks" as inescapable. With few exceptions, the information they conveyed to us about their experiences does not appeal to a scientific means of interpretation, that is, they do not seek to explain (or have explained to them) the events that took place, for example, why they had to be transferred or operated on. Their references are of a metaphysical nature, are more "holistic" and at a more global level than the specific circumstances surrounding their births.

The decisions to consult someone during their pregnancy, or not, are dominated by material considerations that also come into play in their or their family's decision to resort to medical care in the case of complications. Our respondents spoke of their prenatal care as a fairly common practice, but in general they did not refer to a dimension of risk prevention or reduction. They go to their appointments with midwives at the health center when they have time and when they know they have the money to purchase the drugs prescribed, associating appointments with drug prescriptions. Many do so because their husband or family expects them to consult or because, as a young woman living in a suburb of Cotonou and married to a physician told us: "They tell us on the radio, the 'dotos' tell us: a pregnant woman must come to the consultation— for tests of urine, for vaccinations" (10/9/95). But they do not seem to go to prevent their death.

This does not, however, mean that they have no personal apprehensions. Some know women who have died in childbirth, some themselves have had difficulties during previous pregnancies or births,[10] and it is noteworthy that women who had cesareans seem inclined to consider antenatal care from now on as an obligation. In other words, it is not that they are sure they will not have any problems. It is that they do not view these problems as specific risks to be managed and instead give a meaning to eventual difficulties by referring to a metaphysical explanation.

In southern Benin, the cult of *vodun* is very present (Passot 1993). Our informants told us that they waited before revealing their pregnancy or the beginning of their labor because these situations leave them vulnerable to evil spells.[11] This appears conceptually far from the medical prevention of complications but it can be interpreted as an action to avoid the occurrence of problems.

There is another dimension that confirms how different Beninese women's perceptions are from a Western risk-based approach. Several of them while recounting their experience spoke of family planning in the sense that they expressed their desire to have a say when it comes to future pregnancies, in some cases clearly for fear of dying. Among those who indicated that they wished to practice family planning, several claimed that they did not know any methods or how to go about it. The objective was there—birth control or birth spacing—but they had not yet decided how this was to be done. There appeared to be a significant gap between the objective of limiting births (even when it is justified by a fear of dying) and actually using methods to achieve that objective through approaches advocated by family planning programs aimed at avoiding "the risk of pregnancy" and promoting "safe sex."

One cannot, then, conclude that these women unconditionally accept fate. For example, one respondent clearly explained to us how she hoped to avoid another pregnancy because of the pain she had experienced in childbirth. The interpretation these women give for the occurrence of complications or even death is not a denial of agency. They give meaning to the events with their own references.

Women's Experience: Motherhood, the Economic Situation, Health Services

I found that the most interesting aspect of the information gathered from the women concerns their experience of their place in society and within the family insofar as this relates to maternal mortality issues. Their sayings confirm the important role social factors play in determining the way they experience their pregnancies and births; most of these factors are closely connected to their status and the possibilities (or lack of) of their making decisions for themselves. I deal with this issue from three specific angles: the relationship to motherhood, economic factors, and the relationship with health services.

Motherhood: Status and Gender Relations

An understanding of how women experience the complications associated with pregnancy and childbirth, how they face the problems that arise, and what gender relations prevail in their society must precede the introduction of new practices. Their discourse is the most adequate source of information we can rely on to clarify these points. It helps to measure the concordance (or disparity) between their needs, their expectations, and the solutions proposed. We often forget that the meaning given to women's reproductive experiences changes with the cultural context and that any projection in interpretations can be misleading. For example, in Benin, biological reproduction (and the physiological experience) is apprehended as a primarily social event and not as an individual experience, as it is elsewhere (Morsy 1995).

In Benin, as in many other societies, women are viewed foremost as reproducers (WHO 1995b). They are socialized to fulfill this role from a very young age, which partly explains their low educational levels. Motherhood is not only highly valued but expected of all women. A certain sense of inevitability associated with biological reproduction is therefore part of each woman's potential life path.

Family planning, whether to limit or to space births, must be placed in this context; it directly affects what is expected of women. Here too, interpretations refer to divine will. In the words of an illiterate salesperson living in Cotonou with a polygamous husband, it is divine authority that decides how many children a woman has: "They said that you can't just have one child: you don't know how many God sent you to just stop at one— Even after three or four years, if God sends another one, I'll take it and stop there" (9/29/95).

Nonetheless, several women expressed the desire to stop having children or to space them further apart; but they must confront their husbands: "I talk about it indirectly, that we will stop. But, he does not accept, he wants more children" (10/3/95). In one case, a young illiterate woman living in a small village, who had two young children and had lost a third, told us that she would not have any more children (although she was not sure how) and that if her husband left her she was willing to pay the price: "He can't force me to, otherwise I think I'll leave him" (10/18/95). The strength of her will appeared to us totally inflexible. Her motivation was the fear of being cut again. She had experienced an episiotomy and a cesarean.

Another case is worth recounting to further illustrate the point. The woman lived in a suburb of Cotonou and had come very close to death while giving birth. When she was pregnant for the twelfth time, having had four pregnancies end in miscarriage, she was hospitalized. She told us that she had not followed medical advice to stay in the hospital because she had no one to take care of her children. When she gave birth before term, she had to have an emergency cesarean section during a blackout in the hospital. The medical personnel told her that they had operated, not to save her life, but to save the baby, because she had not followed their advice. She had very ambivalent feelings about the pregnancy, which she had hoped to end by refusing medical care. Her husband disapproved of her attitude because he wanted her to have as many children as possible, even though he had a second wife. "I'm the one who suffers," she said. "I had asked before this pregnancy. My husband refused, he refused and every time before giving birth it costs at least 100,000 francs [about US$215], I have to get a cervical ring and medicine every time. I wanted an abortion, but he refused."

She was very critical of her husband, who, in her view, exposed her to death. But because of social pressures she was unable to stand up to him. The cost of her cesarean, however, had made him finally accept that she would not have any more children. But she remained strongly affected by the experience and ended the interview saying: "If there hadn't been a torch that day— I'd be gone. I feel that that day it was between life and death" (9/20/95). She made it clear that had she been a victim of maternal death her husband should have been considered responsible.

Two interacting factors seem to me particularly significant in Benin: the very low level of literacy or schooling, and polygamy. Women's lack of education makes them more dependent on others for health information and creates obstacles when they try to fulfill their own needs or those of their children.

Polygamy also seems to be particularly significant; it has an important effect on gender relations. This effect is apparent in our material and was also suggested by people working in the field. A woman's decision whether to have a child must take into account the prospect that a man may take another wife. While one woman was telling us of her difficulties (including a still-born baby) and of her desire to practice birth control (she had six living children), her husband's aunt joined us and, having heard her words, stated that her niece by marriage had to continue reproducing, otherwise the family had no reason to keep her. More than once, we were told quite clearly that if a woman does not want any more children, her husband will go find another wife. This "threat" clearly conveys the extended family's expectations.

> The ideal of fertility in Benin is based on the conception of family structure. The latter is made up of individuals who trace their line back to the same mythical ancestor. The duty of each person within the structure is to contribute to its survival and continuity. Since each individual is only recognized in relation to a group of relatives that we call family, the motivation to procreate can be interpreted as the need to expand one's group. . . . Procreating is therefore a duty to continue the work of the common mythical ancestor. (Akoto, Guingnido, and Tabutin 1991, 136; my translation)

Nevertheless, family planning programs in Benin, as in other countries with high fertility rates, target women, investing very little in raising awareness among men. While in Benin, I was told of several strategies used by women, often in collusion with health workers, to gain access to contraception without their husband's knowledge, since men were considered totally unaware of the implications of the number of the children they wished to have. It is worth pointing out that men's lack of responsibility for contraceptive practices can also be observed in societies with low fertility rates, such as ours.

I was amazed to see to what extent gender inequalities have a tangible effect on women's health through the dependence they impose on women. This is particularly true when it comes to information.

More than one participant described her ignorance of what happened during her birth, for example, what problems and complications led to her transfer to the hospital: "What causes this, we do not know. What leads to a cesarean, I don't know— I cannot ask such a big question. And I am not alone with the health agent, we are many together" (9/11/95). The husband, however, may have received the information, or at least had access to it, had he so wished.

> My husband told me that if I am going to give birth again, it
> will again be an operation because I do not have a pelvis
> [*bassin*]. My husband says that. I say it is false. He says, he will
> show me the paper, that he went to the hospital. He says that
> it is written on the paper. (10/9/95)

Later on, this woman told us she was convinced her husband was lying to her. We asked several participants whether they had asked questions regarding the nature of their complications or the reason they were transferred or operated on. The majority said no, considering that it was not their place to ask or that their husband was responsible for finding out. "It surprises me but I do not say anything. I do not ask anything from anyone, that's how it is" (10/30/95). This reinforces my previous statement that understanding specific factors as the cause of events does not seem to be part of women's explanatory framework, maybe because they do not estimate they could have changed the course of events.

In concrete terms, women's dependence on others leads to a delay between the appearance of a problem and the search for help, often with disastrous consequences. What plays a role here is the woman's and her entourage's perception of the seriousness of the situation, which makes all the difference. The time factor is decisive when complications arise, for example, in the case of hemorrhages, the main cause of maternal mortality. When hemorrhaging occurs those present must recognize it as a situation that requires help, then they must get transportation and find money for drugs. Furthermore, for many people, the cost of hospitalization (and all the more, the cost of surgery) is forbidding; it is not the woman's decision, and she usually does not have her own income to pay for it.

These facts raise another question at the heart of a comparative approach between the situations of women in industrialized and developing countries, namely, our understanding of their experiences. We know so very little about them, despite the many studies that attempt to identify women's perceptions, knowledge, and practices (WHO 1995c).

The Economic Situation: Dependence and Poverty

The economic factor is central to this whole issue of maternal mortality. Most obvious is its relation to the decision-making process. It cannot be considered independently of the broader context of women's status and their relationship to motherhood. Their lack of income has an impact on their possibilities and actions. With only one exception, the women we spoke with were financially dependent on their husbands for drug-related and medical service expenses. Even those who earned money could not use medical services or purchase medicine without their husbands' permission and contribution.[12] That is why some of them explained that they did not go to their prenatal visits at the health center because there was no money to buy the medicine that would be prescribed.[13] As a woman living in Ouidah, the mother of six children, with two co-wives said: "The reason I didn't go is that my husband only buys what he wants to when he gets a prescription. When three things are prescribed, for example, he only buys two. So if I'm going to take the bother to go all the way there, I find I'm doing it for nothing" (9/25/95).

When women cannot follow the advice of the health agents, they are afraid that they will be reprimanded, so they prefer not to go. Their financial dependence should not, however, be interpreted simply as an expression of men's control over women because it also reflects men's responsibility for reproduction. But its consequences can be very serious. For example, one of our respondents told us that her baby died because her husband refused to purchase the medicine necessary for treating the child. Another woman told us that she had to stay at the hospital for one month while her husband looked for the money needed to pay for the operation.

The economic situation of the overall population must be kept in mind. To the question, "What is the priority in fighting maternal mortality?" the medical director of the largest maternity unit in Cotonou, whom we interviewed, spontaneously answered, "poverty."

By this, she referred not only to the necessary services in case of complications but to the general health status. Anemic women who become pregnant may easily develop pregnancy complications. Under- or ill-nourished, exposed to different pathologies because of difficult living conditions, women of childbearing age are vulnerable when pregnancy takes its toll. Health services cannot prevent all problems and alleviate all pains in such a context. But even so, it seems that these services could do more.

The factors that come into play in seeking and obtaining health care are not only financial or family-related. They also involve women's relationships with the health service personnel.

Health Services: Resistance

Women's relationships with health practitioners are strongly marked by hierarchy. Many of the accounts we gathered are critical of midwives, who are accused of ill-treating patients. The midwives they refer to are the ones that have been trained as professionals, are paid by the state, and work in the health centers and hospitals where they attend women giving birth unless there is a complication. Some women told us that they do not dare to ask questions because they have heard midwives yelling at other women. "First they insult you about this or that. So if I—I don't ask questions, that's why" (10/9/95). "You can rarely ask midwives, they rarely ask you, speak nicely to you, or ask you what is wrong . . . . Sometimes you can even hear someone being hit with a loin cloth" (9/20/95). "The way they treated me, they started beating me— I could not push anymore, they started beating me, beating me. I became upset and I left, my mother found me a taxi to go to the Maternity Lagune" (9/29/95).

It is common knowledge that health professionals treat women rudely (Vlasssof 1994). We were told that this is due to their long work hours and their miserable wages. But differences in educational levels and social class undoubtedly play a role. A study carried out in Niger also confirmed this problem with midwives' attitudes. In fact, I did not expect to hear women in Benin speaking of the lack of respect shown to them in the same terms as others had, both in a survey carried out in Senegal on nurses in a PMI (center for maternal and infant protection) and in a study carried out in Montreal on very poor women (Jaffre and

Prual 1994; Wane 1992; Colin et al. 1992). The accounts all agree on one point: health personnel tend to be critical when women do not abide by their instructions, so women avoid consulting in order not to be blamed. I would add, they resist to protect their dignity. One informant, who has had four pregnancies, described her experiences with midwives:

> Our *dotos*, our newly arrived midwives, don't behave as they
> should, they lack wisdom. When they examine you, for
> example, if you don't act properly, they start insulting you: "Did
> I send you to your husband, did I tell you to go get— " And
> they yell at you. That's why when I go to my appointment and I
> only see young ones, if it's those young midwives, I go home,
> even if I have to wait to be treated, I go home— I can't stand
> being ill-treated and then suffer alone afterwards. (9/29/95).

Another participant said she walked long distances to get to Ouidah even if there was a health center close by. "They deliver well. They do well the injections. But, their way of caring does not please me. Whether things be good or bad, you must welcome us. But, our *dotos* do not want that, that is why we run away" (10/3/95).

The women's accounts indicate that even when services are available, it is not easy to bring women to them. Not only do they need money, but they must trust the quality of services. It is not surprising that many wait until the last minute to go.

Some of our informants commented on the issue of technical interventions without appearing to support the model, although one young urban woman who had chosen to give birth in the hospital and had found it difficult told us: "If they could give injections to speed up the labor, it would be good" (10/16/95). One literate woman working as a technician in communications who had had a second cesarean and whose sister had died after the same operation told us:

> Before, cesareans didn't exist in Africa, eh? When there are
> complications, there are herbal teas, there are amulets, just to
> unblock the way. Whereas now a little problem, when there's a
> snag, they butcher you— In the old days, supposedly, I say
> supposedly, because I wasn't, I wasn't alive— there were
> leaves, herbal teas, our own amulets that could only be given
> to the woman, have her drink maybe, or things like that that
> make the labor go faster and the woman is delivered without
> having to have a cesarean." (9/26/95)

Finally, even if they are treated in an institution where so-called modern medicine is practiced, many of our respondents told us that they consulted traditional practitioners and used traditional medicine. The coexistence of the two systems is clearly evident, and it is interesting to see how women move with ease from one to the other and in general do not appear to consider one more effective than the other: "I went to the *dotos*, they made me some serum, but it did not work. We finally used traditional medicine" (10/3/95). Another informant who had problems with her breasts told us: "I went to the hospital and they prescribed medication that I should spread on my breast. When I started using the medication as prescribed, pain became atrocious. It hurt me more than before. So I went to the herborists who tried to cure me too" (10/30/95).

On this issue, Carol Vlassof notes: "It is reported that women in many cultures prefer traditional healers because they provide meaningful explanations of their illness, whereas modern providers tend to give limited information, instructing women regarding procedures they should follow rather than explaining how the problem can be treated and what steps can be taken to avoid it in the future" (Vlassof 1994, 1254). This remark corresponds to what we heard from Beninese women who reported they did not seek explanations from medical personnel concerning precise events, while proposing a global interpretation referring to their beliefs and representations. Indeed, traditional healers help make sense rather than give reasons based on a scientific discourse and therefore consulting women may feel they have received what we call satisfactory explanations.

When considering transfer of knowledge and of practices, this dimension raises one last question I want to address here: the expertise that is being transferred is largely dependent on technology. The latter has been developed in a particular context and, like the notion of risk, is rooted in a philosophy of control. Biomedical practices and knowledge that dominate in the West have their roots in a philosophy of control over nature and the ideology of progress (Wertz 1981; Arney 1982). This orientation explains the fact that the growing control over pregnancy and childbirth can be interpreted as progress for women and a means of liberating them from the curse of nature (Shorter 1982). It has encouraged the medicalization of these events, particularly when childbirth was moved from the home to the hospital and also through the process by which formerly exceptional procedures have become commonplace. This context of technological developments and the consequences of resorting to technology cannot be ignored when considering their transfer to societies where the representations of procreation and its surrounding differ profoundly.

Unanswered Questions

This field experience, however brief, confirmed two things. The first is the inestimable value of women's accounts as a source of information to better understand a situation such as maternal mortality and to seek solutions to it. Although I was convinced this was true before I stayed in Benin for a few months, I was impressed by the distance between my culture and theirs. The second is the complexity of women's experiences and how they are rooted in gender relations. My understanding of hierarchy greatly evolved during these months, particularly in regard to the mechanisms of socialization and social control that help maintain a domination of women. These two dimensions are most significant when considering the transfer of knowledge and practices.

Concerning the issues raised above, which I consider central to a reflection on actions in the field of maternal mortality, the information gathered in Benin leads me to the following conclusion.

Any approach based on risk and aiming to control reproductive events cannot be considered transferable unless cultural changes are also considered transferable and desired. Women's discourse reveals that their interpretation of events is anchored in a global vision of their society, of their role in that society, and of reproductive events. Introducing modern practices puts into question their interpretation, since it proposes technical control in order to prevent deaths and morbidities in childbirth that they perceive as parts of the event. On what grounds could we propose such a project? In the name of women's health, we can say. But, this laudable goal must not occlude the fact that modern medical practices belong to a different world vision with its premises and corollaries, namely, particular representations of the body, of the individual, of health, of health care and interventions (see Chapters 3 and 8). Being aware that practices and techniques are not neutral and decontextualized suggests that before they can be adopted there is a need for a stage during which the people concerned can be confronted with this vision and enabled to make choices.

Moreover, defining a risk-based approach and medical control as inevitable is an evolutionary and linear perspective that disregards the real situation of women. When transplanted to a context where hierarchy imbues social relations, it can lead to the consolidation of power relations in which women are the losers. We have noted how relations within the family and in the health services put women in a dominated position. If no changes in these relations come with the diffusion of modern medical practices, women might face even more obstacles in their quest to gain some control over their health.

To count on access to education as the keystone to empowerment would also be insufficient. It is a valid move toward confronting the perspectives that lead women to accept situations that are remediable and a way to help them have a better understanding of the issues in keeping with the eventual changes in practices. But education must be used mainly to support women's skills and creativity in finding solutions for themselves. This is the real challenge. Knowledge developed in the West for overseeing pregnancy and childbirth can be offered, keeping in mind its controversial aspects, most notably, the potential for medicalization, but it should be shared and not transferred. I now show the ways in which sharing certain types of knowledge would work differently, and more in favor of the women whose lives the knowledge ends up influencing.

Women have a right to health services and to practices that have proved to be beneficial in the Western world. However, knowing how these may in a certain way "disempower" women if their experiences become controlled by biomedical discourse and practices, we must try to find ways to avoid a reinforcement of unequal gender relations while sharing the benefits of modern medicine. Therefore, knowledge and practice must be appropriated by women on their own terms, "revised and updated" in accordance with local knowledge. This implies support to their status enhancement, which cannot be done only through education.

Another argument for such an approach is that our knowledge and practices were developed and adopted in a context involving changes in the situation of women that go beyond the health service sector (i.e., antenatal or obstetric curative care), namely, education and participation in the labor force. Thus our knowledge and practices must be considered within this context.

Indeed, the many conditions that can be grouped together under the term "social factors that impact on health status" and are known to play a role in maternal mortality are largely determined by unequal gender relations. They must be addressed in order to reduce maternal mortality and morbidity. As mentioned above, poverty is one of these conditions and if it affects the population as a whole it becomes critical when women are not even able to use their meager resources to get care or medication, not to mention being able to become independent from an oppressing husband. Here again, the questions must come from women themselves so that they define what space they wish to occupy and, most significantly, the place they want reproduction to have in their lives. Although education may play a role, there is more to this problem than education. The long road to recognition of legal and economic rights that translate into autonomy when it comes to the age of marriage, family planning, access to economic resources, and access to care are all not incidental to the fight against mortality. In fact, they are central to it. What is the best strategy? Networking between women, of course, but also supporting political discourses and actions that challenge systems founded on women's subservience.

The major problem in effecting such changes is the time delay during which so many lives are lost. The attraction of setting up emergency obstetrical services is real. Even in Benin, such services save lives in the few existing hospitals, and if there were more of them, it would make a difference, as we have seen with the women interviewed; many of them nearly missed dying but survived because they were taken to a hospital. Moreover, by encouraging an active approach, such specialized interventions counteract the attitude of fatality surrounding childbirth. But for services to be used at large, women must have access to them culturally, socially, and economically and must feel respected by those working in them. These conditions cannot be fulfilled if women themselves are not involved in their implementation. In the context of Benin, a woman may not be able to decide for herself to use a health service, may not have access to the financial resources to get there or to pay once she has been treated,[14] or may not want to go to avoid being unwelcome or ill-treated by the staff. This aspect of the changes is all too often forgotten in our context. While supplying services creates a demand, the demand cannot be understood outside of the social context. The mere availability of services is therefore insufficient and may generate adverse effects. They must be usable, and that depends on conditions that are numerous and of different natures.

The current tendency (particularly the promotion of emergency medical practices) may make initiatives focused on health services an isolated solution because they are concrete and pragmatic. That appears to be the most disturbing aspect of establishing an order of priorities for putting an end to situations that fill us with indignation. Can it be assumed that they are clinically and socially effective in the long-term and to a significant degree? I have my doubts. Cesarean sections can save the lives of women with major complications, but they are used as a solution to several problems—for example, young girls' pregnancies—that could have been avoided through social changes. One paradox remains. Prevention of birth complications within the framework of biomedical developments is defined on the basis of its own criteria of medical control. We may wish to share our knowledge, but in doing so, we are supporting a certain type of practice. The desire to export the knowledge we have gained should require us to take a look at its foundations, but also its consequences and its unwanted effects. As Sohier A. Morsy reminds us, an emphasis on maternal mortality may also correspond to another agenda, population control. Awareness is needed to ensure that

> the relationship between women's compromised health and state policies in historical and global contexts [is elaborated]. Otherwise the state and international development institutions will continue to be presented as the promoters of women's well-being, absolved of responsibility for the social production of compromised health, while responsibility remains assigned to "culture" and potentially innumerable discrete variables ranging from those designated "individual" to those labeled "institutional." (Morsy 1995, 173)

Finally, technology transfers, especially in a context such as that of Benin where hierarchy defines relations in the field of health, does not necessarily bode well for women's ability to play a significant role in the management of their experiences. Although a concern with the adverse effects of transferring technologies may seem like a luxury to some, it is only because they are unaware of the cultural roots of medicalization and the role of the medical institution in women's subjection, which is at the origin of a number of alienating conditions. Transferring technology may be an interesting strategy as long as it remains a part of a more global one in which women play an active role. Whether it be the design of health services or their implementation, women should be at the center of the decision-making process. This will be possible only if gender relations are put into question.

Women's forms of resistance, manifested in different strategies such as refusing to go to the health center for prenatal care to avoid disrespect or refusing to abide medical prescription, indicate there is on their part a determination to gain respect and to be autonomous when it comes to their health and reproductive lives. This may be the basis for building on the integration of practices in societies where efficient health services are badly needed, even if it will not exclude all dilemmas and paradoxes we as feminist researchers and activists from the Western world encounter in sharing with our Third World sisters our experiences, our analyses, and our skills.

NOTES

1. Maternal death is the death of a woman while pregnant or within forty-two days of termination of the pregnancy, irrespective of the duration and the site of pregnancy, from any cause related to or aggravated by the pregnancy or its management but not from accidental or incidental causes.

2. One must, however, be careful. Disparities exist between social groups. For example, in the United States, maternal mortality rates are much higher among black women than among white women. See Atrash, Alexander, and Berg 1995.

3. In the beginning of the 1990s, during a public lecture, I was questioned by an African woman who considered my criticisms of the technological invasion of childbirth to be unjust. She felt that I was contributing to the defamation of services that African women wish to see developed in their countries. I would even go so far as to say that she seemed to view my remarks as those of a "spoiled child" who had the luxury of criticizing what others have not even had the opportunity of trying out.

4. Here there is undoubtedly room for epistemological debate on the criteria used in evaluations on the effects achieved in a variety of experiences, particularly the polysemic concept of effectiveness.

5. Overall fertility rate refers to the number of births over the past twelve months divided by the female population between fifteen and forty-nine years of age; the synthetic fertility rate is the average number of children a woman would have in her lifetime based on the pace of childbearing in a given year.

6. The project was carried out between September and December 1995 with women who had given birth in 1995 in one of the three hospitals in the regions of Cotonou and Ouidah. Two of them were located in Cotonou, a large maternity unit and the national hospital, and the other in Ouidah. With the help of Véronique Filippi, a demographic researcher from the London School of Hygiene and Tropical Medicine, the women were selected from among the subjects of a survey on "near missed deaths" for which she was the principal researcher. This study was carried out in collaboration with the Centre de recherche sur la reproduction humaine et la démographie de Cotonou (Cotonou's center for research on human reproduction and demography) and was funded by the United Kingdom's Overseas Development Agency. When the researchers met with the women to fill out the questionnaires, they asked them if they would agree to meet with me for an open interview. They generally accepted willingly. Only one woman who had accepted refused at the time of the interview on her mother's advice. During the interviews, most of which (fourteen) were held in the local language by the sociologists Lydie Kanhonou and Solange Logonou, they expressed themselves freely in response to questions that aimed to evoke their accounts of their last pregnancy and birth. The interviews were tape recorded, then translated when necessary and transcribed verbatim. I also carried out three interviews with physicians and accompanied the investigators in the field several times when they were filling out questionnaires.

7. Since the majority of the women we met with had had complications, our data are, in a certain sense, biased. Their experiences are undoubtedly more negative than those of women who had a normal birth. However, actions aiming to reduce maternal mortality and morbidity specifically target this group of women.

8. My project's main objective was to explore through a sociological study how women's discourse could be used in a public health perspective. A small sample was valid for such a purpose. For a deeper anthropological study of women's experience in Benin society, one may be interested in reading Carolyn Sargent's publications. She remained a few years in the field and interviewed over a hundred Bariba women living in the north on their childbirth practices. Her most important publication on this subject is Sargent 1989.

9. This has been confirmed by the discrepancy between the discourse on risk and the concerns of aboriginal women in Canada who have been and still are faced with practices that are part of another culture. See Kaufert and O'Neil 1993.

10. Three participants told us about women close to them who had died in childbirth.

11. Avoiding problems by hiding one's state is not exclusive to Benin. Margaret M. Oosterbaan and Maria V. Barreto da Costa report the same phenomenon in Guinea-Bissau in Oosterbaan and Barreto da Costa 1995.

12. Most of our respondents earned some money through commercial activities.

13. Medicine refers here to vitamins, but also to other types of medicine; medication is indeed widespread and prescriptions are given at every visit.

14. After giving birth, some women run away from the hospital with their records because they are unable to pay.

8 Anomalous Women and Political Strategies for Aging Societies

Margaret Lock

That's my girl.
She's a natural resource, a renewable one luckily,
because those things wear out so quickly. They don't
make 'em like they used to. Shoddy goods.
                    —Margaret Atwood, "The Female Body"

Since the mid-nineteenth century, female life-cycle transitions in Euro-America have been interpreted with increasing insistence by physicians as a series of events that should be subject to medical management. Although passage through the life cycle is simultaneously a social and a biological process, the focus of attention within medical circles, perhaps not surprisingly, has been confined with increasing intensity to changes in the body physical. The result has been that, aside from a heightened sensitivity to chronological age on the part of many individuals, the subjective experience of maturation and associated changes in human relationships have been rendered largely inconsequential, a situation that is now widely reflected in public discourse, in particular that currently associated with female middle age.

Of course, women have not sat by passively, willing consumers of every new piece of medical technology. On the contrary, the female body has become the site for ever more contentious debate about both its representation and the medical practices performed upon it. Furthermore, these contested meanings are not simply responses to the imperialism of a particular medical "gaze" (in Michel Foucault's idiom), nor are they due entirely to the development of new technologies and an urge to maximize their use (Fuchs 1974). The female body, being a potent but malleable signifier, inevitably becomes a forum around which sex and gender relations are delineated (Butler 1993). At this particular historical moment arguments are most often concerned with the extent to which women will be granted equity in social life (in reality and not simply in name), as well as with the degree of autonomy assigned to individuals in connection with their own bodies, particularly with respect to behaviors having a bearing on reproduction.

The medicalized body, therefore, is not merely the product of changing medical interests, knowledge, and practice. It is at the same time a manifestation of potent, never settled, partially disguised political contests that contribute to the way in which the female body is "seen" and interpreted both by women themselves and in the popular domain (Bordo 1993), by policy makers and professionals working in the health care system (Lock 1993a), and by the pharmaceutical industry invested in the medical management of the female body (Oudshoorn 1994).

In this chapter I address the female midlife transition for which, over the past half century, the end of menstruation has come to be iconic. The French physician Gardanne invented the term *menopause* in the first quarter of the last century to describe the constellation of biological changes associated with the end of menstruation. He did so with the express view of stripping away popular knowledge associated with female middle age and creating a concept limited to the biology of female aging. It took more than a century for this term to filter through the barrier of ignominy associated with aging women, so that subjective experiences at the end of menstruation and critical commentary about medicalization could become a topic for open discussion.

Feminist commentary on medical and associated health care discourse and practices in connection with menopause were sparse until the mid-1970s, and such commentary as there was has been internally contradictory, revealing deep-seated ambiguities arising out of different epistemological stances. One school of thought has asserted that, by reconceptualizing menopause as a disease, physicians actively sought to extend their power, since they put themselves in a position of insisting that all women need medical care at this stage of the life cycle (see, for example, MacPherson 1981). Other writers argued that medical paternalism and condescension encouraged gynecologists to downplay the physical distress that many women experience at menopause by dismissing their complaints as psychological (and therefore not real), thus leaving women to "pull themselves up by their own bootstraps" (Posner 1979, 186). An assumption was shared alike by medical professionals and the majority of commentators from the social sciences, feminist or otherwise, until well into the 1970s, that both "vasomotor" symptoms (the hot flash and night sweats) and "psychological" symptoms (mood alterations, notably depression) were inherent to the menopausal experience. Arguments tended to erupt among those interested in this subject about how common and how severe symptoms were and whether their frequency and variation depended upon social and cultural factors. Only a relatively small number of gynecologists were interested, however, in treating menopausal symptomatology at that time, leaving the door open for criticism by feminists interested in achieving better health care for women at this stage of the life cycle. At the same time, the active promotion of menopause as a diseaselike entity by physicians was criticized by other feminist writers.

Since the mid-1970s debate in the medical world about the significance of menopause has shifted focus. The majority of "expert" gynecologists, largely on the basis of outcomes obtained from medication use, now dismiss all symptoms, with the exception of those they associate directly with lowered estrogen levels (hot flashes and night sweats), as being irrelevant to the menopausal transition. The concept of menopause has been streamlined and normalized in medical usage and is frequently classed as an "estrogen deficiency." Moreover, dominant medical discourse is currently concerned with the postulated long-term effects of lowered estrogen levels on the health of women as they age. The category "postmenopausal" is now applied to all women once past reproductive age who by definition are deemed to be at an increased risk for heart disease, osteoporosis, and other diseases associated with aging. Attention has shifted away from any short-term discomfort that may occur around the time of the end of menstruation, aside from providing symptom relief, and it is the specter of old women in ill health and the burden that this burgeoning population of baby boomers is expected to place on the health care system in the near future that is of primary concern. As I explain, certain feminist activists have responded critically to this new regime of "preventive medicine" currently recommended by representatives of the leading gynecological associations, one of lifelong medication for the majority of women.[1]

To date the bulk of the feminist literature on the topic of menopause, as well as that produced by women's groups and organizations in general, has been written in direct response to the process of medicalization. Its ultimate purpose is usually to produce guidance for individual women as they approach this stage of the life cycle. Although some of these publications deal with the larger context in which medicalization takes place, for example, the culturally infused negative stereotypes that surround aging women in Euro-America (Freidan 1993), the politics of aging is usually dealt with superficially, the concept of menopause, a medical concept, remains unproblematized (but see Greer 1991), the categories of "women," "nature," "culture," and "aging" are not critically examined and appear as unqualified descriptors, and the medical world is treated as a monolithic whole (but see Lock 1985). Furthermore, some of the literature, in particular the best seller by Gail Sheehy, contains several errors that are profoundly misleading (see below).

In this chapter I present a comparative analysis of some of the current discourse about female aging in North America and Japan, in particular that concerned with the end of menstruation. My purpose is to contrast the ways in which female middle age is construed in these two locations, both of which are saturated with scientific knowledge and its practice. The comparison at once makes the permeation of scientific discourse by culture very evident and challenges any totalizing critique of medicine. This should come as no great surprise—the location of bodies in time and space influences both the way they are subjectively experienced and the way they are constructed in medical discourse; the present example clearly reflects differences between Japan and North America in the historical and contemporary production of gynecological knowledge, and in popular attitudes about women's bodies and associated behavior at mid-life. We must go further, however, and pry open the black box of aging itself.

The sociologists Mike Featherstone and Mike Hepworth (1991) argue that representation of the life course is currently undergoing reconceptualization, notably in the social sciences. In place of an inflexible age-based chronology, there is recognition of malleability, of a "process . . . which need not involve a predetermined series of stages of growth" (375). Thus, whatever normative expectations society may retain about an orderly progression through the life course, it is evident, to some researchers at least, that this is not borne out in practice. Despite their commitment to flexibility, Featherstone and Hepworth are unwilling to locate the body in the terrain of the hyperreal. They are quick to remind us, and I would concur, that the physical existence of the body cannot be ignored, and that not only medical but also cultural and political representations of the body will inevitably be constrained and shaped by the body physical. The relationship of nature to culture has to be confronted at some point, therefore, in representations about birth, growth, maturation, and death. This is not to assert, however, that the biological body should be conceptualized as an invariant base upon which culture is layered as so much flotsam (Lock 1993a). Nor should the universalized natural body remain as "the gold standard of hegemonic social discourse" (Haraway 1989, 355).

A good number of years ago, Russell Keat (1986) chastised contemporary philosophers and social scientists for consigning the human body to the supposedly neutral terrain of scientists (24). Today it is abundantly clear that we can no longer afford to take this liberty, if for no other reason than that biomedical technologies—the "artifice of culture," in Strathern's usage (1992)—permit us to go beyond mere representations of nature and to enter the arena of radical reconstruction, so that, as a result of our tinkering, the natural world is made increasingly plastic (Rabinow 1992; Lock 1995). In connection with aging, for example, the hunt is on for the gene or genes that, it is believed, confine us to our biologically programmed "life span potential." Meantime we satiate ourselves with unrefined, experimental technologies that, among other things, permit us to place an egg fertilized in vitro in the body of an endocrinologically hyperstimulated woman who wishes to have a child even though she is past the usual reproductive age. In short, we seek no longer merely to "combat" disease but to wrest control from nature entirely.

There is yet another way, also relevant here, in which it is appropriate to reconceptualize the category of nature and its relationship to culture. On the basis of empirical research in Japan (discussed below) I argue that discourses on aging not only are shaped by unexamined beliefs about the female body and its function in society but also are in part the product of what I term "local biologies." In other words, subjective experience intimately associated with physical changes in the body at the end of menstruation appear to be sufficiently different in North America from those in Japan to produce an effect on (but not determine) the creation of a relevant discourse. The danger of such an argument is, of course, that the Western body remains unproblematized, that the experience of aging in other locations is simply taken as so much variation on the norm, or else as anomalous. However, the creation of nuanced arguments in which recognition is given to both individual and population-based biological diversity with respect to a range of events and experiences has enormous implications for individual health and well-being as well as for decentering a theory of cultured embodiment grounded in Western assumptions of biological universalism.

Differences in the sex ratio at birth, as well as certain toxic responses to medication, foods, alcohol, and so on are well-established examples of regional biological diversity created over many thousands of years to which culturally shaped behaviors appear to have contributed. For example, absence of an enzyme to metabolize cow's milk in most peoples of the world is described as a lactase deficiency, when it is the presence of the enzyme (predominantly in people of European ancestry and among East Africans with a long history of an intimate association with cattle herding) that is the "oddity."

Having set out an argument for local biologies, the implications of which are for an ever finer contextualization with respect to knowledge production and related practices, I must add at once that to remain in the camp of extreme relativism, however well nuanced, is to stop the discussion prematurely. There is, after all, something finite about growing old and facing death that informs all associated narratives and experience, wherever their location in space and time. Moreover, while no metanarrative can be retrieved, the "fact" of the end of menstruation, the timing of which appears to be remarkably uniform in all geographical locations, must inevitably play a part in the creation of discourse about female aging.

One question I address here is why in contemporary Euro-America the end of menstruation has become a synecdoche for middle-aged women in all their variety, who appear in current discourse as an estrogen-starved population, at high risk for hot flashes, future heart attacks, and other diseases of aging. In Japan, despite the presence of a powerful medical profession and an aggressive pharmaceutical industry, discussion about middle age is much less concerned with pathology and gives primary emphasis to care of the elderly. Thus the form and course of medicalization in any location cannot be assumed. Feminist commentary that confines itself to a critique of medicalization, while important, is constrained by the very discourse it seeks to counter, one that limits itself to changes in female biology as the key to the meaning of aging, while associated social and political transformations are relegated to the margins.

Against Nature: Anomalous Female Aging

The "graying" of society is a subject of more than passing interest today to politicians and bureaucrats living in the so-called developed corners of this world, most particularly because the baby-boomers are now well into middle age and approaching the "autumn" of their lives. In North America and Japan, however, the "problem" is not conceptualized in the same way, and middle-aged women, cast in both locations as the leading figures in this drama, have their roles plotted out for them on remarkably different trajectories. Let us first consider North America.

In North America, discourse about middle-aged women, whether that of the medical world or popular accounts, focuses obsessively on menopause and the supposed long-term consequences to health in later life of an "estrogen starved body" (as it is often described). Medical literature, with only a few exceptions, is overwhelmingly concerned with pathology and decrepitude. Thus, the end of menstruation is understood to be the result of "failing ovaries" (Haspels and van Keep 1979,

59), or the "inevitable demise" of the "follicular unit" (London and Hammond 1986, 906). There are other, more positive ways to interpret these biological changes, as at least one gynecological textbook has suggested (Wentz 1988), and a group of concerned women practitioners has sought to take a more "holistic" approach to female middle age (Bell, personal communication), but the dominant discourse continues to be about loss, failure, and decrepitude (Martin 1987).

Why should there be such an emphasis on female decrepitude, for surely aging is an unavoidable process common to both men and women? An article by Gail Sheehy (1991) gives us a clue. She states blithely: "At the turn of the century, a woman could expect to live to the age of forty-seven or eight" (227), a sentiment expressed widely not only in popular literature but also in scientific articles. R. G. Gosden, for example, in a text for biologists (1985), is explicit that the very existence of "post-menopausal" women is something of a cultural artifact, the result of our "recent mastery of the environment" (2). What is not recognized in such arguments is that high rates of infant and maternal mortality have served, until well into this century, to keep mean life expectancies low. Simply paying attention to mean life expectancy masks the presence of older people in all societies, including hunting and gathering economies and those using subsistence farming. Examination of remaining life expectancy once aged forty-five or older shows clearly that after achieving middle age, the majority of people could expect to live to old age throughout most of human history. Coupled with this faulty demography is a second assertion, that the human female is the only member of the class Mammalia to reach reproductive senescence during her lifetime: "With increasing longevity modern woman differs from her forebears as well as from other species in that she can look forward to 20 or 30 years . . . , after the menopause" (Dewhurst 1981, 592). These arguments suggest that the very existence of older women goes against Nature's purpose. A thinly disguised assumption would seem to be that reproduction of the species is what female life is all about, and that we find ourselves in contemporary society with an ever increasing number of perambulating anomalies. What is willfully forgotten in these arguments is that men age too; that the maximum human life span potential is somewhere between ninety-five and over one hundred years; that there is an increasingly challenging literature from biological anthropology that argues that menopause in human females evolved approximately 1.5 million years ago, most probably as a biological adaptation to the long-term nurturance necessary of highly dependent human infants, a dependency not found in apes (Peccei 1995;

Lock forthcoming); and finally that all the systems of our bodies, male and female, with the exception only of the female reproductive organs, age for survival to eighty years of age or more (Leidy 1994).

Nevertheless, middle-aged women are explicitly contrasted with the animal world and found wanting; they are also compared to their detriment with younger, fertile women whose bodies are taken as the standard for women of all ages (Lock 1993a, 38), but of even more significance, perhaps, is that women's bodies differ from those of men. Donna Haraway, writing about nineteenth-century Europe and North America (1989), asserts that "the 'neutral,' universal body was always the unmarked masculine" (357). Simone De Beauvoir was perhaps the first feminist to elaborate extensively about the way in which woman is constructed as "other" and here, in the current literature on aging, we find a striking example of this type of discourse, for received wisdom has it that men have the potential to reproduce successfully until the day they die (despite increasing evidence to the contrary). Paradoxically, mention is rarely made that in the "advanced" societies men do not live on average as long as women (although men's interest groups have begun to discuss this lately), no speculation is put forward about why this should be, and no hint given that women may have some "natural" advantage here; on the contrary, the very longevity of women marks them as potential liabilities.

The Pathology of Aging

It has been postulated since classical times that ovarian secretions produce a profound effect on many parts of the female body, and, although explanations have changed over the years about just how this effect is produced, this assumption is not in dispute. From early this century a few physicians interested in the effects of lowered hormone secretions on aging created a small replacement therapy industry in which whole ovaries were ground up and injected into patients who had undergone early menopause, usually because of surgery (Oudshoorn 1990). This practice was simply a small spin-off, however, from another, larger research project, in which middle-aged men had been injected with ground-up testes as rejuvenation therapy. The pharmaceutical industry did not become involved to any extent in the medicalization of menopause until the 1940s, after the development of synthetic estrogens (Bell 1987). By the late 1930s one or two gynecologists had likened menopause to a deficiency disease—specifically diabetes and thyroid deficiency disease (Shorr 1940)—but, despite the availability of a specific medication to counter the supposed deficiency, very few gynecologists conceptualized menopause as pathology until relatively recently. Instead, most physicians were vociferous in describing the end of menstruation as a normal event and were opposed to the use of estrogens except under extenuating circumstances, largely because of concerns about iatrogenesis (Bell 1987). Only a very small number of women, therefore, were regularly medicated with estrogens before the 1960s.

By the 1970s estrogens were among the top five most frequently prescribed drugs in the United States (Kaufert and McKinlay 1985). Until the mid-1970s estrogens were most frequently used to reduce hot flashes and other so-called vasomotor symptoms associated with the end of menstruation. A sudden and sharp decline in the prescription of estrogens occurred after 1975 when four studies were published in major medical journals linking estrogen replacement therapy to an increased risk for endometrial cancer. A protracted debate has since ensued about how best to "protect" women from the postulated effects of reduced estrogen in the postmenopausal body without causing severe side effects (Kaufert and McKinlay 1985). Writers of these articles apparently share an assumption that the female body will be unable to age in reasonably good health unless regularly fueled with hormones.

> Clinicians abound who believe that the menopause is a physiological event, a normal aging process, therefore estrogen replacement therapy (ERT) is meddlesome and unnecessary. Presbyopia is a normal aging process, but none will deny the need for spectacles. To do nothing other than offer sympathy and assurance that the menopause will pass is tantamount to benign neglect. (Greenblatt and Teran 1987, 39)

From the 1980s, prescription of replacement therapy accelerated so that once again it ranks among the most frequently prescribed drugs, but it is now usually suggested that a second hormone, progesterone, should be added to the medication in order to counter the toxic effects of "unopposed" estrogen. Rather than simply dispensing medication, physicians are now required to weigh up individual "risks" and "benefits," on the basis of which appropriate therapy is selected in consultation with "informed" patients, who are then regularly monitored.

The current medical language describes "target" organs and tissues, and their negative response to "ovarian failure," which includes the pelvic structures (the vulva, vagina, and uterus), breasts, skin, and bones. The heart and cardiovascular system are also implicated, but indirectly, and so too are mental states (although there is little agreement about this particular association). Medical interest in failing ovaries and dropping estrogen levels is no longer, as it was until recently, confined to what are for most physicians, at least, the rather inconsequential symptoms usually associated with menopause, in particular the hot flash. As is becoming increasingly well known, interest has now lighted on the postmenopausal woman, her thirty years of remaining life, and the ongoing "medical management" necessitated by her increased risk for broken bones and a failing heart (WHO 1996).

In the medical literature on menopause it is common to start out with a rhetorical flourish that sets the stage for coming to terms with the superfluity of older women: "It is estimated that every day in North America 3,500 new women experience menopause and that by the end of this century 49 million women will be postmenopausal" (Reid 1988, 25). In a journal for family physicians, the estimated "cost" to society of these potentially decrepit women is explicitly addressed: "An unwelcome consequence of increased longevity, osteoporosis eventually develops in almost all untreated Caucasian women who reach their 80th year. The direct cost of osteoporotic fractures is estimated to be $7 [billion] to $10 billion each year in the United States alone, and the population of postmenopausal women is continually increasing" (Lufkin and Ory 1989, 205).

As this quotation makes patently clear, the concern that drives the production of these figures, veiled as a motivation for physicians to practice preventive health care, is women's cost, once elderly, to society. Moreover, pharmaceutical companies have vested interests in the medicalization of female aging. The profits to be made are highly lucrative and companies in turn place pressure on medical practitioners to purvey hormone replacement therapy (HRT). It is not surprising, therefore, that despite continuing debates about the iatrogenic effects from long-term use of HRT, and unresolved arguments about its effectiveness or otherwise as preventive medication against a range of chronic diseases associated with old age, combined estrogen/progesterone hormone therapy continues to be widely promoted for daily use by virtually all women once they approach menopause. During the decade of the 1990s a medicalized approach has come increasingly to dominate both professional and popular literature about female aging, while socioeconomic, political, and ethnic issues remain poorly researched.

The debate about menopausal women in both the medical literature and at conferences is now carried forward not only by interested gynecologists but also by cardiologists, orthopedic surgeons, geriatricians, breast surgeons, and, above all, clinical epidemiologists who work with physicians in each of the relevant specialties. One article starts out with the statement: "The goal of contemporary hormone replacement is to minimize net predictable lifetime risk; success therefore depends upon quantitative assessments of the net quality of life, of net morbidity and of net mortality" (Mack and Ross 1989). These particular researchers applied a meta-analysis to numerous epidemiological studies and, after totting up the possible risks and benefits of HRT in several different ways to produce a variety of outcomes, asked rhetorically whether there are "any treatment strategies which will provide the valuable benefits while playing it safe." Their conclusion was "probably not." None of the strategies they list—screening out high-risk women, preferentially treating only those most likely to gain some benefit, treating only those with no uterus (one-third of American women over fifty), or using only short-term treatment—"will provide major benefit without risk."

T. M. Mack and R. K. Ross (1989) remind readers that those women over fifty who have not has their uterus removed will be "patently" at risk for cancer, and all patients must be routinely monitored with endometrial biopsies (painful and invasive), as a result of which "large numbers" of them will receive "unnecessary curettage," some under general anesthesia (1818). Mack and Ross close with a caveat similar to others that appear regularly at the end of articles comparing risks and benefits: "Perhaps a prudent course in any event is to assume the role of medical fiduciary rather than that of decision-maker, to insist that the patient fully participate in the choice of therapy, and to make sure that whatever the choice, she explicitly acknowledge the measure of uncertainty" (1818). Other researchers have shown that from a purely economic perspective the benefits of HRT are at best tentative. Milton Weinstein and Anna Tosteson (1990) asked themselves, for example, whether this medication, including the medical supervision involved, is a prudent investment of health care resources. Their article starts out with the usual litany: "In the year 2005 the number of American women between the ages of 50 and 64 will be more than 25 million." They then go on to point out that the national bill for providing HRT and physician monitoring for involved women is estimated to be between $3.5 billion and $5 billion annually. After performing a cost-benefit analysis they reach the conclusion that any possible benefits of HRT must be considered "highly tentative," in terms of both the cost to society and the risk to individual patients (171). Despite these and other cautionary statements, during the 1990s estrogen has been touted as a wonder drug for older women, a medication that will relieve anything from tooth loss, memory loss, Alzheimer disease, osteoporosis, and stroke to heart disease. The fact that unopposed estrogen is no longer recommended for widespread use in women who are naturally postmenopausal, and that there has been no time to establish the effect, if any, that combined hormone therapy has on the diseases of aging usually goes unnoted. So too does the fact that powerful medications are being recommended for up to thirty years of continuous use. The biases embedded in virtually all the epidemiological research, whether it be about estrogen or HRT are usually also overlooked, with the exception of a few concerned organizations and individuals among which is the Women's Health Network in Washington, D.C.

Countering the Hegemony: Women's Responses

Women have not sat silently on the margins while debate about hormone use has taken place. The National Women's Health Network put out a paper in 1989, updated in 1995. For the 1989 publication they too reviewed a substantial portion of the literature on HRT. After stating that they are opposed to the view taken in the majority of articles appearing in medical journals that normal menopause is a deficiency disease, they then point out the blind spots and assumptions that are made in virtually all of the articles they reviewed.

Among other things, the Health Network reminds its readers that oral contraceptive pills used in the 1970s (which contained a progesterone) were associated with an increased risk for stroke and heart attacks. Furthermore, the research widely cited in the literature as evidence of reduced risk for heart disease uses, and continues to use, subjects who are for the most part taking only estrogen. Today most patients are started out with combined estrogen/progesterone therapy, and hence no long-term predictions can be made in connection with present and future generations of women based on the results of survey research conducted thus far. The Health Network also points out that less expensive and "more natural" forms of prevention for heart disease, osteoporosis, and cancer, including dietary changes, giving up cigarette smoking and excessive alcohol use, prevention of falls, and so on are only rarely discussed, and they attribute this to the fact that most researchers are funded by drug companies. Since dietary changes have proven to be successful in significantly reducing the incidence of heart disease among men, arguments along these lines are particularly persuasive.

The Health Network further argues that many women who are now using HRT were exposed when younger to high-dose birth control pills,

and among these women some were given the carcinogenic diethyl-
stilbestrol (DES) while pregnant. The next generation of hormone tak-
ers will have been exposed to a lower-dose pill, but from a younger age.
It is further argued by the Health Network that it took twenty years for
some of the cases of cancer connected with DES use to become manifest,
and that this experience should encourage the exercise of great caution
in connection with HRT (this argument has been countered by the assertion that it was fetal tissue that developed the cancer, and not the
pregnant women who were medicated—and therefore, presumably,
older women have nothing to fear [Greenblatt 1972]).

The Health Network notes that women are not usually told about
the side effects they can expect with HRT use, most notably that hot
flashes usually reoccur when treatment is stopped, and that HRT often
causes what is euphemistically known as "break-through" bleeding,
which not only creates anxiety but entails close monitoring and often
painful medical procedures to establish its cause. (Recent use of smaller
doses of HRT counters this problem in some women.) In addition, bloat-
ing, "the blues," breast tenderness, and headaches are commonly experienced. Because of these symptoms women tend to start and then stop
taking medication, and many fill only one prescription.

As a result of their review, the Health Network concluded that it is
"dangerously misleading" to suggest that the "average" middle-aged
woman will experience better health by taking drugs where the risks
have not been sufficiently examined, and that women are, in effect, being urged to take part in a "risky, uncontrolled experiment without their
fully informed consent" (National Women's Health Network 1989, 3).
One further criticism passed over by the Health Network can be made
of the epidemiological research: Virtually all of the surveys of the impact of ERT and HRT have been conducted with Caucasian middle-
class women, usually with those who have actively sought out medical
care or whose profession is nursing, or alternatively those who live in
middle-class retirement communities in California (Kaufert 1988). Inappropriate extrapolations are then made from the results found among
these populations to all middle-aged women. The studied populations
are not, for example, at high risk for heart disease in the first instance,
as compared to the general population of middle-aged American women.
Moreover, recommended medication regimen and dosages have changed
with time, making the accuracy of results obtained from longitudinal
studies and their relevance for the current cohort of women passing
through menopause exceedingly problematic.

The cumulative cost of medication and gynecological check-ups for individuals is, of course, considerable. Given that the experts strongly recommend that virtually all women take medication and be monitored for twenty years or more after the end of menstruation, it is odd that no attention is paid to the fact that well over half the population of middle-aged American women cannot possibly afford this kind of care. But, it seems, these women are the lucky ones, in that they will not be required to juggle with the head-spinning probabilities and risk-benefit analyses with which a middle-class, largely Caucasian population is expected to cope, in order to make an "informed decision"—in consultation, of course, with their suitably educated physicians. In the 1995 report, the Health Network concludes as a result of its updated survey that hormone therapy is suitable only for those women who experience extreme discomfort at the end of menstruation, and for those who are at very high risk for bone fractures caused by osteoporosis. They do not recommend its use as a preventative measure against heart disease or other conditions.

Despite the impenetrable contradictions in the data, the clamor for individual women to act responsibly, to assess the particular risks and benefits signaled by their bodies, and then, for the majority, to choose HRT, grows ever louder as the population as a whole ages (although at the 1995 meeting of the North American Menopause Society held in San Francisco, a very few of those gynecologists who have been most active in the medicalization of female aging have recently expressed doubts at a press conference about systematic and long-term use of HRT). If we step back a little from the issues associated with the medicalization of menopause, then it becomes clear that, in North America, medical professionals and a good number of women have focused almost obsessively on biological aging, leaving the broader social and political issues that affect the lives of all women relatively unexplored. Moreover, because a focus on biology tends by definition to depoliticize and essentialize the bodies of women, the enormous variation among women's lives and experiences that have a profound influence on aging is not given suitable recognition. With this in mind we turn now to the situation in Japan.

The "Graying" of Japan

The aging society raises many concerns in Japan, too, not the least of which is about a decline in the national economy caused by the burden that the future elders will, it is assumed, place on society. The "graying" of Japan is particularly disturbing because demographic changes that occurred over the course of about one hundred years in Europe and North America have taken only a quarter century in Japan, and some official estimates calculate that, if present trends continue, by 2025 people aged sixty-five and over will make up a remarkable 24 percent of the population, and among the elderly, more than 53 per cent will be over seventy-five years of age (Ōgawa 1988). Again, if present trends continue, it is estimated that there will be more than 2.25 million Japanese suffering from senile dementia by 2025, of whom 68 percent will be women, and more than 2 million people will be bedridden, of whom 62 percent will be women. It is these figures about bedridden and senile elderly, and not the number of menopausal women, that are iconic in contemporary Japan, and, although women are picked out for special mention (not surprising since Japanese women live longer than anyone else in the world), decrepit men too make an appearance in these predictions.

Since the early 1970s when the question of the elderly first began to capture the attention of Japanese policy makers, it has been stated repeatedly that it is preferable for the elderly to be taken care of in their own homes and that family members should be the primary care givers (Kōsei Hakusho 1989). Politicians are concerned that the government is increasingly "expected" by the public to play a larger role in the care of the aging population, and several policy changes have been implemented to reverse this trend, along the lines suggested in the following government document on long-term economic planning:

> The home is extremely important to the aged for a secure life of
> retirement, their health and welfare. In an attempt to form a
> social environment ideal for future living, it will be necessary
> to correctly position the home in society . . . [and] the role
> of people caring for the aged at home will become more
> important. . . . Also, it will be necessary to promote a land
> policy aimed at pressing for three family generations to live in
> the same place or for family members to live within easy reach.
> (Keizai Kikaku Chōhen 1982)

Not even the most conservative of politicians dares to resort to the pre-war term for the extended family (*ie*) to describe what they are promoting, but the intention is nevertheless clear. The "new residence system" goes under the tag of "living together in three-generation households," and it has been suggested that loans should be made available for such families together with the latest devices to help with nursing the elderly at minimum cost. A recent study showed that out of nearly five hundred people nursing aged relatives in their homes over 81 percent were women who averaged fifty-six years of age (*Tokyo Shinbun* 1990). A recent study conducted by Japanese women concluded that given the current poor social welfare policies in Japan the burden of care for the elderly is simply dropped into the laps of younger (that is, middle-aged) women (Fujin Hakusho 1989).

The Doctrine of Motherhood

A widely shared sentiment exists in Japan today to the effect that although the economic "health" of the country is excellent this does not extend to the state of the nation itself, nor to the "spiritual" health of its peoples (Mochida 1980). The conservative government and like-minded intellectuals lament what they describe as a loss of traditional values— in particular the "thinning" of family relationships leading to an undue emphasis on the "Western" value of individualism. The three-generation household, the *ie*, was for three-quarters of a century, from the Meiji Restoration until the end of the World War II, recognized as the official family unit in Japan. In this household are enshrined the ancestors, representatives of moral and spiritual values instilled on their behalf in the younger generation by the adult woman of the household, the "pillar" of the family. Modeled on the samurai system of feudal times, and laced with a little late nineteenth-century European sentiment, the "good wife and wise mother" was expected to discipline herself for service to the household, in particular for the nurturance and well-being, physical and spiritual, of all other family members (Haga 1990). Whereas feudal Japan exhibited an acute sensitivity to class and occupational differences, with the creation of the early modern state, difference was in theory obliterated and Japanese women were appealed to for the first time as a unified body in terms of gendered social roles to be carried out within the confines of the *ie* (Nolte and Hastings 1991).

As part of such a family, a woman reaches the prime of life in her fifties and at that time enjoys the acme of her responsibility, which, although it gradually wanes, is never extinguished unless she succumbs to severe senility or some other catastrophe. Many Japanese women still live in these circumstances, and their days are filled with monitoring the household economy, care and education of grandchildren, and care of dependent in-laws, to which is often added piece work done inside the home or participation in the household enterprise, usually farming or independent business. Although in feudal Japan upper-class women were sometimes described as a "borrowed womb," from the end of the nineteenth century all women came to be thought of primarily as nurturers in addition to economically productive members of society, tasks that they retained throughout their lives, although their specific duties changed through time. Reproduction was obviously important, and the bearing of a son particularly so, but the Japanese have through the years been remarkably flexible about adopting children, as well as adults, into their families should the need arise. Hence, the dominant image of a woman in Japan in recent times has been that of nurturer, a role for which all women are assumed to be "biologically" endowed (Mitsuda 1985). Emphasis is given in this ideology to dedication to a life-long gendered role, and reproduction is rendered less important. Japanese feminists have coined the term *boseishugi* (the doctrine of motherhood) to capture the essence of this ideology.

Social Anomaly: Female Aging and Japanese Modernity

The nuclear household in which approximately 60 percent of Japanese live these days, lacking both enshrined ancestors and the elders, is thought by many commentators to be a fragile "pathological" conglomeration, particularly because the juridical powers of the household head were stripped away at the end of the war, leaving the household devoid of either authoritative or moral voice (Mochida 1980; Eto 1979). Members of the nuclear family—men, women, and children—are thought to be particularly vulnerable to what has been termed "diseases of civilization" or "modernization," including a whole range of neuroses, behavioral disorders, and deviant behaviors. These diseases are made factual by catchy diagnostic labels such as "school refusal syndrome," "high rise apartment neurosis," "moving day depression," "death from overwork," and so on (Lock 1988a). One of them is "menopausal syndrome," a problem believed to have surfaced only in postwar years and that is particularly associated with middle-class "professional" housewives who live in urban environments. When asked if he thought that all women experience trouble at menopause, a Kobe gynecologist answered: "No, I don't think so. Women who have no purpose in life have the most trouble. Housewives who are relatively well off, who have only one or two children and lots of free time come to see me most often. Menopausal syndrome is a sort of 'luxury disease' [*zeitakubyō*]. I'm sure women never used to come running to a doctor before the war with this kind of problem."

A physician who works in the countryside stated emphatically that rural women are much too busy to experience distress at menopause, the implication clearly being that any discomfort they may feel is of minor importance, something that an active and busy woman will "ride over" (*norikoeru*) with ease. Women who are unoccupied, who are not contributing in any obvious way to society, and hence, it is assumed, who have too much time on their hands are likely to be deficient in the will power and endurance that was characteristic of their mothers and generations of Japanese women before them, and it is therefore they who will experience distress at the end of menstruation (Lock 1988b).

The irony of this rhetoric, very evident in popular literature for women, does not pass unnoticed by feminist commentators (Higuchi 1985). Women have systematically been kept out of the full-time work force in postwar Japan despite the fact that large numbers of them regularly put in a full day's work (it is estimated that less than 30 percent of Japanese women are "professional housewives"). By far the majority of employed women are "temporary" blue-collar workers officially classified as part-time who work long hours with no benefits and are subject to hiring and firing as the national economy waxes and wanes. Aside from the helping professions, married women are rarely found in white-collar and professional jobs because enormous social pressure is placed on them to resign once they become pregnant. Being rehired into a "good" position at a later date is virtually impossible, even though most women wish to work for financial reasons. Nevertheless, once their children are raised, housewives are subject to stigmatization because, while the rest of the nation, with the exception only of some of the elderly, is worked to death (at times literally [National Defense Counsel for Victims of Karōshi 1990]), middle-aged housewives, it is assumed, pass their time by playing tennis and making plastic flowers. Under the circumstances, there are some grounds for this claim, provided one is not responsible for sick elders.

In Japan the "homebody" is idealized, she is made into the standard by which all women are measured, but the assumption is that once she becomes middle aged she is likely to become a social anomaly, no longer of obvious productive use beyond occasionally feeding her husband unless she is prevailed upon, as in times past, to carry out her lifelong duties to the extended family. The government, as we have seen, has unveiled plans to ensure that women remain out of the work force by actively encouraging them to fulfill their "natural" duty as unpaid nurses in extended families (and in this manner politicians strive to keep unemployment figures to a minimum, while at the same time avoiding the necessity of providing adequate public facilities for care of the elderly).

Because those who are financially secure are assumed to represent Japanese women as a whole, it is possible to erase the situation of the majority of women (those who must give up paid labor to look after their relatives, often at great cost to the well-being of the family as a whole) from national consciousness. Since many Japanese live to be well over ninety years of age, some daughters-in-law in their seventies find themselves bound over to caring for one or more incontinent, immobile, and sometimes senile relatives. Furthermore, since stroke is the most usual cause of disability among the elderly in Japan, intensive nursing is often required, and men assist very rarely with this onerous duty.

It is, therefore, the debate about home nursing and the three-generation family that takes up the energy of activist women in Japan today. Together with the politically active among the elderly themselves, they question the intransigence of governments national and local on these matters. Against the urgency of this situation the end of menstruation fades into the background, particularly because it has a moralistic rhetoric associated with it—in a country driven overwhelmingly by the work ethic, few people relish being accused, even indirectly, of indolence.

Maturation for Society

Despite a concern about the "graying" of the nation, aging itself is not thought of as an anomaly. Japan is a society exquisitely sensitive to the passing of time and positively wallows, on occasion, in the ephemeral nature of human life. The life course of both men and women was until recently marked and celebrated as a social event; continuity with past generations and the memorialization of ancestors reinforce the notion that each individual is part of an encompassing cosmically ordained order (Smith 1974). Women who are at present age fifty were immersed in this ideology as children, and the majority still embrace it (Lebra 1984; Lock 1993a). Movement through the life cycle is subjectively experienced largely in terms of how one's relationships with other people shift through time, and for women particularly, life is expected to become meaningful according to what they accomplish for others rather than for themselves (Plath 1980, 139). Under these circumstances the end of menstruation is not a very potent symbol. While there is some mourning for the loss of youth and sexual attractiveness on the part of a few women, emphasis is given by most to what is described as the inevitable process of aging itself: to graying hair, changing eyesight, faulty short-term memory, and so on (Lock 1986). Furthermore, these signs of aging, while they obviously represent irretrievable youth, are primarily signifiers for the future—for what may be in store in terms of an enfeebled body, and hence an inability to work and to contribute to society.

Some women do not apparently mark the end of menstruation as part of menopause at all. In a survey I conducted,[2] 24 percent of the sample of women aged forty-five to fifty-five who had ceased menstruating for more than one year reported that they had no sign of *kōnenki* (the term usually glossed as menopause) at all (Lock 1986, 30). In this discourse about aging, therefore, women are not markedly distinguished from men, for the physical changes associated with middle age that are attributed with significance are common to both sexes.

Signs and Symptoms of *Kōnenki*

When over one hundred women were interviewed in their homes about the physical symptoms that they associated with *kōnenki,* nearly 80 percent of the responses were along the following lines:

> I've had no problems at all, no headaches or anything like that . . . I've heard from other people that their heads felt so heavy that they couldn't get up. A few of my friends complain that they don't exactly have pain, but that they just feel generally bad.

> I started to have trouble sleeping when I was about fifty; that was *kōnenki,* I think. Some people have dizziness, headaches, stiff shoulders, and aching joints.

> In my case, my eyesight became weak. Some people get sensitive and have headaches.

> The most common disorders that I've heard about are headaches, shoulder stiffness, and aching joints. Some women get irritable too.

A small number of women, twelve among one hundred, made statements such as the following:

> The most noticeable thing was that I would suddenly feel hot; it happened every day, three times or so. I didn't go to the doctor or take any medication. I wasn't embarrassed and I didn't feel strange, I just thought that it was my age.

Symptom reporting in response to a questionnaire administered to over thirteen hundred Japanese women was low and significantly different from comparable Manitoban and Massachusetts samples (Avis et al.

1993). Commonly reported symptoms included shoulder stiffness, headaches, lumbago, chilliness, aches and pains in the joints, and feelings of numbness. Only 10 percent of the sample as opposed to 31 percent and 35 percent in Manitoba and Massachusetts, respectively, reported experiencing a hot flash in the two weeks prior to answering the questionnaire (Lock 1993a).[3] Night sweats, reported by only 4 percent of the Japanese sample as opposed to 20 percent in Manitoba and 12 percent in Massachusetts, were very infrequent. The "classical" symptoms of menopause, hot flashes and night sweats, are not, therefore, reported to anything like the same extent in Japan as among comparable North American samples.

Over 40 percent of the Japanese women interviewed agreed with the statement made by a Kyoto factory worker: "*kōnenki* starts at different ages depending on the person. Some start in their late thirties and some never have any symptoms; they don't have *kōnenki* at all." The term *shō gai* ("ill effects") has to be added to *kōnenki* ("change of life") before most women start to think in terms of symptoms that could be thought of as distressing.

Creating the Discourse of *Kōnenki*

The end of menstruation has been recognized for many hundreds of years in Sino-Japanese medicine as an occurrence that can leave "stale blood" in the body, the cause in some women of numerous nonspecific symptoms that often last a few years, including dizziness, palpitations, headaches, chilliness, stiff shoulders, a dry mouth, and so on (Nishimura 1981). It was believed that many other events also produce stale blood and associated nonspecific symptoms, and no specific term was created to gloss discomfort associated with the end of menstruation. Toward the end of the nineteenth century, Japanese medicine, under the influence of German medicine, created the term *kōnenki* to convey the European concept of the climacterium. Hideo Nishimura (1981) has suggested that *kōnenki* could, until recently, be used to refer to all of the life-cycle transitions, both male and female, regardless of age. This interpretation is very close to the meaning given to the term *climacterium* as it was used until the middle of the nineteenth century in Europe. Contemporary Japanese has no term that expresses in everyday language the event of the end of menstruation, although there is, of course, a technical term, much as menopause was a technical term in English and little used in daily parlance until as recently as forty years ago.

Similarly, those few Japanese women who experience hot flashes have to convey this experience by stating simply that they "suddenly

become hot," or that they have *nobose*—a term used to express the idea
of a sudden rush of blood to the head associated with vertigo and dizziness, or alternatively *hoteri*, usually used to comment on the flushed
faces that many East Asians experience when they imbibe alcohol. In
other words, there is no specific term that designates a hot flash, despite
the presence of highly nuanced discriminators for body states in the
Japanese language in general.

Part of turn-of-the-century German discourse about the climacterium that made good intuitive sense to the Japanese medical world
was the concept of the "autonomic nervous system." This idea, when it
was first clearly articulated in 1898, caused a stir in medical circles
everywhere (Sheehan 1936), but perhaps particularly so in Japan where
it "fitted" with the holistic physiological approach characteristic of
Sino-Japanese medicine. Later, in the 1930s, when a close association
was postulated between the endocrine system and the autonomic nervous system (Sheehan 1936), Japanese physicians comfortably adopted
this idea and postulated a connection between *kōnenki* and disturbances
in the autonomic nervous system, an association that the majority of
Japanese physicians and women accept today (Lock, Kaufert, and
Gilbert 1988; Rosenberger 1992). The dominant discourse in Japan is one
in which distress is not linked directly to a decline in estrogen levels but
is said to be due to a destabilization of the autonomic nervous system.
Both sexes are vulnerable, but women are thought to be more so than
men because of the added impact of declining estrogen levels.

Another factor that no doubt worked in Japan against the construction of a narrowly focused discourse on the aging ovary and declining
estrogen levels was that Japanese doctors, unlike their Western counterparts, had practiced little surgery before the twentieth century, a specialty that was disparaged by the powerful, physiologically oriented
herbalists of the traditional medical system. Furthermore, anatomy as it
was conceived in Enlightenment medical discourse in Europe had relatively little impact in Japan until the twentieth century, and autopsies
and dissection were not widely practiced. Japanese gynecologists, therefore, did not have first-hand experience of removing and dissecting
many hundreds of ovaries, as was the case for many late-nineteenth-
century European and North American gynecologists (Laqueur 1990)
and their "gaze" remained predominantly physiologically rather than
anatomically oriented.

One other result of the emphasis given in Japan to physiological
changes associated with *kōnenki* has been that until recently the majority of Japanese women, those few who consult with a doctor at this stage

of the life cycle, usually go to see an internist and not a gynecologist, since gynecology is primarily a surgical specialty. Taken together, these differences have ensured that the discourse on *kōnenki* is markedly different from that for menopause in North America. Stiff shoulders, headaches, ringing in the ears, tingling sensations, dizziness, and so on are the symptoms that form the core of the *kōnenki* experience, an experience that is also in part contingent upon "local" biology, since hot flashes and other so-called vasomotor symptoms, assumed to be characteristic of menopause, occur rather infrequently.

It is evident to most Japanese gynecologists that *kōnenki* is not the same thing, either conceptually or experientially, as menopause. The more than thirty physicians I interviewed in Japan believe that hot flashes are infrequently experienced by Japanese women and in any case cause little distress. More than one gynecologist asked why "Western" women are so disturbed by hot flashes. That the hot flash is not the key signifier of distress at *kōnenki* has meant that there has been relatively little incentive over the years for Japanese doctors to prescribe estrogen therapy for symptom relief. Furthermore, the Pill is not available in Japan for contraceptive purposes. Both doctors and women regularly report in survey research that they are concerned about possible iatrogenesis caused by long-term use of the Pill (*Mainichi Daily News* 1987), and this fear extends to the use of HRT, the chemical composition of which is very similar to the Pill, a fact that the majority of Japanese women are well aware of.

The Medical World and *Kōnenki*

In Japan obstetrics and gynecology have not usually been separated in primary care practice, and individual physicians own and run small hospitals where their income is derived largely from deliveries, abortions, and minor surgery. Recently, however, gynecologists find their medical practices growing less lucrative partly because women now choose to have their babies in tertiary care facilities and partly because the abortion rate is going down, thanks to a more sophisticated use of contraception (despite the unavailability of the Pill). Until recently *kō nenki* has not been medicalized to any great extent in Japan, by either internists or gynecologists, but this is changing, in part because of the economic pressures under which many gynecologists in the private practice now find themselves. Some physicians are currently setting up counseling services for middle-aged patients, while others are busy writing books and articles on the subject for popular consumption. Despite these changing practices, however, and the presence of an aggressive pharmaceutical industry, so far relatively little use is made in Japan of HRT, which is prescribed less frequently than are herbal medications (Japan Pharmaceutical Manufacturers Association 1990).

Japanese physicians keep abreast of the medical literature published in the West, and so one could expect in a country such as Japan, which is actively dedicated to preventive medicine, that there might be some incentive to make use of HRT. Here again, local biology plays a part, because mortality from coronary heart disease for Japanese women is about one-quarter that of American women (WHO 1990), and it is estimated that, although Japanese women become osteoporotic twice as often as do Japanese men, nevertheless, this is approximately half as often as in North America (Ross et al. 1991). These figures, combined with a mortality rate from breast cancer that is about one-quarter that of North America, has meant that there is relatively little pressure for Japanese gynecologists to enter into the international arena of debate about the pros and cons of long-term use of HRT, something about which many of them are, in any case, decidedly uncomfortable because of a pervasive concern about iatrogenesis. The first line of resort of Japanese doctors when dealing with healthy middle-aged women is usually to encourage good dietary practices and plenty of exercise. For those with troubling symptoms, herbal medicine is commonly prescribed, even by gynecologists (Lock 1993a). As certain Japanese physicians seek to medicalize *kōnenki* it will interesting to see, not only how successful they are, but also whether symptom reporting by Japanese women is transformed as a result of this medical interest in female aging.

The Politics of Female Aging

Japanese women, although politically second-class citizens, and until recently legally subordinated to men, have traditionally been conceptualized not in opposition to them but in a complementary relationship, particularly in terms of family life. Even when elderly, women were not rendered peripheral but served as vital links between the extended family and the ancestors. The process of aging was thought of as unavoidable, with a focus on physiological changes common to both men and women; aging has not generally been associated with pathology, although a few people have very recently started to think of it this way. Historically, therefore, middle-aged women in Japan were not conceived of as either biological or social anomalies, although changes in the structure of the Japanese family and in working conditions have meant that today "professional" housewives are at risk for being thought of as social oddities at *kōnenki*.

In seeking to understand themselves, the Japanese have for centuries drawn on an ideology of national unity in which the "Japanese" are set off from the "Other," most often in historical times that of the Chinese, or else a generalized "barbarian outsider" from further afield. Since the end of the nineteenth century, with the self-conscious modernizing of Japan, an idealized abstracted culture of the "West" has become the foil for national self-reflection in which Japan was usually pictured as "catching up." But with ever-growing intensity over the past thirty years, since the Japanese economy has become a force to be reckoned with, it is this same "West" (by which today is often understood the worst excesses of the United States) which is drawn on to create the current discourse about the dangers of unbridled individuality leading to the supposed fragility of Japanese families. It is this rhetoric of difference that fuels the moralistic negative discourse associated with *kōnenki*. Thus, aging Japanese women are rarely negatively compared, even implicitly, with men or younger Japanese women, nor is their actual age at issue. It is their social position that makes them targets for action—political rather than medical—and, to bring this about, the current generation of middle-aged women, the first to mature in the postwar years, are represented as different from all the generations of properly disciplined and controlled Japanese women believed to have gone before them from time immemorial. The closer their behavior is thought to be to "Western" women, the more of an anomaly they become.

Many Japanese feminists find themselves in an ambivalent position when arguing about the use of middle-aged women in Japan as unpaid care givers. They usually consider that Japanese women remain exceedingly vulnerable to exploitation given their cultural heritage and the current economic arrangements in Japan. Nevertheless, they are often equally concerned when arguments created by feminists in which values associated with the "West," in particular those of autonomy and individualism, are assumed to have universal application. Many argue that committing oneself to a range of family obligations can be both fulfilling and vital work (Lock 1993b).

The politics of aging, an urgent matter in both Japan and North America, is constructed in both cultural spaces, therefore, out of assumptions about the place of women in society. Although the respective discourses are in part the product of a rhetoric about biological change with its associated risk for distress and even major disease (particularly in North America), this rhetoric is produced from local biologies, historically informed knowledge, and situated social exigencies. Women's experiences at the end of menstruation, also informed by this complex of situated variables, are not universal.

Susan Bordo (1993) has argued that in Euro-America the body has consistently been constructed as something apart from "the true self (whether conceived as soul, mind, spirit, will, creativity, freedom)" (5), and numerous feminists have pointed out that women tend to be seen as bodies, thus prohibiting the possibility for maturation as a fully responsible social self. It is not so surprising, therefore, that in North America attention is paid almost exclusively to individual biology. In Japan, where the idealized "true" self is a product of both body and mind, and where women's bodies are trained above all else to be socially responsible, it is the care that middle-aged women are expected to provide for the elderly, rather than physical decline, that has captured public attention. Any distress women may experience in Japan is likely to be ignored or suppressed in favor of a display of self-control and discipline so that their social duties may continue uninterrupted. Even though the Japanese woman is reduced to the behavioral qualities with which she is "naturally" endowed, however, and not to her anatomical profile, nevertheless, the regulatory norms created about the end of menstruation in both cultural contexts are legitimized as though scientifically grounded.

In these respective discourses the subjective experience of aging is suppressed, assumed to be irrelevant and inaccurate in political arenas where reality is above all quantitatively determined (in North America we still have virtually no information of the subjective experiences of women in mid-life). Cast aside too are the economic constraints under which women live, as well as the fact that many women in North America care for their elderly (Harrington et al. 1985), although not as many as do in Japan. Women in both settings are reduced to a uniform mass, their variety obliterated. These criticisms do not apply only to medical and epidemiological literature; they apply equally to the bulk of the feminist literature (although there are some important exceptions in both genres). Whereas in North America efforts are made to discipline women indirectly, through their internalized sense of individual responsibility to keep fit, in Japan the bureaucratized state enters more directly into the fray. Meantime, the numerous ways in which women confront, modify, resist, manipulate, or ridicule the respective ideologies go unmarked (Lock 1993b). Also largely unnoticed is the position of men in aging societies—few suggestions are given about how their declining bodies should be medicalized, or alternatively, their habits, hygiene, and behavior "reformed" for the benefit of their families (although there are some signs that this is changing a little in North America and northern Europe).

Research into the health of women as they age is, of course, of vital importance. This is an area that until recently has been sadly neglected. But if we in North America are to move beyond the dangerous reduction of women = biology, then an analytic perspective that considers more than the merits and shortcomings of medical knowledge and the medicalization of women's bodies is imperative. When considering questions about the autonomy and agency of women, a comparative perspective is often helpful, for it permits us to glimpse the way in which our concerns tend to be formulated within the bounds of conventional knowledge where inevitably, tacit, unexamined assumptions lie concealed. The purpose of comparative work is not to argue for moral superiority in one location or another. Instead, a feminist approach to, for example, the comparative study of female aging should, I believe, work to reveal assumptions embedded in all types of knowledge production, assumptions frequently common to those who share a common cultural and political heritage, whether they are in powerful positions or not. Failure to set discussion of autonomy and agency in this larger framework of unexamined truth claims about scientific knowledge, female aging, and the place of women in society means that the task of a feminist bioethics remains only half done.

NOTES

1. There are recent signs that these recommendations are being modified in the light of further research, but virtually all North American gynecologists insist that middle-aged patients seriously consider the risks and benefits associated with hormone replacement therapy.

2. A cross-sectional survey was administered to 1,738 Japanese women aged forty-five to fifty-five, inclusively. The sample was divided between factory workers, women who live on and run farms, and full-time housewives. A total of 1,316 usable replies was obtained and the study was comparable with a sample of over 8,000 women in Massachusetts and 2,500 Manitoban women (see Lock 1993a and Kaufert, Gilbert, and Hassard 1988).

3. This difference holds even when account is taken of the very different rates of hysterectomies in the three settings (Lock 1993a).

9

(Re)fashioning Medicine's Response to Wife Abuse

Marilynne Bell
Janet Mosher

Only within the past few decades has violence perpetrated against women within their intimate relationships been recognized as a significant social problem. This recognition of the social prevalence of violence within women's intimate relationships is in large measure attributable to the national and international work of women activists in the "battered women's movement," who created spaces for women to collectively name their experiences of violence. This naming revealed that violence against women in the "privacy" of their homes was not aberrational but pervasive. It also revealed the problematic responses of many institutional and government systems, including the health care system. Studies conducted by both the women's community and health care researchers in the seventies and eighties found again and again that the majority of women did not disclose abuse to health care providers, that the majority of health care practitioners failed to identify the abuse, and that if abuse was identified, practitioners often responded in inappropriate, indeed at times harmful, ways. Since the mid-eighties numerous articles in Canadian nursing, medical, public health, and mental health journals have repeated a similar, and distressing, message; the majority of health professionals are ill-equipped to detect abuse and to respond appropriately (Hanvey and Kinnon 1993).

In the health professions, these findings resulted in a movement of a small group of concerned practitioners to lobby successfully for the development and dissemination of guidelines and protocols for the identification, diagnosis, treatment, and management of abused women (Hanvey and Kinnon 1993). While such reformers also worked, and continue to work, on revising professional education and on other initiatives, protocols and guidelines moved quickly to the forefront of attempts to bring wife abuse within the parameters of the everyday practices of health care practitioners.[1]

In this chapter, we critically examine the response to wife abuse in the context of one health discipline, medicine, under three broad headings: medicalization, standardization, and dichotomization. By medicalization we mean that the social phenomenon of wife abuse is transformed into a medical entity to be treated. This transformation is greatly facilitated by the application of the "medical model" as the means of gaining insight into "patients" lives. We argue that protocols are grounded in, and thus help to sustain, tenets of the medical model. As such, they play a constitutive role in the medicalization of wife abuse. The medicalization of woman abuse is problematic, we argue, not only because it has implications for an individual woman who seeks assistance from a physician, but also because it depoliticizes the issue of abuse.

We also argue that standard calls for the "routine screening" of wife abuse commonly made in medical protocols presuppose a homogenous category, "women in abusive relationships," and are inadequately attentive to the context of a given woman's life or the diversity among women. Routine screening undertaken by a person knowledgeable about wife abuse and how it, and responses to it, are deeply intertwined with a woman's social, economic, and cultural location is likely to result in improved outcomes for women. In the hands of a person without this skill and knowledge, routine screening potentially exposes women to harm. A "standardized" response from a physician without any formal training or experience may result in unintended, yet untoward, outcomes. Both "medicalization" and "standardization" discussions draw on parallels within the criminal justice system's response to wife abuse.

Lastly, we argue that many of the medical protocols draw upon the dichotomization of women as victims or agents that pervades much of the literature on abuse. This dichotomization also reflects inadequate attention to the context of choices for these women. Close attention to context reveals that women abused in their intimate relationships frequently exercise choice, albeit in a world in which their choices are incredibly constrained. They are not passive victims; nor does ascribing "survivor" status insure autonomy in the medical encounter as discussed by Susan Sherwin in Chapter 2.

Background Context

One-third of Canadian women have been physically or sexually assaulted by their marital or "common law" partners (Rodgers 1994).[2] For a significant number of the women surveyed, the assaults began during pregnancy.[3] One-fifth of women who experienced violence at the hands of a previous partner reported that the violence occurred following, or during, separation and in 35 percent of these cases, the violence increased in severity at the time of separation (Rodgers 1994). At least 60 percent (551 of 969), and possibly as many as 78 percent (691), of the women murdered in Ontario between 1974 and 1990 died at the hands of an intimate partner. The most common motive was an offender's anger or rage over an actual or impending estrangement (Crawford and Gartner 1992).

For most women, the physical and sexual assaults perpetrated against them are but one of the many means of control wielded by their abusive partners. Many men exercise power over, and seek to control, their intimate partners by resorting to a range of other tactics: emotional abuse (he puts her down in front of others, humiliates her); isolation (he limits her contact with friends and family); minimalization, denial, and blame (he minimizes the wrongfulness or harm of his behavior or blames her for it); coercion, intimidation, and threats, including the use of weaponry; using the children (he threatens to take them away, or that she will lose custody); exercise of male privilege; and economic power (he denies her access to money or to information about finances).[4]

The Violence Against Women survey found that about half of the reported incidents of violence resulted in injury and of these, 43 percent required medical attention (Rodgers 1994). The immediate and long-term injuries that result from the abuse of women in intimate relationships are well documented. The harms of ongoing abuse include anxiety, depression, chronic headaches, abdominal and pelvic pain, eating and sleeping disorders, and sexual dysfunction (Head and Taft 1995; Heise 1993a; Rodgers 1994). Physical trauma from hitting, slapping, pushing, and shoving includes bruising, contusions, and other nondisabling injuries. Other injuries, such as concussion, bone fractures, inflicted burns, lacerations, and weapon-related injuries, often result in long-standing disability and all too frequently, death. The risk for alcoholism or drug abuse increases fourfold for women following the onset of abuse. Physical or sexual abuse often precedes suicide attempts (Abbott et al. 1995; Stark and Flitcraft 1991). Indeed, some American authors have concluded that physical abuse in intimate relationships is the leading cause of serious injury to women, accounting for more trauma than automobile accidents, muggings, and sexual assault combined (Sassetti 1993).

Multiple explanations exist, some complementary, others clearly not, of the violence perpetrated by men against women in the context of intimate relationships.[5] We do not propose here to offer a comprehensive review of these multiple explanations; we offer instead two broad vantage points, or perspectives, the "feminist" and the "therapeutic." The feminist is the ideological basis from which we work and construct our critical analysis; the therapeutic is integrally connected to the "medical model" and thus, to medicalization.

There is no single, unified feminist account of the violence in women's intimate relationships. But several common threads do run through feminist accounts that make it possible to speak of a feminist vantage point or perspective. Within this perspective attention is focused not upon discrete acts of physical aggression but more broadly on the control (through violence and other tactics) that men exercise over women. The construct of "gender," and its links to an ideological "family" are central within this perspective.

Within this framework, gender is understood to be a social construct, the attributes socially ascribed to the biological categories of male and female. As Seyla Benhabib (1987) describes, gender is "the social-historical, symbolic constitution and interpretation of the anatomical differences of the sexes" (80).[6] Within Western cultures the "symbolic constitution and interpretation" of these anatomical differences has constructed two selves: "woman," who is nurturing, caring, dependent, emotive (irrational), selfless, submissive, and passive and associated with the roles of wife and mother and with the institution of "the family"; and "man," who is aggressive, rational, autonomous, and independent and associated with the roles of worker and leader and the institutions of work and politics. Women are constructed as men's opposite and the attributes associated with each are paired in a dichotomous, hierarchical structure. So, for example, women are dependent, men independent; independence is understood to be antithetical to, the polar opposite of, dependence; independence is valued, dependence is not. Men, and the attributes associated with them, are ranked over and above women and the attributes associated with women. As such, women, and the physical and emotive labor that they frequently invest in the care of children and of other adults in the household, are systematically devalued.

These particular gender constructions are integrally connected to another social construction, the nuclear family. This ideological family is premised upon a gendered division of labor according to the role ascriptions of men and women. Men support the family economically through paid employment; women sustain the family by meeting the daily needs of its members for food, cleaning, and emotional support. This image of the family, as nuclear, nurturant, intimate, and caring is pervasive. Indeed, to call it an image is to challenge its own projection of timelessness and naturalness.

From a feminist perspective, these normative constructs help us to understand men's violence in intimate relationships. Much abuse centers on the enforcement of these particular role expectations: her performance of her role of wife (being submissive and ready to meet his sexual and other needs, keeping the house well, and so on) and his as the "ruler of the roost." Her performance of her role is monitored by her abusive partner and any perceived failure to perform satisfactorily is invoked as a justification for his acts of control, including his physical aggression. He may humiliate her in front of family and friends by criticizing the quality of her food preparation, the cleanliness of the home, the behavior of the children. He may prevent her from accessing employment readiness programs, English-language classes—any and every avenue that might decrease her dependence upon him. He may assault her because he thinks she is flirting with another man, or because she is inadequately sexually responsive to him.

James Ptacek (1988) analyzed how men who batter talk about their violence. He found that they use two verbal strategies: excuse ("I lost control") and justification. The justifications commonly offered centered on finding fault with the woman—she was not a good cook, she was not sexually responsive, she was not sufficiently deferential, she was not faithful—in short, for not being a good wife. As put by one of his respondents, "I should just smack you for the lousy wife you've been." As Ptacek observes, a sense of self-righteousness pervades these comments; justified because their "husband-rights," to use Adrienne Rich's term, had not been met. As Rich describes, husband rights are those "rights men are presumed to enjoy simply because of their gender: the 'right' to the priority of male over female needs, to sexual and emotional services from women, to women's undivided attention in any and all situations" (Rich, quoted in Ptacek 1988).

Given the pervasiveness of these gendered expectations, it is not at all surprising that these same justifications are frequently employed by women to excuse the violence of their partners. For example, in a recent study attempting to identify the needs of immigrant women in the Toronto area, women in focus groups were asked what ideas they had to prevent sexual and physical assaults. Women responded: be a good wife; be a good cook; don't make trouble; be a lady, don't lead them on; don't bother your husband if he's in a bad mood; don't annoy your husband; be submissive (Toronto Advisory Committee on Cultural Approaches to Violence Against Women and Children 1992).

It is important to observe that these role expectations are not simply the expression of individual, subjective preferences. Rather, they are embedded in dominant ideologies and social institutions (medicine, law, religion, politics). So, for example, the justifications abusive men offer are often accepted, and thus reinforced, by therapists, lawyers, judges, physicians, and other health care providers, and their colleagues at work, precisely because these expectations are pervasively circulated, taught, and transferred within Western culture. As Ptacek notes, the vocabulary of male entitlement has been routinized within the culture at large; the justifications men invoke are socially approved categories for avoiding blame (Ptacek 1988). Similarly, historically much in Western law (as written and as interpreted and applied by various legal actors) has been premised upon, and has further entrenched, these particular role expectations, such as the denial to women of the right to contract or to hold property; the denial to women of entry into many professions; and the treatment of women as incompetent witnesses. So too, much in other Western traditions, such as philosophy, reflect views of women's natural irrationality, emotiveness, ability to nurture, and so on, rendering them, by "nature," well-suited (or more strongly, capable only of) the roles of mother and wife.

These normative constructs also help us to understand why many women remain in, or return to, abusive relationships. Frequently she (and often her children) will be materially dependent upon her abusive partner (a dependency sustained in multiple and complex ways by the construct of gender); and her sense of self may be integrally connected to her role of wife and to abandon this role may result in shame, humiliation, and loss of status within her community.

By contrast, within the "therapeutic" framework, isolated acts of physical aggression are typically understood to be the problem that requires explanation and attention. Because attention is focused on discrete acts of aggression perpetrated by individuals, the search for an explanation for why the aggression has occurred is also focused on the individual, in this instance either the perpetrator or the victim. It is assumed that "normal" men do not engage in abusive behavior, which some theoretical models label "deviant" or "abnormal" behavior. Moreover, plausible links between these acts of aggression and other forms of "normal" behavior go largely unexplored.

While earlier this century it was largely assumed that men who abused were "drunken loafers" who engaged in this deviant behavior, more recent data that have demonstrated that violence cuts across class boundaries, and that alcohol is present in only a third of cases, have forced a shift in explanation. It is now much more common to point to various "defects" or "differences" in these men, cited most often as psychological, but also biological, as the "cause" of the violence (Dobash and Dobash 1992). While it is more common now to attribute the cause to defects in the abusive male partner, women do not escape being held responsible for the violence within this framework (until recently, they were often labeled as masochistic). In the medical encounter it is most often the woman in the abusive relationship who presents "the problem" to the physician. Hence, a diagnostic label is affixed to "her" problem (the perpetrator becomes invisible). In either case, it is faulty individual traits and personalities that are seen as the source of the problem (Dobash and Dobash 1992). And in either case, a diagnostic category is assigned, and "treatment" by a professional therapist or counselor (be it social worker, psychologist, physician, or psychiatrist) is understood to be the desired intervention. Acts of physical aggression perpetrated by individual men within their intimate relationships remain completely disconnected from the wider social and political worlds (Dobash and Dobash 1992). Indeed, as Michelle Bograd (1988) has suggested, this perspective conflates the question Why do men perpetrate violence against women in intimate relationships? with What pathology causes men to be violent?

Not surprisingly then, from a feminist perspective, the therapeutic perspective is deficient. Acts of physical aggression are not the result of individual pathology but are connected to other tactics of power and control exercised by men, and more broadly linked to a system of domination, sexism. The therapeutic perspective decontextualizes, individualizes, and depoliticizes the issue of violence against women in intimate relationships. It wrongly conceives of the problem, not as a social problem requiring social and structural change, but as faulty individual traits and personalities requiring therapy (Dobash and Dobash 1992).

Dominant Medical Practices

Given the extent of the harm that women in abusive relationships sustain, it is not surprising that abuse is a strong predictor of physician visits and health care costs (Heise 1993a). Indeed, some studies indicate that women in abusive relationships are more likely to seek assistance from a family physician or health care facility than any other community service (Hoffman et al. 1990; Dobash, Dobash, and Cavanagh 1985). If the current trend in the government defunding of community services for abused women continues, it is reasonable to project that increasingly, women will turn to physicians for assistance since physicians may be the only resource available to them.

A Nova Scotia study found that 45.8 percent of women surveyed had seen a physician after the last assault and most women reported a past history of seeking relief through physicians (Davis and MacNevin 1989). Another study found that 80 percent of the abused women surveyed had reported their injuries at least once to a physician and 40 percent had sought medical attention on at least five occasions (Hanvey and Kinnon 1993). One survey of women with histories of abuse cited one-fifth having had more than ten visits a year for medical services (Bowker and Maurer 1987). Studies suggest that one in five women presenting to emergency departments for care and one in four presenting with physical trauma do so as a consequence of violence from their intimate partner (Abbott et al. 1995; Bates et al. 1995).

Women do not often make unsolicited disclosures of the abuse (Campbell and Landenburger 1995; Trute, Sarsfield, and MacKensie 1988). As might be anticipated from our discussion of the normative constructs of "gender" and "family," many abused women feel shamed and humiliated about the abuse. Many fear that they will be judged as responsible, or as incompetent or inadequate, having failed in their responsibilities as wives and mothers. Approximately 25 percent of the women responding to the Violence Against Women Survey had told a doctor about the abuse (Rodgers 1994). In a Toronto study of pregnant women, of the twenty-four women who received medical treatment for abuse, only one had told her prenatal care provider of the abuse (Stewart and Cecutti 1993). Two studies interviewing women in transition houses found much higher rates: approximately 50 percent of women who visited physicians after a violent episode had disclosed the violence as the cause (Perth County, Ontario; Colchester County, Nova Scotia).[7]

The research to date suggests that the majority of physicians routinely treat only the presenting complaint—be it physical or psychological or both—and most often fail to identify or if identified fail to address its underlying source, the abuse (Sugg and Inui 1992; Stark, Flitcraft, and Frazier 1979; Sas, Brown, and Lent 1994). Studies in Canada and the United States have suggested that the identification of abuse in emergency departments ranges from very few to between 40 and 50 percent. Similarly, studies reveal that many family physicians dramatically underestimate the numbers of women in their practices who are, or have been, victims of intimate violence (Sas, Brown, and Lent 1994; Ontario Medical Association, Committee on Wife Assault 1991; Trute, Sarsfield, and MacKenzie 1988; Brown and Sas 1994; Ferris and Tudiver 1992; Ferris 1994).

It is critically important to observe that disclosure or identification of the abuse does not necessarily translate into more appropriate responses by health care providers. One study, for example, found that identification of the abuse had little impact on whether physicians prescribed psychoactive or psychotropic drugs—drugs that expose women to greater danger by reducing their ability to protect themselves and their children, by creating conditions for the development of addictions, and by putting in a woman's hands the means to take her own life.[8] Three in five abused women received prescriptions for such medications, and the majority said that the physician did not explain the side effects. These same physicians recommended that the women take a hot bath, get out more, or take a break from the kids (all forms of minimization and denial) or, alternatively, leave their husbands. Also of note in this study is that many women reported looking to physicians for initiative and assistance, that they had turned to physicians for relief, and for "rescue" (Davis and MacNevin 1989; Head and Taft 1995).[9]

Other studies report as well that the majority of women experience negative responses from their physicians. These include: simply ignoring the disclosure; offering negative attitudinal responses that draw upon the widely accepted justifications reviewed earlier; normalizing the abuse; suggesting that the woman disclosing is neurotic; and breaching confidentiality by raising a woman's disclosure with her abusive partner (Head and Taft 1995; Hanvey and Kinnon 1993). Women report that physicians do not comprehend their predicaments and do not provide validation of their experiences (Hoffman et al. 1990; Dobash, Dobash, and Cavanagh 1985). "Many abused women who seek help from the health care system experience their contact with the 'helping' professions and systems as another form of abuse. These women are doubly victimized by violent partners and by practices and procedures that are insensitive to their needs" (Hanvey and Kinnon 1993).

Those providers who fail to address the source of the presenting complaints—or fail to understand the relevance of abuse when disclosed—potentially expose women to greater harm. These failures may lead to a medical response, such as the prescription of psychoactive and psychotropic drugs, that exposes women to greater danger. They may result in not identifying the gravest threat to fetal outcome. They may lead to the revictimization of women through the assignment of inappropriate psychiatric labels, wherein the woman herself is seen as the source of the problem. Evan Stark and Anne Flitcraft found that in early encounters with health professionals the source of the trauma is often simply unspoken and only the presenting complaint "treated." In time, if an abused woman makes repeated visits for medical attention and it becomes apparent that "treatments" to date have failed—indeed her

condition may have worsened as a result of on-going abuse—she herself is named as the source of her trauma. She becomes subject to referrals to psychiatry, is labeled as suffering from a psychiatric disorder,
and potentially becomes subject to punitive interventions, such as psychiatric hospitalization (Stark, Flitcraft, and Frazier 1979; Stark and Flitcraft 1982; Hoff and Rosenbaum 1994). The failure to identify, or respond appropriately, may mean that some women will become more
despairing and isolated, their abuse having gone unacknowledged and
unaffirmed by a significant authority figure. And for some women, they
will learn by these failures to distrust physicians and to avoid medical
assistance for their injuries (Head and Taft 1995). Nonidentification of
the abuse reinforces the view that the abuse is private, shameful (not
something to be spoken about), and irrelevant to women's health status. As such, it serves to recreate in the medical setting the perpetrator
denial psychology present in the domestic abuse setting (Warshaw
1989, 1994; Stark, Flitcraft, and Frazier 1979).

It is important to note that a sizable number (approximately 30 percent in the few studies we found that address this issue) of women do
report positive responses by their physicians after making a disclosure
(Head and Taft 1995; Ferris 1994). What women found most helpful and
what they most desired from their physicians were support, validation,
and good referrals. Respectful attentiveness to her story, confirmation
that it is credible and believed, and assistance according to her needs are
crucial (Head and Taft 1995; Malterud 1992). As we discuss more fully
in "Evaluating the Protocol Response," these various components of
positive responses—which are often recited in protocols and guidelines—appear deceptively simple and easy to deliver. We argue, however, that words and actions that are supportive or validating cannot be
reduced to a formula but must be shaped in response to each woman
and "where she is" at any given time. Ascertaining this is a complex undertaking, requiring critical interrogation of one's own assumptions
and stereotypes, an openness to change, and an ability to engage across
significant social and cultural experiences, understandings, and values.

Exploring the Reasons for Nonidentification and Inappropriate Responses

It is important to discern the reasons for the low rates of detection and
for the problematic responses of some physicians, since any strategy to
affirmatively change practices and norms must surely be grounded in
an understanding of these reasons. There are, no doubt, several con-

tributing factors: social norms, the structure and philosophy of medicine, lack of skill and knowledge, the structure of the health care system; and personal experiences of abuse (Hanvey and Kinnon 1993; Ontario Medical Association, Committee on Wife Assault 1991).

The attitudes of physicians are, of course, subject to the characterizations of woman abuse arising from broader societal attitudes and beliefs concerning the sanctity and privacy of family, women's role and position in society, male privilege, and public tolerance of abuse. Indeed, it would be bizarre to assume that physicians as a group might escape these pervasive lessons of dominant socialization processes. Hence it is not at all surprising that many physicians, like others, will normalize the abuse, blame women for it, or accept uncritically many stereotypes about who abuses and about abused women. These stereotypes act as strong screening devices, preventing out even suspicions of abuse in particular contexts, while reading it into others. So, for example, stereotyping results in suspicions of abuse running higher for low-income or racialized communities (who are stereotyped as more violent) than for white, middle- and upper-income families (Sugg and Inui 1992). So, too, the "truths" providers hold about families limit their ability to hear or see beyond them and thus will impede the identification of abuse. For example, if one highly values family "privacy" and believes families to be warm and nurturant, the likelihood of "seeing" abuse, even when the signals are quite evident, is low. Thus the "truisms" about woman abuse that providers hold, but rarely articulate, are relevant to nonidentification and inappropriate responses.

The Supreme Court of Canada has acknowledged the pervasiveness of particular myths about women in abusive intimate relationships that frequently operate to women's disadvantage. Madame Justice Wilson observed as follows:

> The average member of the public (or of the jury) can be
> forgiven for asking: why would a woman put up with this
> kind of treatment? Why should she continue to live with such
> a man? How could she love a partner who beat her to the point
> of requiring hospitalization? We would expect the woman to
> pack her bags and go. Where is her self-respect? Why does she
> not cut loose and make a new life for herself? Expert evidence
> is necessary to dispel the common belief that battered woman
> are not really beaten as badly as they claim; otherwise they
> would have left the relationship. Alternatively, some believe
> that women enjoy being beaten, that they have a masochistic
> strain in them. (*R v. LaVallee*, 1990)

We should not, then, be surprised that some physicians dismiss violence in intimate relationships as a "private" matter, contend women are exaggerating or are in some way to blame for the abuse, or go so far as to believe the abuse is deserved.

The attitudes and practices of most physicians will be shaped not only by these norms of the dominant culture but also by the structure and philosophy of medicine. As we argue throughout this book, a significant dimension of the ideological worldview of the medical community (and indeed of those outside of it) is that of medicine as a science. As such, medicine is frequently portrayed as a rational and predictable undertaking that yields answers (treatments, cures) for most everything. Its rationality and predictability are predicated upon categories of organic disease. Information about the lived world is systemically translated and organized into these categories. Information, whatever its source, is sifted by physicians for "relevance," with relevance being determined by reference to pre-existing categories of organic disease. Information that does not fit a category, such as information related to social and political location, is screened out if proffered and certainly not encouraged. The unit of analysis is the individual, and the source of the "problem" located within the individual (see Chapters 2, 3, and 5). The predominant metaphor of the body is one of an efficient machine, functioning in isolation from a determinant social order (Stark, Flitcraft, and Frazier 1979). The biomedical model reduces people's lives to medical "cases," stripped of social context and reduced to medically relevant facts (Smith 1990; Warshaw 1989, 1994; Dobash and Dobash 1992; Gondolf and Fisher 1989). As Carol Warshaw (1994) describes, the medical model transforms people with lives and agency of their own into patients who fit medical or psychiatric diagnostic categories that can be readily manipulated and controlled.[10]

The implications of this conceptual structure, or method of gaining insight into patients' problems, in the context of abuse are multiple. The biomedical model contributes to the common practice described above, wherein physical and mental injuries—the manifestations of abuse upon the body and mind—are often simply treated without the abuse being identified, or if identified, not regarded as relevant. This occurs because, as noted, the focus of the biomedical inquiry is upon the individual. The manifestations of the abuse upon the body, or the mind, lie within the medical gaze; a "fractured arm" or "depression," for example, are the diagnoses made. But what is occluded is the social context: the abuse in women's live, the cause of these injuries. Yet physician understanding of the cause of the injury here, as in other medical contexts, is vitally important for sound diagnoses and the determination of appropriate treatments and referrals.

The translation of lived experience into a medical event within the context of wife abuse is well demonstrated by Carol Warshaw's work (1989). Warshaw retrospectively reviewed emergency room data generated by nurses and physicians on women whose injuries were highly indicative of having been caused by abuse. She found that rarely was explicit information about the abuse recorded or integrated into the diagnosis or the discharge plans. The records were characterized by disembodied language (no relationship was described, no mention was made of who hit whom), concretization of the pathopsychological mechanisms of injury (without attribution to the perpetrator as the source of the injury), and an overall focus on the treatment endpoint. These "habits," she argues, result in the obfuscation of the reality of the injury and the circumstances of the abuse. Warshaw argues not only that the text of the medical records reflect physicians' need to conduct a medical history but also that the standard medical descriptive format limits the ability of physicians even to see the abuse.

If the abuse is identified, the medical model may come into play in another manner. Recall that within the therapeutic approach to the etiology of abuse, individual pathology is understood to be causative. This approach to the etiology of violence is firmly grounded in the medical model; abuse is explained by reference to individual deficits. Hence, it is possible that the woman may be assigned a psychiatric label, "personality disorder," for example, that attributes responsibility for the abuse to her pathology.

In addition to the impact of social norms and the philosophy and structure of medicine, physicians and others also repeatedly point to the lack of training as a significant factor in underidentification and inappropriate responses. As Marybeth Hendricks-Matthews (1992) observed, the vast majority of health care providers have had minimal exposure to the nature of abuse, the needs of women who have been abused, and the role of health care professionals in providing support (see also Sugg and Inui 1992; Sas, Brown, and Lent 1994).

Finally, a physician's own experiences of abuse are an important factor. Consider, for example the physician who has never experienced abuse or violence, and whose experiences of "family" have been positive. It may be very difficult for him or her to see violence in the life of a woman "patient" whose life, in other important respects, is similar to his or her own. Or the reality of abuse may be too close to home, because the physician herself has experienced abuse. In one study, 31 percent of female physicians and 14 percent of male physicians acknowledged their own experiences of violence (Sugg and Inui 1992). And, of course, some male physicians themselves will be perpetrators of abuse within their intimate relationships and the denial, justifications, and mini- mization strategies that they employ at a personal level are likely to be manifest in their professional lives as well.

Evaluating the Protocol Response

As noted at the outset there has been, over the past decade, a prolifera- tion of protocols and guidelines (frequently appearing in articles in pro- fessional journals) on the identification, "diagnosis," "treatment," and "management" of woman abuse. Many proponents of these guidelines and protocols see them as vehicles to assist in the transformation of the attitudes and practices of physicians. Others have expressed scepticism about the worth of standards of practice guidelines, and protocols, not- ing that there is currently no effective means to enforce them (at least not in the context of private practices) (Hanvey and Kinnon 1993). A fre- quent rejoinder here is to argue that we must then fashion ways of more effectively translating the protocols or guidelines into practice. But whether this is a worthwhile pursuit surely depends upon an affirma- tive answer to a prior question of whether the protocols and guidelines, assuming they can indeed be translated into practices, are likely to alter practices in a manner that better meets the needs of abused women. This prior, broad question is the focus of our inquiry. We address it by con- sidering three pervasive features of many current protocols and guide- lines: medicalization, routinization, and dichotomization.

Medicalization

Medicalization is not simply the reduction of wife abuse to a bio- medical label as a syndrome or a disorder. It is more aptly conceptu- alized as a complex process in which a social phenomenon becomes (re)constituted as a medical entity (see Chapter 5). It is important to recognize that wife abuse potentially becomes medicalized both when it is acknowledged (for example, through a protocol response that includes "therapeutic" explanations of the etiology of violence, or through protocols that explicitly analogize abuse to existing cate- gories of organic disease) and when it goes unacknowledged by the medical community (for example, when abuse goes unidentified, or if identified, is treated as irrelevant, when a women seeks medical as- sistance). Given the concerns about the application of the medical model in cases of abuse identified in the preceding section, one would think that countering these tendencies within medical practice would be a central goal of reform objectives. But a close examination of several protocols and guidelines suggests that many are firmly grounded within a biomedical framework. In the various protocols and guidelines it is common to describe "wife abuse" as just like other categories of organic disease, a "true medical condition," a "chronic syndrome"; to claim that it is "eminently treatable"; and to cast physicians into the familiar role of savior. Physicians are told, for example, that they can break the cycle of violence and that by listening to a woman tell of her experiences they take the single most important step in ending violence. The language of "diagnosis," "treatment," and "curability" are pervasive. These sorts of claims appear even in those guidelines and protocols that simultaneously go to some lengths to explain that wife abuse is the result, not of individual pathologies, but rather of a multitude of social, structural, and ideological factors.

> It is therefore hoped that every physician who reads this, especially those who feel too overwhelmed or poorly equipped to address the problem, will come to understand and accept that he or she can break the cycle of violence and profoundly impact the health of thousands of families and thus, society at large. . . . Caring for battered women . . . is actually relatively simple to learn and implement. . . . Physicians have not been educated to understand woman battering as a true medical condition. [It is a] continuing syndrome of chronic emotional, psychological and socially isolating abuse. . . . Wife abuse is best understood as a chronic syndrome that is characterized not by the episodes of violence that punctuate the problem but by the emotional and psychological abuse that the batterer uses to enforce and maintain control over his partner. . . . How do physicians learn to diagnose and treat? Like many other medical maladies, wife abuse is best understood as a syndrome that has a natural history, well recognized signs and symptoms and an established set of guidelines for diagnosis and intervention. The physician must simply ask, the single most effective tool for combating wife abuse. (Sassetti 1993, 289–91)

In seeking to garner the attention of medical practitioners who have ignored the issue of abuse, we find the claim that woman abuse is "just like other medical maladies" poignant. To claim it is just like other medical maladies is to reframe abuse as something that *is* the physician's business, that *is* within his or her authority and expertise, and that *is* diagnosable and treatable. It appears to provide an answer to the physicians who made the following comments:

> When I have somebody coming in with a problem, I want to solve the problem. Diagnose it and treat it and put it behind them then and there. That is being a doctor. Putting it into the medical model. But the problem here is that the medical model doesn't work with wife abuse.

> I feel totally impotent about what to do. . . . If you don't know how to deal with the problem, you don't want to find it.
> (Brown, Lent, and Sas 1993, 188)

Much of the literature now tells these physician that they can, indeed, put abuse into a medical model; that they can diagnose it, treat it, and even end it. But the physician quoted above is right; physicians are relatively impotent. Abuse and a woman's response to it are complex ("a can of worms"), and not amenable to "treatment." Woman abuse is not like many other "medical maladies"; although it often gives rise to mental and physical harm it is always something other than or more than a medical issue. Reframing woman abuse as "like other medical maladies" continues to put women at risk of misdiagnosis and of the inappropriate ascription of psychiatric labels. More globally, it perpetuates the transformation of a complex social problem into an issue of individual pathology or disorder requiring treatment; in other words, it perpetuates the medicalization of abuse.[11]

It is worth reflecting upon how easily feminist reform strategies can come to collude with nonfeminist understandings of abuse; how notwithstanding the critique of the therapeutic, biomedical perspective by feminists, unwittingly many feminists have themselves pursued arguments and strategies that lend credence and viability to therapeutic, biomedical discourses and practices (Ferraro 1996). Consider, for example, feminist reform strategies in the criminal law. Many feminists argued that "wife assault" (a term chosen self-consciously to fit a criminal justice paradigm) was like other assaults as a strategy to reform a recalcitrant legal system. They argued for charges to be laid and prosecuted vigorously, and for courts to impose significant sentences. In a parallel maneuver to the medical context, they argued, not for the medicalization of wife abuse, but for its "juridicalization" (that we understand it as a legal entity and respond to it as such). In these campaigns (which themselves have become central to feminist agendas), many feminists have come to focus upon discrete acts of physical aggression, perpetrated by individual men. Increased rates of conviction and incarceration (or sentences mandating therapy) have been problematically equated with improved outcomes for women (Martin and Mosher 1995). As Kathleen Ferraro (1996) notes, domestic violence discourse establishes parameters of acceptable male domination within relationships; *Criminal Code* misconduct is used to draw a line separating unacceptable and acceptable male domination in families. Male authority in general is upheld and other forms of domination and control (which many women report are as harmful as physical aggression) are ignored. Intervention is focused upon individual men, not upon structural transformation; attention has drifted from "male domination and social transformation to criminalized acts" (86).

Thus, what we can observe in practice, on the ground so to speak, is slippage from a feminist perspective into a therapeutic or biomedical perspective. As such, many of the important insights of feminists into the realities of women's lives—of how the construct of gender creates appropriate aggressors and passive victims, of how the roles of wife and mother and the attendant responsibilities for care of others are policed and enforced by men, and of the many ways in which these responsibilities render women vulnerable to abuse—are given little attention. Similarly, attempts to shape medical responses to woman abuse by treating it as a medical entity to be diagnosed and treated potentially occlude the social and structural roots of violence against women, by offering limited individual ministrations at best, in lieu of the fundamental social and structural reforms necessary if we are to truly take seriously the violence in women's lives, and thus women's value as persons.[12]

This is not to suggest that there is no role for physicians to play, individually or collectively. As a political voice, the medical profession (and other health care professions)—-whose voices are relatively powerful—can play a role in not permitting the state to engage in the pretense that violence against women is being seriously addressed when (re)constructed as a medical or legal entity and responsibility for it delegated to the medical or criminal justice systems. It can insist on the structural and social reforms necessary to truly improve women's health status. So, too, the profession ought to speak out on the declining public resources available for abused women (welfare, housing, support, counseling, etc.) that make it nearly impossible for physicians to even make referrals. At the level of the individual practitioner, as we develop more fully below, she or he has a responsibility to become knowledgeable about abuse, to engage in critical, self-reflective practice, and to listen and hear the stories of women.

Standardization

Primary care, psychiatry, and obstetrics have called upon their members in recent years to routinely screen for abuse. Protocols and guides to practitioners offer suggestions to facilitate disclosure: direct questioning and posters, buttons, and brochures condemning intimate violence are probably the two most common.[13] Coupled with these in some articles in professional journals is the claim that routine screening takes very little time and is really an easy and straightforward procedure.

Calls are pervasive for physicians to routinely screen for wife abuse by integrating questions about woman abuse into the intake interview and in subsequent visits where appropriate (Chez 1994; Sassetti 1993; Ontario Medical Association, Committee on Wife Assault 1991; Trute et al. 1988; Sas, Brown, and Lent 1994; Stewart and Cecutti 1993; Elliott and Johnson 1995). The benefits claimed by many authors are similar to those that follow:

> By asking questions about battering, the physician gives the abused patient permission to understand she is not alone, that violence is unacceptable, and that she has the right to be safe and to seek viable alternatives. . . . The entire interaction can take as little as 10 seconds and no more than 5 minutes. The time spent can save a life. (Chez 1994)

> When physicians ask about violence, they not only make violence a health care issue but also indicate to the patient that they are potential allies and resources. Then physicians become part of the empowerment that is essential in the resolution of the violence and the patient's healing. (Elliott and Johnson 1995, 118)

Various authors and protocols propose specific questions for inclusion, for example: How do you and your partner resolve disagreements? Have you been hit or hurt by anyone in the last year? (Stewart and Cecutti 1993). When you were a child did you witness parental violence, that is, your father beating up or scaring your mother? How would you feel if he ever hit you? Some people feel frightened when arguing with their husbands, can you recall similar feelings? (Sas, Brown, and Lent 1994).

One rationale here appears to be that practices, and indeed attitudes, may be transformed by demanding of physicians that they screen for abuse.[14] Here, it may be instructive to contemplate possible parallels to developments within the criminal justice system. As many women and women's advocates have claimed, police officers' responses to situations of women abused in intimate relationships have been far from desirable; like many physicians, they too have drawn upon commonly invoked justifications and rationalizations ("it's a private matter"; "she deserved it"; "it's his right") and have failed to provide an adequate response. Many reformers rationalized that the only way to change behaviors was to mandate such changes by dramatically reducing discretion in charging. Many also reasoned that attitudinal changes would follow these required behavioral changes or practices. Mandating charges also seemed to be a way of transforming beliefs about the nature of "real" police practice, a way of making wife abuse "real" police business. Women pressed successfully for the creation of "mandatory charging" policies, requiring police to lay charges whenever probable grounds existed for believing an offense had occurred. Experience with this strategy to date suggests, however, that practices and more so, attitudes, are deeply resistant to change. Many police officers continue to find ways of avoiding the policy altogether; they interpret "probable grounds" to believe an offense has occurred in ways that discount women's words (for example, to refuse to lay a charge if it is "her word against his"); make gratuitous sexist comments; or offer inappropriate advice (Farge and Rahder 1991; Valverde, MacLead, and Johnson 1995). The lesson here may well be that we ought not to expect protocols, standards of care expressed in guidelines, or pleas from professional associations to go any great distance in changing attitudes or practices or ideas about what constitutes "real" medicine (itself a problematic aspiration in the light of our discussion of medicalization).

This lesson is crucially important since it seems entirely plausible that asking the sorts of intake questions proposed will indeed generate increased disclosures. Much of the literature seems to assume that increased identification of abuse alone can be equated with improved outcomes from women. But how is it that the routine asking of questions alone will give a woman "permission to understand that she is not alone," will convey to her that the violence is unacceptable, or will necessarily position the physician as a resource toward her empowerment, as the above statements claim? In the light of the known reality that a sizable proportion of the profession responds inappropriately to disclosures of abuse, is it not equally plausible that what may follow in the wake of a disclosure is disbelief, paternalism, or negative judgments about her conduct? And if so, do increased rates of disclosure represent increased harms, rather than gains, for women? How is it that we could expect affirming, empowering responses from a group who has not escaped patriarchal socialization and has been schooled in the medical model as a means of organizing and understanding knowledge about the human body?

As noted, women are reluctant to disclose to their physicians because of shame, humiliation, and fears that their physicians will make negative judgments about them or hold them responsible for the abuse. But other fears are also at play—for example, fear of retaliation should her abusive partner learn she has disclosed, fear her children may be apprehended by a child protection authority, and a fear of further entrenching stereotypes of her culture. This means that a disclosure almost inevitably entails risk for her. Hence, calls for routine screening, to the extent that they do facilitate disclosures, put a woman at risk. At risk that her physician will, as some women have reported, breach her confidence and tell her abusive partner. At risk that her physician will take it upon himself or herself to call the police. At risk that she will suffer negative judgments, will not be believed, will be assigned a psychiatric label. At risk that a children's aid society will be contacted, and the subsequent investigation expose her to retaliation from her intimate partner for disclosing and to the potential removal of her children.[15]

While some authors and guidelines simply propose a series of questions for incorporation, others offer suggestions about how the physician respond to disclosures. The difficulty here is that women's experiences of, and responses to, abuse vary dramatically. Moreover, any given woman's experiences, interpretations of them, and responses to them are not static. Hence, advice to physicians risks being either too vague or overly prescriptive and potentially inappropriate. Some examples might help to illustrate these concerns. The literature commonly tells physicians to be "supportive," but this is not terribly illuminating; what particular women will find supportive will vary widely, although it may well be possible to identify responses that are uniformly unsupportive. Physicians are commonly counseled to tell abused women that the conduct of their intimate partners is "criminal behavior." While this naming of behavior may be appropriate, one can easily imagine circumstances where it would be tremendously problematic. The abuse has often occurred in the context of a relationship of love and commitment and has been perpetrated not by someone the woman calls a batterer or a criminal but her husband, lover, life partner (Mahoney 1994). As Jacqulyn Campbell (1992) notes, "it is a relatively long way into the process of abuse before women actually label themselves as 'assaulted,' 'abused,' or even more threatening, 'battered'" (466). The renaming of the conduct as criminal and the woman herself as abused or battered may not, in fact, validate her experience, or offer her support. The literature also routinely suggests that women be told that laws exist to protect them; some go further and suggest that the physician direct women to call the police. In fact, there is no sound basis for the claim that laws exist to protect women—while some women are protected, many others are harmed when they resort to law—either because of retaliation from their abusive partners or because of the revictimization that they experience within the civil and criminal justice systems, or both (Martin and Mosher 1995).

Of further concern are the representations that the inquiry and response are relatively straightforward and take little time—a maximum of five minutes as claimed by one author. No doubt these representations attempt to head off the concerns often expressed by physicians that to "open this can of worms" is time consuming and complex. These concerns expressed by physicians, we believe, are well grounded, because actually hearing and validating a women's account and responding in an empowering way is a complex and challenging task. A responsible standard of care employed by a medical practitioner needs to be learned in an environment where attitudes and values are critically examined and discussed, where experienced mentors can respond and model approaches.[16]

Victim-Agent Dichotomy

Women abused in intimate relationships are frequently stereotyped in popular culture as helpless, passive victims, unable to perceive what is in their best interests. In the extreme, women who remain in abusive relationships have been described, and in some circumstances diagnosed, as suffering from "learned helplessness." This theoretical construct, first advanced by the psychologist Lenore Walker (1984), posits that after repeated and unsuccessful attempts to modify the behavior of an abusive partner, women come to believe that no matter what they do, nothing will change. Over time, they become helpless—a form of psychological impairment—and fail to see, or to take advantage of, actual avenues or resources for change.[17]

The language in protocols and guidelines uses both victim and survivor (agent) positioning in describing women presenting for medical assistance. While the majority of the protocols, guidelines, and articles that we have reviewed avoid the label "battered woman syndrome" (quite a few do use the language of "syndrome," however), nevertheless the imagery of abused women as passive and helpless, and explanations for their behavior as rooted in pathology, are pervasive. The Ontario Medical Association material on wife abuse says, for example, because these women often suffer from low self-esteem due to chronic abuse, they may chose a course of action the physician considers inappropriate" (Ontario Medical Association, Committee on Wife Assault 1991).

This tendency to stereotype women as passive victims and to deny ascriptions of agency or rationality to their conduct is rooted in a broader phenomenon: the dichotomization of victimization and agency. As Martha Mahoney (1994) argues, within this framework, each is defined by the absence of the other: an agent is one who does not experience victimization (is self-directed); the victim is one who experiences no agency (is other-directed, that is, both directed by another, and other regarding). The conception of agency generally at work within this dichotomy is one of an atomistic, self-interested individual, with no emotive or other relational connections. This frame of victimization and agency, and the particular meanings attached to each, obscures the many acts of agency in which abused women engage. To see these acts of agency one needs to shift outside of the victim-agent dichotomy and attend to the conditions of constraint under which women exercise choice.

As noted, many women are materially dependent upon their abusive spouses, and in the context of the retrenchment of the welfare state, access to any (let alone adequate) state support has become increasingly difficult. As noted, many fear authorities such as child welfare (their children may be apprehended), or immigration (they may be deported) should the violence become known. Many fear an escalation of violence should they disclose or leave and astutely perceive that society will not offer them adequate protection. As noted, not only does violence frequently escalate after separation but at the time of separation women are at greatest risk of being murdered by their intimate partners. Many racialized women fear that drawing attention to their abusive partners will reinforce stereotypes about the communities to which they belong and which they love and value. Many fear racist responses, particularly from the police, directed against themselves or their partners and actively seek to protect "their men" from such responses. Many fear the loss of their status as wives and mothers within their communities and blame themselves when their relationships do not match the ideology of the nurturant family that they, themselves, have come to value deeply. While this may reflect the internalization of the patriarchal ideologies and practices described earlier, failure to conform to them will have real costs (both material and psychological) for many women.

While these fears, and the risks of harms materializing should one disclose the violence or leave the relationship, vary according to one's social location, all women make the decision to stay, to leave, or to seek help in a world in which "choices" are incredibly constrained. It is also abundantly clear that "exit" may well expose some women to greater harm than remaining. Thus, remaining, rather than a manifestation of a "victim's" failure to take action because of her impaired psychological state, may simply be the best choice for an agent who occupies a world of few options.[18]

While it is no doubt true that a woman who is repeatedly and violently assaulted is a "victim," she is simultaneously much, much more. She may be a caring and courageous mother who takes incredible precautions to ensure that her children do not witness the abuse and do not suffer harm as a result. She may work diligently to try to locate resources for her family to help end the abuse (Head and Taft 1995; Gondolf and Fisher, 1989). She may leave temporarily as part of a strategy to bring about change in her partner. She may have made several unsuccessful attempts to locate supports and decided that further attempts would be futile. She will likely make countless decisions and take countless actions (Gondolf and Fisher 1989; Campbell and Landenburger 1995).

She is not a person who does not exercise agency; she makes choices, albeit in a world of few options. She is likely, however, a person without autonomy in the sense articulated by Susan Sherwin in Chapter 2, in that the conditions under which she exercises choice are so constrained that she has little, if any, scope to proactively shape her life. So, too, in some instances, her ability to proactively shape her life with regard to her own needs, rather than those of her abusive partner, may have been stunted by the harm caused to her sense of self by ongoing abuse.

As noted earlier, the language, theoretical positioning, and "management" vernacular in protocols, guidelines, and professional journals frequently ends up overtly and covertly portraying women as victims. They commonly lapse into paternalism, giving directions that suggest there is only a single, appropriate course of action—"direct her to call the police" (Sassetti 1993). Yet simultaneously much of this literature counsels against paternalistic responses, warning physicians not to become caught up in the desire to "rescue." Articles and protocols frequently stress that decisions are the woman's to make. Thus, women are presented simultaneously as victims in need of rescue, and as autonomous agents who choose from a range of options and whose choices ought to be respected; as occupying both poles of the victim-agent dichotomy. The more recent literature does then reflect something of the complexity of "choice" and decision making in the context of woman abuse but seems to be simultaneously caught at both ends of the victim-agency dichotomy; women who are abused are presented both as victims (who do not exercise agency) and agents (who do not experience victimization).

This is an important issue in the context of medical practice because neither of the two dominant models of decision making—paternalism and informed consent (themselves reflective of victim/agent dichotomization)—is appropriate. Paternalism presupposes that women are incapable of making decisions in their own best interest, that another knows better than the woman herself what ought to be done in particular circumstances—a troubling proposition given the failure of many physicians to grasp the realities of the circumstances of abused women. Informed consent as a model of decision making presupposes a generic decision maker who simply requires "information." This decision maker is one who is accustomed to making decisions and has confidence in his or her ability to do so. The "information" required to make an "informed" decision is assumed to be evident (see Chapter 2). While acknowledging that information might have to be repackaged in modest sorts of ways to meet the particular capacities of a decision maker, in the main, the informed consent model generates a generic package of information for a generic decision maker. This model too is inattentive to the contextual realities of women's lives. A third model is necessary, one that transcends the victim/agent dichotomy and that recognizes women as capable actors who may require assistance in making decisions and taking control of their lives (Campbell and Landenburger 1995).

Protocols and guidelines, standing on their own, seem incapable of transforming the practices and attitudes of those physicians who at present either do not identify abuse or, if they do, respond inappropriately. Protocols are often premised upon—they buy into, rather than resist or challenge—characterizations and understandings of abuse that are fundamentally unhelpful (and sometimes harmful) to women. Through their reliance upon the medical model, they promote therapeutic and biomedical, not feminist, understandings of, and insights into, abuse and, in so doing, promote the medicalization of wife abuse. They treat women as a generic category of persons, and abuse as a "simple" matter, and in so doing fail to attend to the complexities of women's lives. They are caught in the victim-agent dichotomy, in which women are assumed to be either, or both, pathologized victims or full agents.

While one could fashion protocols that do resist medicalization, that warn of the dangers of "standardization," and that offer concrete models of decision making that move beyond the victim-agent dichotomy (and some protocols and guidelines do go some distance on this matters), simply moving in this direction leaves two fundamental issues untouched. First, it is clear that protocols—even those that resist medicalization, and so on—will not effect much positive change in the hands of a person unskilled in using them. Thus, a crucial piece of work to be done is the "skilling" of physicians (an issue we address in more detail below). Protocols also leave untouched the issue of the political responsibilities of the medical profession. A responsibility to resist the transformation of abuse into a medical entity. A responsibility not to let the state sidestep its obligations by treating abuse as either a medical or a legal entity requiring no fundamental redistributions in social power. A responsibility to understand that medicine holds no "cures" for abuse, but that women require knowledgeable, affirming, and supportive medical attention in addition to access to housing, to counseling, to advocacy, to economic independence. And a responsibility to use the power of its political voice to demand that all of the these resources be in place for women.

What then are the skills that physicians need to learn? They need to learn to listen and to hear the realities of women's lives. This necessitates "a good faith effort to hear the other" and "requires vulnerability and humility, and a willingness and ability to leave the security of one's own beliefs, feelings, and frame of reference" (More 1994; More and Milligan 1994). It requires, as Lorraine Code (1994) argues, "finding out who [the woman seeking assistance] is in the pertinent respects, resisting stereotypes and swift categorizations." The resistance to stereotypes begins with an acknowledgment of one's own partiality, with confronting one's own assumptions and stereotypes about who is abused and who abuses and about the capacities of women who have been abused by their intimate partners. It requires articulating one's assumptions about why women are abused and opening these assumptions to critical inquiry for both the individual practitioner and the health care system. In no small measure, it requires a genuine openness to change: of one's assumptions, beliefs, and frequently of the "truths" that one holds dear. For some, this includes giving up patriarchal assumptions about the privacy of the family, of families as nurturant and caring, and of women as often unreliable, irrational, and vindictive.[19]

It requires attention to the social, and indeed often distressingly oppressive, circumstances of a patient's life (Candib 1994). It requires leaving the security and comfort of the medical model, engaging with, and attempting to understand the circumstances that oppress and constrain and about which, frequently, the physician can do relatively little. This includes attention to the intersections of various axes of oppression. It requires acknowledging the perspectives, and indeed wisdom, of those outside medicine, including the woman herself. It does not entail the abandonment of critical challenges to other points of view. Thus, in no small measure, it requires giving up one's power over others and the power to fix the problem, and in their stead, embracing a commitment to the empowerment of others (Candib 1994). It does not lend itself to prescription. It is an art, infinitely nuanced in response to subjectivity, not a science.

Its cultivation requires the experience of actually having one's assumptions and truths about wife abuse challenged. Consider circumstances where what is said by the patient—"I am a helpless victim"—is completely compatible with the physician's view of women living in abusive relationships—"you are a helpless victim." While the physician in this example may be open to challenge and to change, nothing in these circumstances prompts challenge or change in either the physician or the patient. One can imagine that situations of correspondence between physician- and patient-held beliefs and assumptions about violence might be quite common, since both are likely to be influenced by patriarchal views. To state this differently, it is unreasonable to presuppose that challenges to patriarchal, racist, classist, or otherwise troubling assumptions and views about violence against women in intimate relationships will necessarily come from patients. Thus, it is imperative that physicians' beliefs, assumptions, and "knowledge" claims be systematically addressed through educational processes. Only then might physicians be able to respond appropriately to the needs of women abused in intimate relationships.

NOTES

1. When we refer to protocols and guidelines, we have in mind not only protocols prepared by professional associations and circulated to their members, and those developed by particular health care institutions, but also the guidelines, and more broadly the "guidance," offered to physicians through professional journals.

2. In 1993, Statistics Canada conducted a nationwide survey, the "Violence Against Women Survey," of 12,300 women over the age of eighteen. Women were asked, among other things, about their experiences of physical and sexual

assault as defined by the *Criminal Code* from the age of sixteen (Statistics Canada, 1994). Other studies indicate that the rates of *Criminal Code* violence may well be higher for women with disabilities and for aboriginal women (Dis-Abled Women's Network, n.d.; Ontario Native Women's Association 1989).

3. In the Violence Against Women Survey, 21 percent of the women surveyed reported being abused during pregnancy. Forty percent of these women reported that the abuse began during their pregnancy (Rodgers 1994). In a study by Stewart and Cecutti (1993) 6.6 percent of the pregnant women surveyed reported abuse during the current pregnancy.

4. The categories are taken from the "Power and Control Wheel" developed by the Duluth Domestic Violence Intervention Project (Pence and Paymar 1986). The Violence Against Women Survey also questioned women about many of these same forms of abusive behavior (Statistics Canada 1994).

5. Several articles provide a topology of these theories (see Johnson 1996; Campbell and Landenburger 1995).

6. As Kathryn Morgan notes in Chapter 5, these ascribed differences are often portrayed as natural.

7. These findings underscore one of the difficulties in doing research on the abuse of women in their intimate relationships. Women in transition houses represent a population that has been repeatedly studied, since they are easier for researchers to access than those who do not deal with social agencies. Women in transition houses are a selected-out population in that they have likely experienced escalating violence, have sought resources, and have been motivated to go to the transition house for safety. These realities may account for the difference between the lower disclosure rate in the general population, as compared with the disclosure rate among women using transition houses.

8. Of the twenty women interviewed in a study by Head and Taft (1995), every one of them had her symptoms dealt with medico-pharmaceutically by a physician at some point.

9. The hope of "rescue" is based in the fallacious, but understandable, assumption on the part of the woman that the physician will have some power or legal authority over the perpetrator and be able to "do something" to end the violence. As discussed below, some guidelines promise to physicians precisely this power to end the violence.

10. It is important to appreciate that while biomedical patterns of thought and practice are pervasive they are not all-encompassing. Many physicians manage to work with categories of disease without stripping their patients' lives of context. But even those physicians who are not ordinarily wedded to the "disease-centered" approach, may well revert to the medical model of care when they perceive the problem to be "opening a Pandora's box" (Ferris and Tudiver 1992).

11. See Chapter 5 for a full discussion of medicalization.

12. It is important to observe that at the same time that significant numbers of health care practitioners fail to identify abuse, or fail to see it as relevant to health care, there has been a proliferation of mental health professionals (psy-

chologists, psychiatrists, social workers) firmly wedded to the medical model, specializing in the "diagnosis" and "treatment" of abusive men and of abused women. Indeed, the currency of such labels as "battered woman syndrome," and of such theories as the "intergenerational transmission of violence," speak to the tremendous influence that mental health professionals, and biomedical patterns of gaining insight, have had upon our "common sense" understandings of intimate violence.

13. In one study, women reported that brochures in the waiting room or "stop abuse" buttons worn by medical staff prompted them to make disclosures (White 1991).

14. The means and intensity of the requirement to screen could vary, from moral persuasion, to professional pressure, to making the matter a subject of codes of professional conduct and subject to discipline by the professional governing body.

15. Disclosures of physical or sexual abuse, or of the neglect of a child, puts even the most woman-positive physician in a bind. She or he may feel a duty to the child to protect him or her from harm, and making good on this duty may require a breach of confidence. In most jurisdictions, this moral duty is accompanied by a legal duty, obliging the physician to report the abuse to child welfare authorities. Yet at the same time one's duty to the woman—both to respect her confidence and to protect her from harm (the harm of exposing her to retaliatory violence, the harm of losing her children) may conflict with the duty to the child. This dilemma is exacerbated by the reality that child welfare interventions tend to pit mothers against their children, rather than to support and protect women so that they might more effectively mother their children (Sheeran 1996). As more jurisdictions move toward the incorporation of child abuse definitions that include the witnessing of domestic violence by a child, physicians (and others) are increasingly put in this bind.

16. Positive predictors for physicians to screen and respond appropriately to interpersonal violence are as follows: medical school training that includes a curriculum on domestic violence; in-training supervised clinical experience with wife abuse victim-survivors, and site placement with social agencies working in the field of domestic violence. These predictors also correlated with physicians' expressed comfort when working with this patient population. While more women physicians expressed comfort with both screening for and responding to wife abuse, no gender difference was found in patient satisfaction if physicians demonstrated comfort with wife abuse during the medical encounter. Hence, we recommend that some form of supervised training in this field be required in addition to published protocols.

17. "Learned helplessness" draws life from the medical model; it attempts to make sense of women's actions through the individualistic, psychologized lens of the medical model. While clearly abuse often results in detrimental psychological consequences, the problem with this approach (as with the application of the medical model more generally) is that it treats abuse as an in-

dividual problem and occludes the social and structural factors—the material realities of women's lives—that often virtually entrap some women in abusive relationships.

18. While in the early days of abuse protocol development it was recommended that women leave, we now know that leaving brings with it the risk of escalating abuse, including stalking and homicide, and that abuse continues to take place in childcare transfers after separation. Hence, leaving is no longer the standard recommendation. Assessing risk potential and safety, apprising the woman's own perception of her relative risk and needs is essential. Yet some provincial protocols sit in place, with leaving as a fundamental recommendation. At a minimum, then, protocols need some form of revision accountability and updating as we learn about the unpredicted, yet present, attendant harms in some of the recommendations.

19. Various manifestations of these views have been documented in surveys that ask physicians why they do not inquire about abuse.

10 Reframing Research Involving Humans

Françoise Baylis
Jocelyn Downie
Susan Sherwin

In spring 1994, in the wake of several research-related controversies,[1] the Tri-Council Working Group, involving Canada's three major national funding agencies—the Medical Research Council (MRC), the Natural Sciences and Engineering Research Council (NSERC), and the Social Sciences and Humanities Research Council (SSHRC)—was convened at the initiative of the Ministry of Health and the Ministry of Industry and Commerce. The goal was to develop a common set of ethics guidelines (not legislation) that would govern research involving humans in Canada.[2] The task initially set by the chair, however, was "more circumscribed, namely, to revise the '87 [MRC] guidelines where necessary" (Working Group on Ethics Guidelines for Research with Human Subjects 1994, 7). In fall 1994, the Tri-Council Working Group (hereafter, the Working Group) issued a call for input on its task.

Now, whereas many academics believe that they should try to remove themselves from the influence of any special interests in the pursuit of some abstract ideal of "truth," feminists believe that interestedness is more effective in inquiry than disinterestedness, and that knowledge is not incompatible with political and emotional interests. In our view, doing ethics well requires express moral commitments that are clearly visible when addressing ethical issues. Ethics is far more than an intellectual exercise or an application of certain philosophical skills; it is an effort to determine what sorts of behaviors are to be encouraged and what sorts condemned. For us, it also includes a commitment to promoting what is morally right and correcting what is morally wrong. Further, in our view, it is only when ethicists engage in public debate and attend to the implications of their positions in actual policy that they are likely to develop sufficient understanding of the issues in question to decide on morally appropriate practices.[3] Thus, members of the Feminist Health Care Ethics

Research Network (hereafter, the Network), rejecting the view that ethical theory and political activism are and must remain distinct activities, chose to respond to the call for input and thereby to engage in the political process initiated by the Working Group (Baylis 1996). While our Network was organized around research activities, we determined that our research agenda required us to take the opportunity offered by the Working Group to influence the guidelines for research involving humans, from a feminist perspective.

In this chapter we document the work of the Network as we participated in the public consultation process in an effort to ensure that the concerns of women and others who are systematically oppressed in society were not overlooked. First, we provide an overview of the theoretical views that informed the Network's participation. Second, we outline several specific feminist concerns regarding research involving humans. Third, we summarize and review the Network's various attempts to engage in the policy-making process. Then, in closing, we focus on the themes of the book—autonomy, agency and politics—and reflect briefly on the substance and process we discuss.

Theoretical Framework

Our conception of a feminist approach to the ethical questions associated with research involving humans is rooted in both feminist ethics and feminist epistemology. Feminist ethics explores questions about political relations as well as interpersonal ones. Unlike traditional (nonfeminist) ethics, which tends to focus on interactions among individuals (such as between physician and patient or researcher and subject) in isolation from the context in which they are situated, feminist ethics promotes an awareness of the various ways in which people's interpersonal relationships are also structured by larger social patterns; power attaches to people as members of social groups and not merely as a consequence of their own efforts in the world. Feminist ethics is especially concerned with systematic patterns of oppression in a society. This perspective encourages us to consider how expectations are derived from deeply entrenched social patterns that structure social institutions and practices. It also helps us to appreciate how these institutions and practices help to maintain oppressive patterns, for example, by serving some groups' interests at the expense of others. Finally, because it is ultimately committed to challenging and eliminating oppression, feminist ethics asks us to consider how these institutions and practices can be modified to reduce their oppressive impact and increase their liberatory potential.[4]

As such, feminist ethics provides us with a framework for review-ing the norms that govern research involving and affecting women and members of other oppressed groups in a way that invites us to consider how research practices have harmed women and others (individually and collectively). By raising the familiar feminist questions "Whose in-terests are served?" and "Whose interests are harmed?" the ways in which research has historically tended to serve the interests of privi-leged social groups and to subordinate those of oppressed groups is made visible. Further, feminist ethics' commitment to social change en-courages us to consider how current research practices might be re-formed to better serve the interests of those who have been disadvan-taged, and thus to improve their health status. Appealing to a concept of social justice that involves not only fair distribution of identifiable and quantifiable benefits and burdens in society but also fair relations among social groups (see Young 1990), feminist ethics allows us to see the sorts of institutional changes necessary if the conduct of research is to meet the standards of justice that it should.

Feminist epistemology encourages us to challenge the traditional dis-tinction between active researcher-participant and passive object of study.[5] The traditional view is rooted in the belief that accurate scientific observation must be conducted by disinterested parties who study "pure" data that is "free" from the influence of personal interests. Partic-ular interests and desires on the part of either the researcher-participant or the subject-participant are commonly thought to pose a risk of distor-tion since either or both parties might consciously or unconsciously ma-nipulate the process and thereby skew the research results. Such interest-based distortion is considered to be especially risky in the case of subject-participants because they are typically assumed to be unknowl-edgeable about the technicalities and requirements of the research process. Hence, if subject-participants have reason to prefer one outcome to another, it is feared that they will modify their behavior or reports to represent that outcome. It is also thought that even highly trained researcher-participants—who are well schooled in the importance of maintaining neutral, dispassionate postures, who appreciate the need to remain open to whatever results appear, and who are thoroughly com-mitted to the necessity of minimizing the effect of their own preferences on their observations by erasing the details of their own status in the process of data collection—run the risk of unconsciously contaminating data whenever they have a personal stake in detecting one outcome over others. Hence, for generations scientists have been trained in the ideol-ogy of "the scientific method," which requires them to approach their work under norms of objectivity understood to mean that they conduct their research with no preferences about the outcome(s) that results. This approach encourages them to discount the specificity of their own locations and concerns and it obscures rather than addresses the particular nature of each scientist's distinct agency in the research process.

Feminist epistemologists have been critical of such interpretations of objectivity (Harding 1991). They have argued that researcher-participants are seldom truly indifferent to the outcomes of their studies and that the inevitable personal interests involved are most dangerous when denied rather than made explicit. Science is not a value-neutral activity in practice, nor should it aspire to be. The demands of disinterestedness do promote, not better science, but rather science that preferentially serves some interests and neglects others while blocking efforts to expose that fact by denying and thereby hiding the interests that are operative. When the determinate interests are those of the dominant group(s) in society, they seem to be both natural and general since they blend seamlessly with the cultural dominance of those groups in all spheres of activity. It is only the particular interests of marginalized groups (i.e., those who are subject to oppression) that appear to be "special interests" that threaten to complicate or contaminate otherwise "pure" scientific methods. Feminist epistemology helps us to understand the importance of challenging the underlying assumptions about the conduct of research in order to ensure that research programs not perpetuate patterns of privilege and oppression but rather break down such forms of injustice. In such ways, scientific research can help to promote the well-being and autonomy of members of oppressed groups.

Some Feminist Concerns Regarding Research Involving Humans

In this section, we apply the theoretical underpinnings of feminist ethics and epistemology more directly to concrete problems with research involving members of oppressed groups, and in particular women. These issues are discussed with particular (but not exclusive) attention to biomedical and pharmacological research, under the following headings: exclusion and underrepresentation, exploitation, and research priorities.

Exclusion and Underrepresentation

The exclusion and underrepresentation of women subject-participants is, at this time, the most visible and widely debated issue concerning women in the research process. As Rebecca Dresser (1992) notes, women's exclusion is "ubiquitous." For example, using age-standardized mortality rates, coronary heart disease is the leading cause of death among North American women (Wilkins and Mark 1992) and yet, a study sponsored by the National Institutes of Health (NIH) "showing that heart attacks were reduced when subjects took one aspirin every other day was conducted on men, and the relationship between low cholesterol diets and cardiovascular disease has been almost exclusively studied in men" (Dresser 1992, 24). Two-thirds of the elderly population are women (on average women live eight years longer than men) and yet, "the first twenty years of a major federal study on health and aging included only men." In fact, until quite recently, issues pertinent to women and aging have been seriously understudied. Women suffer from migraines up to three times as often as men and yet, "the announcement that aspirin can help prevent migraine headaches is based on data from males only." Women are the fastest growing AIDS population and yet, "studies on AIDS treatment frequently omit women." Women, not men, get uterine cancer and yet, "a pilot project on the impact of obesity on breast and uterine cancer [was] conducted . . . solely on men."[6] A direct consequence of this sort of exclusion is that the data necessary for making choices regarding prevention and treatment for women are unavailable and must be inferred from data collected about men, even though there are important physiological and psychosocial differences between men and women that make such inferences problematic.

In addition to the problem of complete exclusion, there are the related problems of significant underrepresentation and the failure to undertake appropriate gender-based analyses of the research data. Many of those who contest the claim that women have been excluded from research fail to appreciate that the issue is not just the inclusion of some women but the inclusion of women in numbers proportionate to the population expected to benefit from the research results. Of equal concern is the way in which the data are collected and analyzed. In many instances in which women are included in research, the research is not designed to look for anything that is specific to women, or to specific groups of women (e.g., those who are elderly, pregnant, or poor).

In recent years the principle of inclusion and representation has been accepted by North American policy makers. In the United States, the NIH and the Federal Drug Agency (FDA) recently passed guidelines concerning the inclusion and representation of women and minorities in most clinical research studies.[7] And, on September 25, 1996, a policy statement regarding the inclusion and representation of women in clinical trials during drug development was issued by the Drugs Directorate of Health Canada. The policy explicitly requires "the enroll-ment of a representative number of women into clinical trials for those drugs that are intended to be used specifically by women or in popula-tions that are expected to include women" (Drugs Directorate, Health Canada 1996, 2). Not surprisingly, however, political change has brought political resistance. This resistance is manifested in at least three ways. Some deny the claim that women have been excluded from and under-represented in research; others deny that the exclusion and underrep-resentation of women has harmed women; and others attempt to justify the exclusion and underrepresentation.[8]

The first form of resistance to the principle of required inclusion and representation is evident in the widespread movement among researcher-participants and others to deny that women have ever been (improperly) excluded from or underrepresented in research. This claim is difficult to rebut because data regarding study composition typ-ically are not reported in a manner that would facilitate the requisite analysis.[9] In the United States, at least, this was the finding of the Insti-tute of Medicine Committee on Ethical and Legal Issues Relating to the Inclusion of Women in Clinical Studies (Mastroianni, Faden, and Fed-erman 1994), which had considerable resources at its disposal to address this very issue. The committee concluded that the full data were unavailable. It did find, however, examples of federal policies and particular protocols that had the effect of treating female subject-participants differently from male subject-participants. It also found ev-idence of gender inequity in at least two significant areas of research: coronary heart disease and AIDS (Mastroianni, Faden, and Federman 1994). In these areas of study, the exclusion and underrepresentation of women were deemed to be significant because of known important dif-ferences between men and women in the disease presentation, progres-sion, and response to trial interventions. Whereas in some areas of re-search it is possible (and appropriate) to extrapolate data from one gender to another (e.g., studies on antibiotics), with cardiovascular and AIDS research the gender-based disparities are such that data from male-only studies cannot be appropriately generalized to females.

The second form of resistance to the principle of required inclusion and representation is the denial of the harm resulting from exclusion and underrepresentation. But consider, for example, the exclusion of women from many of the studies on cardiovascular disease that have signifi-cantly influenced both prevention and treatment: MRFIT, Coronary Drug Project (CPD), Lipid Research Clinic, and the Physician's Health Study (Healy 1991). This exclusion has been harmful to women in at least two ways. First, it has resulted in "insufficient information about preventive strategies, diagnostic testing, responses to medical and surgical therapies, and other aspects of cardiovascular illness in women" (Wenger, Speroff, and Packard 1993). Second, as a result, women have been offered less effective or ineffective interventions. For example, the Physician's Health Study (a male-only study) found that an aspirin every other day reduced heart attacks. Subsequent data has shown, however, that while aspirin is an effective primary preventative for men, it is not so for women (McAnally, Corn, and Hamilton 1992). Consider also, the exclusion of women from AIDS research. As late as 1991, there were "virtually no published, prospective data on the natural history of HIV infection in women or IVDUs [intravenous drug users]." Furthermore, "as with the natural history, the literature to date on the clinical management of HIV infection [was] necessarily based almost exclusively on reports involving male patients" (Modlin and Saah 1991, 39). As the disease may manifest itself differently in women than men (Modlin and Saah, 1991), there is no doubt that as a result of the male bias in the research, women's health care has been seriously compromised. Clearly, resulting knowledge gaps have limited women's ability to make informed choices about their health care and thus unjustly limited their ability to exercise full autonomy in the affected areas.

A similar male-bias prevails in occupational health research. A recent example is a study by Jack Siemiatycki and colleagues (1989) on cancer risks associated with certain occupational exposures. When challenged to defend the decision to exclude women from the research, Siemiatycki simply stated, "It's a cost-benefit analysis; women don't get many occupational cancers" (cited in Messing 1995, 231). But Siemiatycki's analysis is invalid. Because of the exclusion of women from occupational health research, we simply do not know the incidence of occupational cancers among women. The absence of knowledge that he and others perpetuate through exclusionary studies is harmful to women because it is confused with absence of occupational cancers and then used to justify continued exclusion of women from relevant research. And, lest one think this is an isolated incident in the realm of occupational research, it is worth noting that 73 percent of all research funded by the Quebec Institute for Research in Occupational Health and Safety during its first six years of operation involved absolutely no women workers (Tremblay 1990).

Further, in the realm of psychological research, we find the influential Kohlberg studies on moral development (1984). As Carol Gilligan demonstrated (to name his most influential critic), Lawrence

Kohlberg's work left invisible an entire supplementary, if not alternative, approach to moral decision-making. As with the other examples discussed above, the harms of the exclusion went beyond invisibility. In this case, they extended to what Kathryn Morgan (1987) has characterized as "moral madness."

It is telling that many of the researcher-participants who deny the exclusion and underrepresentation of women in research are among those who object to the provisions aimed at insuring adequate inclusion and representation. Arguably, this undercuts their denial of such exclusion and underrepresentation. If indeed women have not been excluded from or underrepresented in research, and thus special provisions to insure their appropriate inclusion and representation are unnecessary, then why the vigorous objections to initiatives that presumably would only codify existing practice? If, on the other hand, these initiatives do demand changes in current practice, the objections of researcher-participants seem to suggest that they do indeed prefer to conduct their studies without the complications that may be created by including women in the subject-participant population. These complications may include dealing with the hormonal changes of the menstrual cycle (and the possible use of exogenous hormones) and the need for a larger subject-participant population to insure statistical significance, as well as the tracking of data along more variables.

The final form of resistance to the required inclusion and representation of women involves attempts to justify the exclusion and underrepresentation. For example, it is argued that women can be appropriately excluded from research that examines male-specific conditions. While there is no disagreement with this claim, disagreement arises when the justification for excluding women extends to research on conditions that occur disproportionately in males (e.g., spinal cord injuries) or research using a male population simply for reasons of convenience. Also suspect are claims based on the importance of a homogeneous research population, the need to protect women and fetuses from research harms, and the increased costs associated with the participation of women (see, for example, Baylis 1996).

Consider first the claim that "good science" requires the use of a homogeneous research population. In the realm of the biomedical sciences it is argued, from the perspective of researcher-participants, that "the more alike the [subject-participants], the more any variation can be attributed to the experimental intervention" (Dresser 1992, 25). On this basis it is argued that including women in specific research protocols unnecessarily "complicates" the research. Such "complications" are deemed unnecessary because women and men "have more biological similarities than differences" (Piantadosi and Wittes 1993, 565). Now, most often when women are excluded from research it is on the basis of stipulated inclusion-exclusion criteria. At times, however, they are included in the original subject-participant population and their data is later removed (i.e., not included in the final analysis). One striking example (among many) of the scientific elimination of women from a study is the research by Gladys Block and colleagues on cancer among phosphate-exposed workers in a fertilizer plant. One-hundred-and-seventy-three women were included among the thirty-four hundred subject-participants. Their data was eliminated from the research results with the sole comment that "females accounted for only about 5% of the study population, and were not included in these analyses" (Block et al. 1988, 7298).

There are several possible responses to the argument that researchers must keep the sample uniform. First, even if there are legitimate scientific reasons for studying populations that are as "uniform" as possible, it does not follow that the homogenous group to be studied should be white males. If women and men "have more biological similarities than differences" such that it is sufficient to study one gender, why assume that "the white male is the normal representative human being"? (Dresser 1992, 28). Second, it is well-documented that, in at least some areas of health care, drug trials for instance, there is good reason to believe that women and men will respond differently to the study intervention. Factors such as body weight, body surface, and ratio of lean to adipose tissue can affect optimal doses as can the greater concentration of steroids in men's bodies, the differences in hormones, the use of artificial hormones by women (for birth control, control of menopausal symptoms, fertility treatments), and so on. Vanessa Merton (1994) writes: "Without good science that includes the full range of human subjects, patients who depart from the white male norm will not have the advantage of good clinical medicine—medicine that addresses their problems and works safely and effectively for them" (276). Focusing on one type of human physiology reduces the generalizability of the experimental data and thus reduces the scientific utility of the research. The "best" approach should surely be linked to the promise of benefit to society (broadly construed).

Consider now the specter of miscarriages and birth defects. Reference is frequently made to concerns about women who are or who could become pregnant while enrolled in clinical trials. This view is problematic in that it is both overinclusive and underinclusive. It is overinclusive because, in the name of protection for potentially pregnant women and their fetuses, all women lose opportunities to improve their health and possibly extend their lives. Complete exclusion of women subject-participants is an unnecessarily blunt instrument to accomplish the goal of fetal protection. This approach is also underinclusive because it ignores the fact that research participation can carry reproductive risks for men as well as women. For example, it is possible that the research intervention will genetically damage the sperm or, in the alternative, that a new substance will bind to the sperm without affecting motility. If the sperm is able to effectively fertilize an ovum, this could result in birth defects in the offspring. And yet, the specter of birth defects is not used to justify a blanket exclusion of men. It should also be noted here that only a very small class of clinical studies are relevant to fetal well-being.

Finally, consider the claim of the prohibitive cost of inclusion. One of the main reasons for the powerful resistance to the principle of inclusion is the fear that inclusion requirements will increase the costs of particular studies and hence make them more difficult to conduct. Unless there are known important gender differences, it is argued that there is no need to assume the additional costs of including women subject-participants. The short response to this is that when there is no anticipated statistical difference between men and women, it is appropriate to include both and inappropriate to exclude either. Such inclusion allows for the possibility of recognizing unanticipated differences provided that gender is coded for. More important, one must recognize that a potential increase in the financial cost of conducting a particular trial is not the only cost associated with the equal participation of men and women in research. As Merton (1994) notes, the question that must be asked is "cost to whom?" (273). Typically the costs considered are those borne by the researcher-participant (e.g., costs associated with recruiting and retaining a larger subject-participant population and costs associated with tracking and analyzing data along more variables), not those borne by the persons whose health may be negatively affected by the absence of relevant health data. While it is likely that a principle of inclusion will involve some additional costs to the researcher-participants, these are legitimate costs to be incurred for the benefit of the subject-participants.

The Risk of Exploitation

It is important not to translate the call for greater research attention toward women and other oppressed groups into a wholesale endorsement of the use of members of oppressed groups as subject-participants in all studies. Clinical trials often expose subject-participants to significant risk, discomfort, or inconvenience without offering any special benefits to either the subject-participants or the groups from which they are recruited. Many shameful events in the history of clinical research testify to the ease with which researcher-participants have exploited the vulnerability of oppressed or devalued members of society for the ultimate benefit of others.

The Nazi studies on concentration camp residents and the Tuskegee syphilis study are two of the most notorious examples in this category (Grodin 1992; Jones 1981). A more contemporary example of exploitation, one involving the exploitation of women, is the contraceptive research in the United States on minority populations (e.g., Enovid studies on Puerto Rican and Mexican American women [Hamilton 1996]), and in the Third World (e.g., Norplant studies in Bangladesh, Sri Lanka, the Philippines, the Dominican Republic, Chile, and Nigeria [Hamilton 1996]). There is also the suggestion that experimental AIDS vaccines be tested in high-risk populations in the Third World such as prostitutes in Thailand (Hamilton 1996).

While most ethics guidelines recognize the need to take special precautions with certain groups, such as children, prisoners, and very ill patients, none seem to have appreciated that members of oppressed groups also face unacceptable risks of exploitation in a society that values them less highly than members of other groups and so is more inclined to expose them to risk. To guard against such exploitation, clinical studies that propose to recruit women or members of other oppressed groups should be required to demonstrate that the results produced will be of specific benefit to the individuals or to the group in question (see Sherwin 1992, 159–65).

We recognize that some feminists are wary of this principle because it seems to invite paternalistic approaches to women's participation in research. Their argument against it might run as follows: it allows others to decide whether women should be invited to participate in certain studies; it implies that women are not capable of making such decisions for themselves; there is no reason to assume that women are any less qualified than other competent potential subject-participants to make these decisions independently and no need for special protections to be built in for them as they are for members of groups thought incompetent to make such decisions; and, moreover, given the historical tendency to exclude women from studies that promise benefits to the participants and to women generally (as discussed above), it is a mistake to build in a principle that serves as a license to disregard our first principle (of inclusion) and allows perpetuation of the historical pattern of exclusion of women from research.

We are sympathetic to this concern but ultimately are not convinced by the argument. We believe it rests on an individualistic view of autonomy that we reject in favor of a more nuanced relational approach (see Chapter 2). Specifically, we believe that it is important to keep in mind the role that oppression plays in the choices made by members of oppressed groups as potential research subject-participants. Members of oppressed groups experience a far greater risk of exploitation than members of more privileged groups. In our view, the oppression of women is so deeply entrenched in our culture that it often goes unnoticed and women's training in self-sacrifice could mean that many women would be overly compliant with researcher-participants' efforts at recruitment and retention of women subject-participants. Hence, we believe it remains necessary to take steps to ensure that the exploitation of women is not operating in research contexts.

Two additional but closely related issues must be considered in the context of exploitation: first, the lack of clear distinctions between therapy and innovative practice on one hand and research and innovative practice on the other; and second, the resultant lack of norms for innovative practice.[10] Research, unlike innovative practice, is governed by regulations and guidelines that require peer review (before the initiation of the study or the publication of its results), detailed disclosure of information to prospective subject-participants regarding potential harms and benefits, and careful monitoring and the implementation of other precautionary measures to reduce the risk of harm. In contrast, less rigorous controls exist for conventional therapies, and still less for innovative practices.

Historically, many interventions have been developed and offered to women as innovative practices without adequate prior research to establish their safety and efficacy. Consider, for example, contraceptives (Dalkon Shield, early doses of birth control pills), drugs prescribed in pregnancy (DES, thalidomide), and the ever-expanding practices in the area of new reproductive technologies. As a result of the failure to adequately research these "innovations" many women have been seriously harmed. Therapy, research, and innovative practice must be carefully distinguished and innovative practices must be subject to careful scrutiny. Moreover, when dealing with practices offered solely to members of an oppressed group it is especially important to rigorously scrutinize the proposed practices.

Research Priorities: What They Are and Who Sets Them

The research agenda regarding the health needs of women and members of other oppressed groups has historically neglected many important questions. For example, even though the links between poverty and illness are well known, health research often focuses on ways of responding to illness rather than avoiding it in the first place. Also, it is noteworthy that many clinical studies explore expensive, highly technological innovations, even though such treatments will be economically inaccessible to most people in the world. In sharp contrast to the neglect of many of the health needs of women, there has been a substantial body of research directed at gaining control over women's reproduction. In this area, women have received a disproportionately large share of research attention, and, as a result, women must now assume an unfair share of the burden, risks, expenses, and responsibility for managing fertility, because that is where the knowledge base is. The concentration of medical attention on women's reproductive role not only assumes but also reinforces the conventional view that women are, by nature, to be responsible and available for reproductive activities; it also legitimizes, reinforces, and further entrenches such views and the oppressive attitudes that accompany them.

This unacceptably narrow research focus underscores the importance of moving the control of the research agenda from the hands of an elite group of knowledgeable scientists to a more democratically representative group. In our view, the prevailing norms, according to which research subject-participants are reduced to passive objects of study, is unacceptable. Along with Sandra Harding (1991), and other feminist scholars, we propose that research be pursued as a collegial activity; under this model, subject-participants and researcher-participants collectively negotiate the terms of participation and the goals of the activity. We believe that it is both possible and desirable to conduct scientifically valid research that involves subject-participants in the initial formulation of the research questions to pursue and the method of study, as well as the decision about whether to participate once all the terms of participation have been set. Provided that an effort is made to involve subject-participants with diverse perspectives and experiences, such engagement need not undermine the research endeavor or the validity of the research results. Relational autonomy demands that members of oppressed groups, in particular, be made active participants in the process of determining research priorities and approaches. Restricting a group's involvement to the opportunity to consent to or refuse subject status on a predetermined project retains the focus on agency alone, and not the more encompassing notion of relational autonomy.

We recognize the moral and epistemological value of efforts aimed at reversing the traditional research pattern in which researcher-participants and those who support their work (funding agencies, publishers, colleagues), who are predominately drawn from the most privileged sectors of society (white, male, middle class), decide what research projects to pursue and who to recruit to participate in them and on what terms. In place of the traditional pattern we envision a research program that is designed to ensure that the least powerful and most vulnerable participants—those who are, at best, typically afforded the opportunity only to agree or refuse to participate in a set protocol—gain an opportunity to ensure that the research to be pursued is responsive to their interests and needs.

From Theory to Practice

Our aims, as the Network, were to ensure that the new ethics guidelines governing research with humans give prominence to these feminist values and contain specific proposals to make them operational. This goal required multiple decisions about how best to influence the process and have an impact on the group charged with establishing the new guidelines.

Creating the Space

As noted, in fall 1994 the Working Group issued a public memorandum inviting submissions from all interested parties. The initial deadline for submissions was December 15, 1994, and the projected completion date for the new research guidelines was spring 1995. With the call for input, the Working Group released seven questions for consideration and an issues paper outlining seventeen sections to be addressed in the revised guidelines.

It was very clear from the beginning that our vision of the appropriate task for the Working Group was much broader than the one it had envisioned for itself. The specific questions asked, the time line set, and private conversations with some members of the Working Group all indicated that initially the Working Group was planning simply to tinker with the existing MRC Guidelines, making minor corrections here and there and broadening the scope of the Guidelines to make them relevant to the other two granting agencies. By defining its mandate as (modestly) revisionary, rather than visionary, it seemed clear that the Working Group planned to avoid addressing many of the deep questions surrounding research involving humans, questions that tend to be invisible to those who do not adopt a feminist perspective.

The changes we sought in the ethics guidelines had to do with fundamental assumptions about research activity; hence, they required significant rethinking of the whole field of research ethics. Addressing our concerns would, therefore, require a longer time than initially envisioned and a far more open debate than the Working Group planned. Our first objective, then, was to encourage the Working Group to broaden its mandate and to allow for greater public input into its deliberations; in other words, we began by seeking to change a process the Working Group had tried to impose.

We lobbied for these procedural changes at an open forum the Working Group held in November 1994 at the annual meeting of the Canadian Bioethics Society (CBS). In the discussion period, we called for more time and more opportunity for public participation in the process. We also raised concerns about: (1) the moral framework for the revised guidelines (i.e., despite the generally recognized insufficiency of the principles of autonomy, beneficence, nonmaleficence, and justice,[11] it appeared that these principles might nevertheless be taken as the moral framework for the revised guidelines); (2) the need to attend to the political, social, and cultural context of research involving humans (e.g., Who determines what counts as research? and Who sets the research agenda?); and (3) the need for a broader conception of health and research methods. Happily, this intervention was well received by those present and our concerns were featured in an official communiqué sent to the Working Group on behalf of the CBS by its president. There was widespread consensus in the bioethics community that the process should not be rushed and that the Working Group should seek significantly more input from across the country. The deadlines were subsequently relaxed and we had concrete evidence that the process could be changed.

The First Official Submission to the Working Group

We determined that the best way for us to influence the Working Group's substantive deliberations was to prepare an official submission that would identify and explain the concerns we thought relevant from the perspective of feminist ethics.[12] More broadly, we thought it important to offer a feminist critique of the way the Working Group had defined its agenda and also to indicate concretely how our concerns could be addressed by modifications to existing guidelines. In spring 1995, the submission was completed and circulated to all members of the Working Group. In addition, subsections of the submission (parts 1 and 2) were circulated to others, including CBS participants who had indicated an interest in receiving a copy of our final text. Our submission was structured in part in response to the agenda set out by the Working Group in the original memorandum inviting public comment (Working Group 1994) and in part according to our own understanding of how the issues should be framed for the Working Group. By combining our own sense of how to shape the discussion with an openness to responding in the terms invited by the Working Group, we acknowledged the specific context in which we were working for change. This could be seen explicitly in the structure of our submission. Part 1 of our submission briefly spelled out our theoretical perspective and made explicit the breadth of the revisions we sought, and the ethical basis for such a broad approach. In part 2 of the submission, we turned our attention to the specific questions posed by the Working Group:

1. Do you use the current Guidelines of one of the Councils in planning and conducting your research? If not, why not? If you do, in what way do you use them?
2. What needs to be changed to make current Guidelines more useful and relevant?
3. What difficulties, if any, do you experience in the ethical review of research proposals? How should these difficulties be addressed?
4. What problems, if any, exist in obtaining informed consent for research?
5. What issues about the functioning of Research Ethics Boards (REBs) should the Guidelines address?
6. Have you encountered research-related issues that concern you? Please give examples and how you solved them.
7. What format for the Guidelines would be most useful for you? Please provide examples.

We did not attempt to answer all of these questions. Rather, we focused narrowly on question 2, the only question we could identify that would capture the broad range of concerns we wanted addressed. We structured our response to include several general comments followed by a discussion of specific concerns regarding women in research studies. Three general themes emerged: the risk of underrepresentation and exclusion, the risk of exploitation, and the risk of exclusion from the process by which research decisions are made and carried out.

In part 3 of our submission we considered some of the topics the Working Group had identified as foci for their discussions under the following subheadings: I. The Context of Research Involving Humans and

Research Ethics;[13] II. Areas of Research Involving Humans;[14] and III. Process Issues.[15] In particular, we expressed very strong reservations about section 10, Genetic Research, and Section 11, Embryos and Fetuses.

Finally, in part 4 of our submission, in an effort to make sure that our theoretical concerns would be translated appropriately into the revised research guidelines, we systematically worked through the existing MRC Guidelines to show how these could be modified to be more attentive to feminist concerns. We identified the site of each of our proposed changes and we offered an explanation or justification for each suggested revision. We thought this level of detail was necessary because we had been given to believe that the Working Group would only be tinkering with the existing MRC Guidelines and we believed that if we actually provided draft text that our suggested revisions were more likely to be understood and adopted. Thus, parts 1 and 4 represented our efforts to reframe the discussion from the limited focus proposed by the Working Group; as "bookends," they framed our responses to both the specific questions posed by the Working Group and those introduced by the Network.

In the months that followed, several members of the Network presented various aspects of our first submission to various audiences.[16] In general, the responses to the presentations and to the written submission were enthusiastic and encouraging.

The First Unofficial Submission to a Member of the Working Group

In the fall 1995, at the initiative of one member of the Working Group, we were invited to comment on a draft of the subsection on populations at risk of exclusion from or exploitation in research. In our report back to the member of the Working Group we made several specific suggestions.[17] Following the format dictated by the Working Group, we proposed eight revised guidelines in which we insisted on the importance of including women in clinical trials in adequate numbers, forbidding research that excludes or underrepresents women without ethically compelling justification, prohibiting the exploitation of women (especially disadvantaged women), and not using pregnancy or childbearing potential as an automatic exclusion criterion. On this last issue, we also attempted to outline some of the relevant considerations in proceeding with research involving pregnant and fertile women.

The Second Official Submission to the Working Group

In March 1996, the Working Group published a draft "Code of Conduct" and invited public comment. We were pleasantly surprised to find that the document was sensitive to many of the issues we had raised in our first official submission. In particular, it did include references to inclusion of women and other disadvantaged groups (though they did not fully appreciate the complexities of this requirement). As well, we noted that much of our "unofficial submission" to a member of the Working Group was included almost verbatim. The areas in which disagreement remained, however, were quite telling. Most notable was the Working Group's decision to (1) adopt a philosophical framework that relied on the three or four principles approach to bioethics; (2) remain silent on the distinctions between therapy, research, and innovative practice, (3) allow researcher-participants to require that all women in particular studies be on contraceptives; and (4) ignore the larger political, social, and ethical questions concerning control of the research agenda. These and other concerns were again noted in our second submission to the Working Group.[18]

It seemed that both formal and informal strategies had had some effect, but the limits to our influence around issues of power and control were telling and worrisome.

The Second Unofficial Submission to a Member of the Working Group

After public release of the first draft document, the Working Group was reconstituted. Among other changes, one member was added who did explicitly feminist research. This newly constituted group proceeded to make extensive revisions to the draft Code previously circulated. Once again, at the initiative of another member of the Working Group we were invited to comment on work in progress that overlapped with our area of interest. In an effort to assist this person and to advance the concerns of women we offered a number of suggestions.[19] For example, we indicated that the proposed section on inclusiveness should carefully distinguish between two very different sorts of problems—insufficient inclusion and inappropriate inclusion. In discussing the first of these problems we pointed out that the objective is not only to ensure that equal numbers of men and women are recruited as research participants but also to ensure that there is appropriate subgroup analyses of the data so that one may identify relevant differences. On the second issue, we argued that women and other members of disadvantaged groups should not bear an unfair share of the burden of research participation, or be excluded from an appropriate share of the benefits of research.

In addition, we registered a serious concern about several omissions: (1) the continued inattention to the differences between research, therapy, and innovative practices and the need for more rigorous review of innovative practices offered as therapy when they should be subject to research review; (2) the ongoing silence on the question who controls the research agenda; and (3) the absence of a separate section on women as research participants that would discuss unique issues such as research involving women of childbearing potential, pregnant women, and lactating women.

The External Review Process

In the final phase of the project, the Working Group invited five scholars to a meeting in Toronto to serve as external reviewers. Each reviewer was provided with a second draft of the Code, now titled "Code of Ethical Conduct for Research Involving Humans (February 1997)."[20] A member of the Network (FB) was among the invited reviewers, but not in this capacity. Nonetheless, many of the Network's general concerns were raised in both the written submission and the verbal presentation. Particular attention was paid to the section originally titled "Exploitation or Exclusion" and later retitled "Justice and Inclusion in Research." This section now included only two prescriptive clauses concerning women, both of which were seriously flawed. The first clause stipulated that women be included in research "when possible and appropriate." Significantly, no such exception qualified the previous prescriptive clause that required the inclusion of members of social, cultural, and racial groups. The other prescriptive clause about women stated that, "presumably fertile women and those who are pregnant or breastfeeding should not be automatically excluded as research participants." Elsewhere in the document, however, there was implicit permission for researchers to insist on the use of hormonal contraception. Previous objections to this permissive stance in the earlier draft had clearly fallen on deaf ears. Any optimism we might have felt upon seeing the first draft Code was dashed by the second draft.

It now appeared that fundamental ethical change was unlikely to emerge from this process despite the presence of feminist voices. It seemed clear that other, more powerful voices (both within and without) were influencing the Working Group's deliberations and the broad conceptual shift we had hoped for seemed more elusive than ever.

The Working Group's Final Version of the Code

The final draft of the Code was completed and submitted to the three councils in May 1997 and a final version was released to the public in July. Given our disappointment with both the first and second drafts, we approached the task of reviewing the final version with considerable hesitation. We expected this version of the Code would also fail to effectively address issues relevant to the exploitation and neglect of women in research. We were more than pleasantly surprised. The changes made were little short of extraordinary.

We do not know the cause of the remarkable shift in the approach taken by the Working Group and we do not claim exclusive credit for the positive changes (many others lobbied the Working Group). We do, however, want to carefully document some of the changes that have led us to believe that the considerable effort devoted to this project was worthwhile.

From the outset, we argued against the moral framework proposed for the revised guidelines, namely, the four-principles approach to bioethics (autonomy, beneficence, nonmaleficence, and justice). We described other, richer, theoretical approaches that could provide the foundation for the Code. While the Working Group remained steadfast in its commitment to the principles approach, the following passage appears in the final version:

> Besides the four basic principles discussed, there are other
> ways of approaching the ethics of research involving humans.
> . . . Another approach that researchers and REBs will find
> helpful is in terms of reflecting on relationships of power and
> socially structured allocations of privilege and status. Feminist
> researchers and ethicists have been concerned with such
> relationships and the ways in which they perpetuate disad-
> vantage and inequality. This type of approach to ethics can be
> extremely illuminating in examining the diverse research
> agendas of various parties and in dealing with prospective
> participants who have been systematically disadvantaged.
> (13–14)

Second, we repeatedly asked the Working Group to address the ethics and politics of who sets the research agenda. Despite earlier indications from members of the Working Group that this issue was beyond their mandate, the final version includes the following:

> With this second concern about distributive justice in research
> [the inappropriate exclusion of women of child-bearing age], it
> is not nearly as easy to focus on researchers and REBs as it is
> for the first type of concern (appropriately benefiting and not
> overburdening research participants). There are multiple
> agents involved in setting "the research agenda," that is, the
> general direction of current and future research: attitudes and
> beliefs of colleagues, availability of funding, technology and

infra-structure, and multiple diverse and sometimes conflicting demands by research institutions and society. This is not to deny that individual researchers and REBs have a role to play in the fair distribution of the benefits and burdens of research; rather, it is easier to avoid specific harms in areas under one's own control than to bring about a larger social good (in this case, a fairer distribution of the general benefits of research).

Finally, our greatest efforts were expended on the problem of exclusion and underrepresentation of women and other oppressed groups in research. The final version of the Code acknowledges this problem and takes a strong stance on the inclusion of women and other members of oppressed groups as subject-participants. In a discussion of the social harms and benefits of research, it states:

> In recent years, one area of social benefit that has deservedly received increased attention has been the inequitable distribution of the benefits of research to various groups, whether defined by gender, age, illness or social status. If members of particular groups (e.g., women, the elderly or immature children) are excluded as research participants, or are seriously under-represented, then it is quite likely that these groups will not only fail to reap the benefits of research, but they may also suffer from misapplication of outcomes of such research to their unique situations. (17)

Elsewhere, this issue is discussed in greater detail.

> Historically, women have been excluded as research participants. The justifications for this exclusion have included fear of damage to the foetus including teratogenicity, the confounding influence of hormonal cycles, and fear of liabilities of research sponsors. Women have also been excluded because of a failure to recognize that certain diseases and conditions might affect men and women differently.
>
> The exclusion of women as research participants also raises serious concerns regarding the generalizability and reliability of the data collected. Research data on, for example, drug dosages, device effects, treatments, cultural norms, moral development, and social behavior obtained from male-only studies likely will not be generalizable to women. As a result, data necessary for the treatment or understanding of women often must be inferred despite important differences which may render such inferences inaccurate. When women, or any group, are excluded from research studies, they may be

deprived of the possible benefits that come from participating
as research subjects, and may suffer as a result. The inclusion
of women in research is essential if men and women are to
equally benefit from research. Careful attention to these issues
is essential to both justice and the quality of research.

Article 6.3
   **Researchers and REBs must endeavor to distribute
equitably the potential benefits of research. Accordingly,
depending on the themes and objectives of the research,
researchers and REBs must:**
   **a) select and recruit women from disadvantaged social,
ethnic, racial and mentally or physically disabled groups;
and**
   **b) ensure that the design of the research reflects
appropriately the participation of this group.**

While some research is properly focused on particular
populations that do not include women or only include very
few women, in most studies women should be represented in
proportion to their presence in the population affected by the
research. In designing and implementing research projects,
particular attention also should be paid to the need to include
women of colour, women who are members of cultural or
religious minorities, and women who are socially or otherwise
disadvantaged. (VI-3–VI-4; emphasis in original)

On the controversial matter of research involving fertile or pregnant
women, the final version states that "No women should be automatically excluded from relevant research" (VI-4).

   These excerpts illustrate the remarkable transformation evident between the first and second drafts and the final version of the Code, and
this transformation accounts for the sense of accomplishment experienced by the Network. While some of our concerns were not addressed
to our satisfaction—for example, innovative practices are not automatically subject to research review—we believe that with the final version
of the Code the interests of women in Canada are now better protected
and, indeed, promoted than they have been in the past.

Reflections on Autonomy

Our interactions with the Working Group provided us with an opportunity to put our theorizing about agency and autonomy into practice.
As Sherwin argues in Chapter 2, the traditional understanding of au-

tonomy ignores the broader social and political contexts in which nominally autonomous choices are made by others, particularly those who are vulnerable to abuse or exploitation. That is, the conventional understanding of autonomy ignores the oppressive circumstances in which individuals are invited to exercise choice. A richer understanding of autonomy, one that does not merely equate autonomy (self-governance) with agency (the making of "reasonable" choice, choice that is rational under the circumstances) is needed. This understanding of autonomy that acknowledges the interdependence of individuals and attends to the social relations and political structures that limit self-governance, Sherwin names relational autonomy.

Relational autonomy challenges rather than accepts the prevailing social conditions that limit choice and effectively perpetuate oppression. Hence our concern, as regards the issue of research involving humans, with ensuring that women and other oppressed groups not be unjustly excluded from, or exploited in, research. We repeatedly demanded of the Working Group that women and members of other oppressed groups be active participants in research as both subject- and researcher-participants, to ensure that the research agenda and individual research protocols would not continue to be skewed in favor of the most privileged segments of society. Our aim was to promote women's relational autonomy in all phases of the research process and to draw attention to the connections between research and autonomy-related health practices.

Second, relational autonomy often requires a change in the framework for action by challenging built-in limitations. This accounts for our efforts to maximize the effectiveness of our own voices by pursuing a variety of strategies in addressing the Working Group. We did not accept the limitations on our participation in the policy-making process imposed by the Working Group. Specifically, we resisted the stipulated time frame for the revision of the guidelines, we challenged the proposed mandate of the Working Group and the authority of the Working Group to limit the scope of the discussion, and, finally, we consciously chose not to limit our efforts to the submission of written documents, as was expected. In addition to preparing official submissions, we gave public lectures on this topic at academic and professional meetings, we initiated and pursued private conversations in the "corridors of power," and, in what might be considered an unusual move, we sought to make the process we were engaged in transparent by publishing the details of our ongoing interactions with the Working Group in a peer reviewed journal (Baylis 1996). All of this activity was conducted not only as an academic endeavor but also as a self-consciously political maneuver.

Thus, at the end of this process, we look back and see that the issues of agency and autonomy informed our analysis of the regulation of research involving humans as well as our political action decisions. This conclusion confirms our belief in the value of theoretical reconceptualizations of such concepts as autonomy as well as our belief in the inseparability of ethical theory and political activism. Although we can never know what specific interventions contributed to the improvements between the first and second drafts of the Code and the final text, we know that change is possible, and we leave this project with a renewed sense of optimism about participation in the policy-making process. While this can be an enormously frustrating and difficult experience, as we have learned, it can also be a rewarding and constructive one.

Postscript

The saga continues. As we go to press, the "Code of Ethical Conduct for Research Involving Humans" that was released to the public in July 1997 has itself been revised. In January 1998, a document titled "Tri-Council Policy Statement on Ethical Conduct for Research Involving Humans" was circulated to the three sponsoring councils for review and a final decision regarding adoption. A number of significant changes were made to the document, but as these were introduced after the time of writing, an analysis of these changes could not be included in this chapter. For the record, we regret to report that much of the text we have quoted from the 1997 Code as accomplishments does not appear in the latest draft. Especially discouraging is the fact that there is no longer any reference to feminist ethics as a legitimate alternative ethical approach; an ethic of care is mentioned, as is communitarian ethics. While there are vague references to approaches that place priority on human relations, that analyze power, and so on, there is no explicit discussion of social justice. Public policy in ethics, as in health matters, is still not sufficiently tuned to feminist insights and concerns. Much work remains to be done. We hope that our analyses will help to guide activity in the ongoing struggle.

NOTES

1. See, for example, Division of Research Investigations 1993; Angell and Kassiner 1994; Cowan 1994.

2. Prior to this initiative, NSERC, which has the largest research budget of the three agencies, had not developed its own ethical guidelines for the research that

it funded. The other two councils had had such guidelines since the late 1970s. MRC developed its original guidelines in 1978 (Medical Research Council of Canada, *MRC Report No. 6: Ethics in Human Experimentation* [Ottawa: Ministry of Supply and Services Canada, 1978] and these were subsequently revised in 1987 (Medical Research Council of Canada, *Guidelines on Research Involving Human Subjects* [Ottawa: Minister of Supply and Services Canada, 1987]. SSHRC adopted its first ethics guidelines in 1979 when it became independent of the Canada Council, at which time the Report of the Consultative Group on Ethics (Report of the Consultative Group on Ethics *The Canada Council, Ethics* [Ottawa: Canada Council, 1977] was officially endorsed. In 1980, the Ad Hoc Committee on Ethics was established and revised guidelines were published in a booklet in 1981 (Social Sciences and Humanities Research Council of Canada, *Ethics: Guidelines for Research with Human Subjects* [Ottawa, 1981]. The content of these ethics guidelines has since been reordered and reformatted, and minor editorial changes have been introduced for clarification. The substance, however, has remained unchanged. The guidelines are reprinted annually in the annexes of the SSHRC applicant guides.

3. In Sherwin 1996b the argument is developed about why efforts to identify concepts and choose morally adequate policies cannot be complete if ethicists confine themselves to purely philosophical exercises.

4. See Sherwin 1992 for an elaboration of these claims.

5. Where appropriate, we use the expressions "subject-participant" and "researcher-participant" rather than the traditional terms "subject" and "researcher." We do this, despite the somewhat unwieldy nature of these expressions, because of negative connotations associated with the term *subject*, which implies passivity, and positive connotations associated with the recognition that both researchers and subjects are participants in the research endeavor.

6. All examples are taken from Dresser 1992.

7. The new NIH Guidelines ("NIH Guidelines on the Inclusion of Women and Minorities as Subjects in Clinical Research," 59 *Fed. Reg* 14508 [March 28, 1994]) require the inclusion of women and minorities in all NIH-funded research in numbers that would permit a valid analysis of significant differences in responses. The new FDA requirements ("Guidelines for the Study and Evaluation of Gender Differences in the Clinical Evaluation of Drugs," 58 *Fed. Reg.* 39406 [July 22, 1993]) encourage the inclusion of women at all stages of clinical trials of drugs to be licensed in the United States, whereas their policy of the previous decades had virtually excluded women who might be or become pregnant.

8. For a discussion of the recent U.S. backlash against feminist critiques of health research see Baylis 1996, 235–39.

9. This being said, it is interesting to note that in 1995 an assistant to the MRC Advisory Council on Women and Clinical Trials searched the MRC archives in an effort to address this issue. He was able to retrieve 37 of the 129 MRC-funded clinical trials since 1985. He found that 15 of these proposals made no reference to gender. One specified all male subject-participants (this was a study on knee surgery funded in 1991). Fourteen proposals specified all female subject-participants (all of

these studies were about reproduction and breast cancer). Five excluded women of childbearing potential. Only two required proportional gender representation.

10. For a discussion of the differences between research, therapy, and innovative practice see Baylis 1993, 52–53.

11. See DuBose, Hamel, and O'Connell 1994; Englehardt 1996; Jonsen and Toulmin 1998; Pellegrino and Thomasma 1993; Sherwin 1992; Singer 1993.

12. Original submission: SSHRC-Supported Strategic Research Network on Feminist Health Care Ethics, Susan Sherwin et al., "Submission to the Tri-Council Working Group on Guidelines for Research with Human Subjects," March 9, 1995. See http://www.dal.ca./law/hli.

13. This included sections: 1. The Research Context, 2. Research Ethics, and 3. Applying the Ethics to Research.

14. This included sections 4. Research That Deals with Collectivities, 5. Population Studies/Epidemiology/Health Services Research, 6. Research That Deals with Clinical Problems, 7. Research That Deals with Behavior, 8. Research That Deals with Biomedical and Bioengineering Problems, 9. Research That Deals with Subjects Who Cannot Give Consent, 10. Genetic Research, 11. Research Involving Embryos and Fetuses, and 12. Research Driven by Industrial Needs.

15. This included sections 13. Accountability, 14. Research Ethics Boards (REBs), 15. Monitoring, 16. Processing Private Sector Research, and 17. Educational Issues.

16. These include Jocelyn Downie, "Women in Research Studies: A Feminist View," Joint Centre for Bioethics at the University of Toronto, February 1995; Françoise Baylis, "'Confusion Worse Confounded': Revising Canada's Research Guidelines," University of Manitoba, May 1995; Baylis, "Ethical and Social Issues Regarding Research Involving Women," MRC Advisory Council on Women in Clinical Trials, Toronto, May 1995; Downie, "Feminist Analysis of Women and Research," Canadian Bioethics Society, Vancouver, November 1995; and Susan Sherwin, "Translating Values into Facts: Making the Links Between Feminist Ethics and Social Change," Canadian Society for Women in Philosophy, University of Western Ontario, November 1995.

17. Interim unofficial draft of the relevant subsection of the research guidelines: "Populations At Risk of Exclusion from or Exploitation in Research." See http://www.dal.ca/law/hli.

18. Second submission: SSHRC-Supported Strategic Research Network on Feminist Health Care Ethics, Susan Sherwin et al., "Comments on the Draft Code of Conduct for Research Involving Human Subjects," July 5, 1996. See http://www.dal.ca/law/hli.

19. Interim unofficial draft of relevant subsection of the research guidelines: "Inclusiveness and Integrity in Research Relationships." See http://www.dal.ca/law/hli.

20. Tri-Council Working Group, "Code of Ethical Conduct for Research Involving Humans" (Ottawa: Minister of Supply and Services, Canada, February 1997). See http://www.dal.ca/law/hli.

References

Abbott, Deborah S. 1985. "This Body I Love." In *With the Power of Each Breath: A Disabled Women's Anthology*, ed. Susan E. Brown, Debra Connors, and Nanci Stern. San Francisco: Cleis Press.

Abbott, J., R. Johnson, J. Koziol-McLain, and S. R. Lowenstein. 1995. "Domestic Violence Against Women: Incidence and Prevalence in an Emergency Department Population." *Journal of the American Medical Association* 273(22): 1763–67.

Abramson, Zelda. 1990. "Don't Ask Your Gynecologist If You Need a Hysterectomy. . . ." *Healthsharing* 11(3): 12–16.

Adams, Diane L., ed. 1995. "Introduction." In *Health Issues for Women of Color: A Cultural Diversity Perspective*. Thousand Oaks, Calif.: Sage.

Adelson, Naomi. 1991. "'Being Alive Well': The Praxis of Cree Health." In *Circumpolar Health 90: The Proceedings of the 8th International Congress on Circumpolar Health*, ed. Brian Postl, Penny Gilbert, Jean Goodwill, Michael E. K. Moffatt, John D. O'Neil, Peter A. Sarsfield, and T. Kue Young. Winnipeg: University of Manitoba Press.

Akoto, Eliwo, Julien G. Guingnido, and Dominique Tabutin, eds. 1991. *L'état et le devenir de la population du Bénin*. Porto Novo: Centre de Formation et de Recherche en Matière de Population, Université du Bénin, Ministère de l'Éducation et Unité de Planification de la Population, Direction du Plan, Ministère du Plan et de la Restructuration Économique.

Alcoff, Linda, and Elizabeth Potter, eds. 1993. *Feminist Epistemologies*. New York: Routledge.

Alcoff, Linda, and Laura Gray. 1993. "Survivor Discourse: Transgression or Recuperation?" *Signs: Journal of Women in Culture and Society* 18(2): 260–91.

Alexander, Sophie, and Mark J.N.C. Keirse. 1989. "Formal Risk Scoring During Pregnancy." In *Effective Care in Pregnancy and Childbirth*, ed. I. Chalmers and M. Enkins. Oxford: Oxford University Press.

Altekruse, Joan M., and Sue V. Rosser. 1992. "Feminism and Medicine: Cooptation or Cooperation?" In *The Knowledge Explosion: Generations of Feminist Scholarship*, ed. Cheris Kramarae and Dale Spender. New York: Teachers College Press.

Angell, Marcia, and Jerome P. Kassirer. 1994. "Setting the Record Straight in the Breast Cancer Trials" *New England Journal of Medicine* 330(20): 1448–49.

Annau, Catherine. 1992. "The Canadian Birth Control Movement in an International Perspective." Master's thesis. McGill University.

Anonymous. 1993. "Inside the Royal Commission." In *Misconceptions: The Social Construction of Choice and the New Reproductive and Genetic Technologies,* ed. Gwynne Basen, Margrit Eichler, and Abby Lippman. Prescott, Ont.: Voyageur Publishing.

Antony, Louise, and Charlotte Witt, eds. 1993. *A Mind of One's Own: Feminist Essays on Reason and Objectivity.* Boulder: Colo.: Westview Press.

Aristotle. 1994. *Generation of Animals.* Excerpt in *Philosophy of Woman: An Anthology of Classic to Current Concepts,* 3d ed., ed. Mary Briody Mahowald. Indianapolis, Ind.: Hackett Publishing.

Arms, Susanne. 1975. *Immaculate Deception: A New Look at Women and Childbirth in America.* Boston: Houghton Mifflin.

Arney, William Ray. 1982. *Power and the Profession of Obstetrics.* Chicago: University of Chicago Press.

Arnup, Katherine. 1994. *Education for Motherhood: Advice for Mothers in Twentieth-Century Canada.* Toronto: University of Toronto Press.

Arnup, Katherine, Andrée Lévesque, and Ruth Roach Pierson, eds. 1990. *Delivering Motherhood: Maternal Ideologies and Practices in the Nineteenth and Twentieth Centuries.* London: Routledge.

Asch, Adrienne, and Gail Geller. 1996. "Feminism, Bioethics, and Genetics." In *Feminism and Bioethics: Beyond Reproduction,* ed. Susan Wolf. New York: Oxford University Press.

Ash, Mitchell G. 1994. "Human Capital and the Discourse of Control." In *Genes and Human Self-Knowledge,* ed. R. F. Weir, S. C. Lawrence, and Evan Fales. Iowa City: University of Iowa Press.

Aspen. 1996. "Muscle Fetish." In *Pushing Limits: Disabled Dykes Produce Culture,* ed. Shelley Tremain. Toronto: Women's College Press.

Atkinson, Paul. 1985. "Strong Minds and Weak Bodies: Sports, Gymnastics, and the Medicalization of Women's Education." *British Journal of Sports History (Great Britain)* 2(1): 62–71.

Atrash, Hani K., S. Alexander, and C. J. Berg. 1995. "Maternal Mortality in Developed Countries: Not Just a Concern of the Past." *Obstetrics and Gynecology* 68(4, pt. 2): 700–705.

Atwood, Margaret. 1994. "The Female Body." In *Minding the Body,* ed. P. Foster. Toronto: Doubleday.

Avis, Nancy E., Patricia A. Kaufert, Margaret Lock, Sonja McKinley, and Kerstin Vass. 1993. "The Evolution of Menopausal Symptoms." *Ballière's Clinical Endocrinology and Metabolism* 7:17–32.

Babbitt, Susan. 1993. "Feminism and Objective Interests." In *Feminist Epistemologies,* ed. Linda Alcoff and Elizabeth Potter. New York: Routledge.

————. 1996. *Impossible Dreams: Rationality, Integrity, and Moral Imagination.* Boulder, Colo.: Westview Press.

Babcock, Marguerite and Christine McKay, eds. 1995. *Challenging Codependency: Feminist Critiques.* Toronto: University of Toronto Press.

Baier, Annette. 1985a. *Postures of the Mind: Essays on Mind and Morals.* Minneapolis: University of Minnesota Press.

————. 1985b. "What Do Women Want in a Moral Theory?" *Nous* 19(1): 53–63.

Bair, B., and S. E. Cayleff, eds. 1993. *Wings of Gauze: Women of Color and the Experience of Health and Illness.* Detroit: Wayne State University Press.

Balsamo, Anne. 1997. *Technologies of the Gendered Body: Reading Cyborg Women.* Durham, N.C.: Duke University Press.

Bannerji, Himani. 1995. "RE: Turning the Gaze." In *Thinking Through: Essays on Feminism, Marxism, and Anti-Racism.* Toronto: The Women's Press.

Barinaga, Marcia. 1991. "Sexism Charged by Stanford Physician." *Science* 252: 1484.

Barker-Benfield, G. J. 1977. *The Horrors of the Half-Known Life: Male Attitudes Toward Women and Sexuality in Nineteenth-Century America.* New York: Harper.

Bar On, Bat-Ami. 1993. "Marginality and Epistemic Privilege" In *Feminist Epistemologies,* ed. Linda Alcoff and Elizabeth Potter. New York: Routledge.

Barroso, Carmen. 1994. "Building a New Specialization on Women's Health: An International Perspective." In *Reframing Women's Health: Multidisciplinary Research and Practice,* ed. Alice J. Dan. London: Sage.

Bartky, Sandra Lee. 1988. "Foucault, Femininity, and the Modernization of Patriarchal Power." In *Femininity and Foucault: Reflections of Resistance,* ed. Irene Diamond and Lee Quinby. Boston: Northeastern University Press.

————. 1990. *Femininity and Domination: Studies in the Phenomenology of Oppression.* New York: Routledge.

Basen, Gwynne. N.d. *On the Eighth Day: Perfecting Mother Nature I, II.* Toronto: Studio D, National Film Board. Videocassette.

Basen, Gwynne, Margrit Eichler, and Abby Lippman, eds. 1993. *Misconceptions: The Social Construction of Choice and the New Reproductive and Genetic Technologies.* Prescott, Ont.: Voyageur Publishing.

Bassett, Mary T., and Marvellous Mhloyi. 1994. "Women and AIDS in Zimbabwe: The Making of an Epidemic." In *Women's Health, Politics, and Power: Essays on Sex/Gender, Medicine, and Public Health,* ed. Elizabeth Fee and Nancy Krieger. Amityville, N.Y.: Baywood.

Bates L., S. Redman, W. Brown, and L. Hancock. 1995. "Domestic Violence Experienced by Women Attending an Accident and Emergency Department." *Australian Journal of Public Health* 19(3): 293–99.

Batt, Sharon. 1994. *Patient No More: The Politics of Breast Cancer.* Charlottetown, P.E.I.: Gynergy Books.

Baylis, Françoise. 1993. "Assisted Reproductive Technologies: Informed Choice." In *New Reproductive Technologies,* Royal Commission on New Reproductive Technologies. Ottawa: Ministry of Supply and Services.

————. 1996. "Women and Health Research: Working for Change." *Journal of Clinical Ethics* 7(3): 229–42.

Beauregard, Micheline, and Maria De Konick. 1991. "Savoir occulté, soins ignorés, institutions à redéfinir: Un programme de recherches féministes en santé des femmes." *Recherches féministes* 4(1): 1–9.

Becker, Marshall H. 1986. "The Tyranny of Health Promotion." *Public Health Reviews* 14:15–25.

Bell, C. C., E. J. Jenkins, W. Keo, H. Rhodes. 1994. "Response of Emergency Rooms to Victims of Interpersonal Violence." *Hospital and Community Psychiatry* 45(2): 143–46.

Bell, Nora Kizer. 1989. "Women and AIDS: Too Little, Too Late?" *Hypatia* 4(3): 3–22.

Bell, Susan. 1987. "Changing Ideas: The Medicalization of Menopause." *Social Science and Medicine* 24:535–43.

Belloc, N. B., and L. Breslow. 1972. "Relationship of Physical Health Status and Health Practices" *Preventive Medicine* 1:409–21.

Bem, Sandra. 1974."The Measurement of Psychological Androgyny." *Journal of Clinical and Consulting Psychology* 42(2): 155–62.

————. 1993. *The Lenses of Gender: Transforming the Debate on Sexual Inequality.* New Haven, Conn.: Yale University Press.

Benhabib, S. 1987. "The Generalized and Concrete Other." In *Feminism as Critique*, ed. S. Benhabib and D. Cornell. Minneapolis: University of Minnesota Press.

Benoit, Cecelia. 1989. "Traditional Midwifery Practice: The Limits of Occupational Autonomy." *Canadian Review of Sociology and Anthropology* 26(4): 633–49.

Benson, Paul. 1991. "Autonomy and Oppressive Socialization." *Social Theory and Practice* 17(3): 385–408.

————. 1994. "Free Agency and Self-Worth." *Journal of Philosophy* 91(12): 650–68.

Berer, Marge. 1994. "The Quinacrine Controversy One Year On." *Reproductive Health* 4:99–106.

Berner, L. S. 1995. "Prophylactic Oopherectomy: A Supreme Court Decision?" *Journal of Women's Health* 4:121–23.

Bhayana, Bhooma. 1994. "Healthshock." In *On Women Healthsharing*, ed. Enakshi Dua, Maureen FitzGerald, Linda Gardner, Darien Taylor, and Lisa Wyndels. Toronto: The Women's Press.

Biggs, Leslie. 1983. "The Case of the Missing Midwives: A History of Midwifery in Ontario from 1795–1900." *Ontario History* 75(1): 21–36.

Billings, P. R., M. A. Kohn, M. de Cuevas, J. Beckwith, J. S. Alper, and M. R. Natowicz. 1992. "Discrimination as a Consequence of Genetic Testing." *American Journal of Human Genetics* 50:476–82.

Biology and Gender Study Group. 1989. "The Importance of Feminist Critique for Contemporary Cell Biology." In *Feminism and Science*, ed. Nancy Tuana. Bloomington: Indiana University Press.

Birke, Lynda. 1982. "From Sin to Sickness: Hormonal Theories of Lesbianism." In *Biological Woman: The Convenient Myth*, ed. Ruth Hubbard, Mary Sue Henifin, and Barbara Fried. Cambridge, Mass: Schenkman Publishing Co.
———. 1986. *Women, Feminism, and Biology: The Feminist Challenge*. New York: Methuen.
Birke, Lynda, and Ruth Hubbard, eds. 1995. *Re-Inventing Biology: Respect for Life and the Creation of Knowledge*. Bloomington: Indiana University Press.
Bleier, Ruth. 1984. *Science and Gender: A Critique of Biology and Its Theories of Women*. New York: Pergamon Press.
Block, G., G. Matanoski, R. Seltser, and T. Mitchell. 1988. "Cancer Morbidity and Mortality in Phosphate Workers." *Cancer Research* 48:7298–303.
Bloom, F. E. 1995. "Editorial: Biomedicine 96: A New Partnership." *Science* 270:1279.
Bograd, Michelle. 1988. "Feminist Perspectives On Wife Abuse." In *Feminist Perspectives on Wife Abuse*, ed. K. Ylló and M. Bograd. Newbury Park, Calif.: Sage.
Bordo, Susan. 1987. "The Cartesian Masculinization of Thought." In *Sex and Scientific Inquiry*, ed. Sandra Harding and Jean F. O'Barr. Chicago: University of Chicago Press.
———. 1990. "Feminism, Postmodernism, and Gender Skepticism." In *Feminism/Postmodernism*, ed. L. Nicholson. New York: Routledge.
———. 1993. *Unbearable Weight: Feminism, Western Culture, and the Body*. Berkeley and Los Angeles: University of California Press.
Boston Women's Health Book Collective. 1976. *Our Bodies, Ourselves: A Book By and For Women*. New York: Simon and Schuster.
———. 1992. *The New Our Bodies, Ourselves: A Book By and For Women*. New York: Touchstone/Simon and Schuster.
Bowker, L. H., and L. Maurer. 1987. "The Medical Treatment of Battered Wives." *Women and Health* 12(1): 25–45.
Braidotti, Rosi. 1994. *Nomadic Subjects: Embodiment and Sexual Difference in Contemporary Feminist Theory*. New York: Columbia University Press.
Brown, J. B., B. Lent, and G. Sas. 1993. "Identifying and Treating Wife Abuse." *Journal of Family Practice* 36(2): 185–91.
Brown, J. B., and M. D. Sas. 1994. "Focus Groups in Family Practice Research: An Example Study of Family Physicians' Approach to Wife Abuse." *Family Practice Research Journal* 14(1): 19–28.
Browne, Susan E., Debra Connors, and Nanci Stern, eds. 1985. *With the Power of Each Breath: A Disabled Women's Anthology*. San Francisco: Cleis Press.
Browner, Carole H., and Joanne Leslie. 1996. "Women, Work, and Household Health in the Context of Development." In *Gender and Health: An International Perspective*, ed. Carolyn Sargent and Caroline Brettell. Upper Saddle River, N.J.: Prentice Hall.
Browner, Carole H., and Nancy Press. 1996. "The Production of Authoritative Knowledge in American Prenatal Care." *Medical Anthropology Quarterly (Special Issue on Authoritative Knowledge)* 10(2): 141–56.

Buckley, Suzann. 1979. "Ladies or Midwives: Efforts to Reduce Infant and Ma-
    ternal Mortality." In *A Not Unreasonable Claim: Women and Reform in Canada,
    1880s–1920s*, ed. Linda Kealey. Toronto: The Women's Press.

Burke, M., and H. M. Stevenson. 1993. "Fiscal Crisis and Restructuring in
    Medicare: The Politics and Political Science of Health in Canada." *Health
    and Canadian Society* 1:51–80.

Burtch, Brian. 1994. *Trials of Labour: The Re-Emergence of Midwifery*. Montreal and
    Kingston: McGill-Queen's University Press.

Butler, Judith. 1993. *Bodies That Matter: On the Discursive Limits of "Sex."* New
    York: Routledge.

Butler, Sandra, and Barbara Rosenblum. 1991. *Cancer in Two Voices*. San Fran-
    cisco: Spinsters Book Co.

Bynum, Carolyn Walker. 1980. "Did the Twelfth Century Discover the Individ-
    ual?" *Journal of Ecclesiastical History* 31(1): 1–17.

Campbell, J. C. 1992. "Ways of Teaching, Learning, and Knowing About Vio-
    lence Against Women." *Nursing and Health Care* 13(9): 465–70.

Campbell, J. C., and K. Landenburger. 1995. "Violence Against Women." In
    Women's Health Care: A Comprehensive Handbook, ed. C. I. Fogel and N. Fu-
    gato Woods. London: Sage.

Campbell, Margaret [Mary Howell, pseud.]. 1973. *Why Would a Girl Go Into Med-
    icine?* New York: Feminist Press.

Campbell, Richmond. 1994. "The Values of Feminist Empiricism." *Hypatia* 9(1):
    90–115.

Campling, Jo, ed. 1981. *Images of Ourselves: Women with Disabilities Talking*. Lon-
    don: Routledge and Kegan Paul.

Canada. 1991. *Family Violence in Canada (FVC)*. Ottawa: Health and Welfare
    Canada, National Clearinghouse on Family Violence.

Canada. 1993. "The Violence Against Women Survey." Statistics Canada, Min-
    istry of Industry, Science and Technology, Catalogue 11–001E.

Canadian Advisory Council on the Status of Women. 1995. *What Women
    Prescribe: Report and Recommendations*. From the National Symposium
    "Women in Partnership: Working Towards Inclusive Gender-Sensitive
    Health Policies," Ottawa, May.

Candib, L. M. 1992. "Violence Against Women as a Gender Issue." In *Violence
    Education: Towards a Solution*, ed. M. Hendricks-Matthews. Kansas City:
    The Society of Teachers of Family Medicine.

———. 1994. "Reconsidering Power in the Clinical Relationship." In *The Empa-
    thetic Practitioner: Empathy, Gender, and Medicine*, ed. E. Singer More and M.
    A. Milligan. New Brunswick, N.J.: Rutgers University Press.

Caplan, Paula. 1993. *The Myth of Women's Masochism*, 2d ed. Toronto: University
    of Toronto Press.

———. 1995. *They Say You're Crazy: How the World's Most Powerful Psychiatrists
    Decide Who is Normal*. Reading, Mass.: Addison-Wesley.

Carlson, Angela Licia. 1998. "Mindful Subjects: Classification and Mindful Disability." Ph.D. diss., University of Toronto.

Carovano, Kathryn. 1994. "More Than Mothers and Whores: Redefining the AIDS Prevention Needs of Women." In *Women's Health, Politics, and Power: Essays on Sex/Gender, Medicine, and Public Health*, ed. Elizabeth Fee and Nancy Krieger. Amityville, N.Y.: Baywood.

Chambliss, L. R., C. Bay, and R. F. Jones. 1995. "Domestic Violence: An Educational Imperative." *American Journal of Obstetrics and Gynaecology* 172: 1035–38.

Charte d'Ottawa sur la promotion de la santé. 1986. "Organization mondiale de la santé." Copenhague: Bureau Régional pour l'Europe.

Chesler, Phyllis. 1972. *Women and Madness*. Garden City, N.Y.: Doubleday.

Chez, R. 1994. "A Guest Editorial: Physician Identification of Battered Women." *Obstetrical and Gynecological Survey* 49(10): 663.

Clarke, Adele. 1990 "Controversy and the Development of Reproductive Sciences." *Social Problems* 37(1): 18–37.

Coburn, D., and J. M. Eakin. 1993. "Sociology of Health in Canada: First Impressions." *Health and Canadian Society* 1:83–110.

Coburn, D., and B. Poland. 1996. "The CIAR Vision of the Determinants of Health: A Critique." *Canadian Journal of Public Health* 87(5): 308–10.

Code, Lorraine. 1991. *What Can She Know? Feminist Theory and the Construction of Knowledge*. Ithaca, N.Y.: Cornell University Press.

———. 1994. "'I Know Just How You Feel': Empathy and the Problem of Epistemic Authority." In *The Empathetic Practitioner: Empathy, Gender, and Medicine*, ed. E. Singer More and M. A. Milligan. New Brunswick, N.J.: Rutgers University Press.

———. 1995a. "How Do We Know? Questions of Method in Feminist Practice." In *Changing Methods: Feminists Transforming Practices*, ed. Sandra Burt and Lorraine Code. Peterborough, Ont.: Broadview Press.

———. 1995b. "Incredulity, Experientialism, and the Politics of Knowledge." In *Rhetorical Spaces: Essays on Gendered Locations*. New York: Routledge.

Cohen, J. 1997. "The Genomics Gamble." *Science* 275:767–72.

Cohen, Leah, and Constance Backhouse. 1979. "Women and Health: The Growing Controversy." *Canadian Women's Studies* 1(4): 4–10.

Colin, Christine, Francine Ouellet, Ginette Boyer, and Catherine Martin. 1992. *Extrême pauvreté, santé et maternité*. Montreal: Éditions Saint-Martin.

Collins, Patricia Hill. 1990. *Black Feminist Thought: Knowledge, Consciousness, and the Politics of Empowerment*. New York: Routledge.

Colodny, Nikki. 1989. "The Politics of Birth Control in a Reproductive Rights Context." In *The Future of Human Reproduction*, ed. Christine Overall. Toronto: The Women's Press.

Comacchio, Cynthia R. 1993. *Nations Are Built of Babies: Saving Ontario's Mothers and Children*. Montreal and Kingston: McGill-Queen's University Press.

Commission nationale pour l'intégration de la femme au développement. 1994. *Évolution de la situation de la femme au Bénin.* National report, Cotonou, Benin.

Coney, Sandra. 1988. *The Unfortunate Experiment: The Full Story Behind the Inquiry into Cervical Cancer Treatment.* Auckland, N.Z.: Penguin Books.

———. 1994. *The Menopause Industry: How the Medical Establishment Exploits Women.* Alameda, Calif: Hunter House Books.

"Conference on the Future Direction of Health Care: The Dimensions of Medicine." 1975. Report on conference sponsored by the Blue Cross Association, the Rockefeller Foundation, and the Health Policy Program, University of California. New York, December.

Conley, K. 1993. "Toward a More Perfect World: Eliminating Sexual Discrimination in Academic Medicine." *New England Journal of Medicine* 328:351–52.

Connor, James. 1989. "Minority Medicine in Ontario, 1795 to 1903: A Study of Medical Pluralism and Its Decline." Ph.D. thesis, University of Waterloo.

Connors, Debra. 1985. "Disability, Sexism, and the Social Order." In *With the Power of Each Breath: A Disabled Women's Anthology,* ed. Susan E. Browne, Debra Connors, and Nancy Stern. San Francisco: Cleis Press.

Conrad, Peter. 1992. "Medicalization and Social Control." *Annual Reviews in Sociology* 18:209–32.

———. 1994. "Wellness as Virtue: Morality and the Pursuit of Health." *Culture, Medicine and Psychiatry* 18:385–401.

Conrad, Peter, and J. Schneider. 1980. "Looking at Levels of Medicalization: A Comment on Strong's Critique of the Thesis of Medical Imperialism." *Social Science and Medicine* 14A:75–79

Corea, Gena. 1985a. *The Hidden Malpractice: How American Medicine Mistreats Women.* New York: Harper Colophon Books.

———. 1985b. *The Mother Machine: Reproductive Technologies from Artificial Insemination to Artificial Wombs.* New York: Harper and Row.

———. 1992. *The Invisible Epidemic: The Story of Women and Aids.* New York: Harper Perennial.

Cottrell, Barbara, Stella Lord, Susan Prentice, and Lise Martin, eds. 1996. *Research Partnerships: A Feminist Approach to Communities and Universities Working Together.* Ottawa: CRIAW.

Council for Responsible Genetics. 1990. "Documents: Position Papers." *Issues in Reproductive and Genetic Engineering* 3(3): 287–95

Cowan, John Scott. 1994. "Lessons from the Fabrikant File: A Report to the Board of Governors of Concordia University." Paper prepared at Corcordia University.

Crawford, M., and G. Gartner. 1992. *Woman Killing: Intimate Femicide in Ontario, 1974–1990.* Ontario: Women We Honour Action Committee.

Crawford, Robert. 1977. "You Are Dangerous to Your Health: The Ideology and Politics of Victim Blaming." *International Journal of Health Services* 7(4): 663–80.

———. 1979. "Individual Responsibility and Health Politics in the 1970s." In

Health Care in America: Essays in Social History, ed. Susan Reverby and David Rosner. Philadelphia: Temple University Press.

————. 1980. "Healthism and the Medicalization of Everyday Life." *International Journal of Health Services* 10(3): 365–88.

————. 1984. "A Cultural Account of 'Health': Control, Release, and the Social Body." In *Issues in the Political Economy of Health Care,* ed. John B. McKinlay. New York: Tavistock Publications.

————. 1994. "The Boundaries of the Self and the Unhealthy Other: Reflections on Health, Culture, and AIDS." *Social Science and Medicine* 38(10): 1347–65.

Currie, Dawn H., and Valerie Raoul, eds. 1992. *The Anatomy of Gender: Women's Struggle for the Body.* Ottawa: Carleton University Press.

Dalmiya, Vrinda, and Linda Alcoff. 1993. "Are 'Old Wives' Tales Justified?" In *Feminist Epistemologies,* ed. Linda Alcoff and Elizabeth Potter. New York: Routledge.

Darwin, Charles. 1874. *The Descent of Man,* 2d ed. rev. London: John Murray.

Davis, A., and A. MacNevin. 1989. "Battered Wives and Medical Service: An Exploratory Study of Wife Assault Victims' Experiences in Nova Scotia Health Delivery Settings." *Atlantis* 15(1): 123–35.

Davis, Dona L. 1983. *Blood and Nerves: An Ethnographic Focus on Menopause.* St. John's, Nfld.: Institute of Social and Economic Research, Memorial University.

————. 1996. "The Cultural Constructions of the Premenstrual and Menopause Syndromes." In *Gender and Health: An International Perspective,* ed. Carolyn Sargent and Caroline Brettell. Upper Saddle River, N.J.: Prentice Hall.

Davis, Kathy. 1993. "Cultural Dopes and She-Devils: Cosmetic Surgery as Ideological Dilemma." In *Negotiating at the Margins: The Gendered Discourses of Power and Resistance,* ed. Sue Fisher and Kathy Davis. New Brunswick, N.J.: Rutgers University Press.

————. 1995. *Reshaping the Female Body: The Dilemma of Cosmetic Surgery.* New York: Routledge.

Davis-Floyd, Robbie E. 1992. *Birth As an American Rite of Passage.* Berkeley and Los Angeles: University of California Press.

————. 1994. "The Technocratic Body: American Childbirth as Cultural Expression." *Social Science and Medicine* 38(8): 1125–40.

————. 1996. "The Technocratic Body and the Organic Body: Hegemony and Heresy in Women's Birth Choices." In *Gender and Health: An International Perspective,* ed. Carolyn F. Sargent and Caroline B. Brettell. Upper Saddle River, N.J.: Prentice Hall.

Davis-Floyd, Robbie E., and Elizabeth Davis. 1996. "Intuition as Authoritative Knowledge in Midwifery and Homebirth." *Medical Anthropology Quarterly (Special Issue on Authoritative Knowledge)* 10(2): 237–69.

Davis-Floyd, Robbie E., and Carolyn Sargent, eds. 1996a. *Childbirth and Authoritative Knowledge: Cross-Cultural Perspectives.* Berkeley and Los Angeles: University of California Press.

————. 1996b. *Medical Anthropology Quarterly (Special Issue on Authoritative Knowledge)* 10(2).

DeBruin, Debra A. 1994. "Justice and the Inclusion of Women in Clinical Studies: A Conceptual Framework." In *Women and Health Research: Ethical and Legal Issues of Including Women in Clinical Studies, vol. 2,* ed. Anna C. Mastroianni, Ruth Faden, and Daniel Federman, Institute of Medicine. Washington, D.C.: National Academy Press.

Dekeseredy, W., and R. Hinch. 1991. *Woman Abuse: Sociological Perspectives.* Toronto: Thompson.

De Koninck, Maria. 1981. "Accoucher ou se faire accoucher: Rapport synthèse." *Bulletin de l'Association pour la Santé Publique du Québec* 5(1).

————. 1988. "Femmes, enfantement et changement social: Le Cas de la césarienne." Ph.D. thesis, Université Laval.

————. 1990a. "L'Autonomie des femmes: Quelques réflexions bilan sur un objectif." *Santé mentale au Québec* 15(1): 120–33.

————. 1990b. "La Normalisation de la césarienne: La Résultante de rapports femmes/experts." *Anthropologie et sociétés, culture et clinique* 14(1): 25–41.

————. 1996. "The Reproductive Body: From Medicalization to Biomedical Management." Paper. Département de médecine sociale et préventive, Université Laval.

De Koninck, Maria, and F. Saillant. 1981. *Essai sur la santé des femmes.* Quebec: Conseil du Statut de la Femme.

De Koninck, Maria, and Marie-Hélène Parizeau. 1991. "Réflexions sur les techno-sciences et l'instrumentalisation dans la procréation humaine." *Service social* 40(1): 12–30.

Delaney, Janice, M. J. Lupton, and Emily Toth. 1976. *The Curse: A Cultural History of Menstruation.* New York: Mentor.

DeMarco, Carolyn. 1989. "Medical Malepractice." *Healthsharing* 10(4): 10–13.

Deutsch, Helene. 1984. "The Menopause." *International Journal of Psychoanalyis* 65(1): 55–62.

Dewhurst, John. 1981. *Integrated Obstetrics and Gynecology for Postgraduates.* Oxford: Blackwell Scientific Publications.

Dillon, Robin. 1992. "Toward a Feminist Conception of Self-Respect." *Hypatia* 7(1): 52–69.

Diprose, Rosalyn. 1994. *The Bodies of Women: Ethics, Embodiment, and Sexual Difference.* New York: Routledge.

————. 1995. "The Body Biomedical Ethics Forgets." In *Troubled Bodies: Critical Perspectives on Postmodernism, Medical Ethics, and the Body,* ed. Paul A. Komesaroff. Durham, N.C.: Duke University Press.

DisAbled Women's Network. N.d. "Violence Against Women Fact Sheet." DisAbled Women's Network, Toronto.

Division of Research Investigations. 1993. "Investigation Report: St. Luc Hospital." Office of Research Integrity, Report no. 91–08, Rockville, Md.

Dobash, R. P., and R. E. Dobash. 1979. *Violence Against Wives*. New York: Free Press.

———. 1992. *Women, Violence, and Social Change*. New York: Routledge.

———. 1995. "Reflections on Findings from the Violence Against Women Survey." *Canadian Journal of Criminology* 37(3): 457–84.

Dobash, R. P., R. E. Dobash, and K. Cavanagh. 1985. "The Contact Between Battered Women and Social and Medical Agencies." In *Private Violence and Public Policy: The Needs of Battered Women and the Response of the Public Service*, ed. J. Pahl. Boston: Routledge and Kegan Paul.

Dodd, Dianne. 1982. "The Canadian Birth Control Movement, 1929–1939." Master's thesis, University of Toronto.

———. 1983. "The Hamilton Birth Control Clinic of the 1930s." *Ontario History* 75(1): 71–87.

———. 1985. "The Canadian Birth Control Movement: Two Approaches to the Dissemination of Contraceptive Technology." *Scientia Canadensis* 9(1): 53–66.

———. 1991. "Advice to Parents: The Blue Books, Helen MacMurchy, MD, and the Federal Department of Health, 1920–34." *Canadian Bulletin of Medical History* 8(2): 203–30.

Donchin, Anne. 1998. "Understanding Autonomy Relationally: Toward a Reconfiguration of Bioethical Principles." *Journal of Medicine and Philosophy* 23.

Donnison, Jean. 1977. *Midwives and Medical Men: A History of Inter-Professional Rivalries and Women's Rights*. London: Heinemann.

Donovan, Leslie A. 1987. "Recurrences." In *With Wings: An Anthology of Literature by and About Women with Disabilities*, ed. Marsha Saxton and Florence Howe. New York: The Feminist Press at the City University of New York.

Doress, Pamela Brown, Diana Laskin Siegal, and the Midlife and Older Women Book Project. 1987. *Ourselves, Growing Older*. New York: Simon and Schuster.

Douglas, Mary. 1990. "Risk as a Forensic Resource." *Daedalus* 119(4): 1–16.

Doyal, Lesley. 1994. "Women, Health, and the Sexual Division of Labor: A Case Study of the Women's Health Movement in Britain." In *Women's Health, Politics, and Power: Essays on Sex/Gender, Medicine, and Public Health*. ed. Nancy Krieger and Elizabeth Fee. Amityville, N.Y.: Baywood.

Dreifus, Claudia, ed. 1977. *Seizing Our Bodies: The Politics of Women's Health*. New York: Vintage Books.

Dresser, Rebecca. 1992. "Wanted: Single, White Male for Medical Research." *Hastings Center Report* 22:24–29.

———. 1996. "What Bioethics Can Learn from the Women's Health Movement." In *Feminism and Bioethics: Beyond Reproduction*, ed. Susan M. Wolf. New York: Oxford University Press.

Driedger, Diane, and April D'Aubin. 1991. "Discarding the Shroud of Silence:

An International Perspective on Violence, Women, and Disability." *Canadian Woman Studies/ Les Cahiers de la femme* 12(1): 81–83.

Driedger, Diane, and Susan Gray, eds. 1992. *Imprinting Our Image: An International Anthology by Women with Diabilities.* Charlottetown, P.E.I.: Gynergy Books.

Drugs Directorate, Health Canada. 1996. "Inclusion of Women in Clinical Trials During Pregnancy." Ottawa, September 25.

Dua, Enakshi, Maureen FitzGerald, Linda Gardner, Darien Taylor, and Lisa Wyndels, eds. 1994. *On Women Healthsharing.* Toronto: The Women's Press.

DuBose, E. R., R. Hamel, and L. J. O'Connell. 1994. *A Matter of Principles? Ferment in U.S. Bioethics.* Valley Forge, Pa.: Trinity Press International.

Duden, Barbara. 1993. *Disembodying Women: Perspectives on Pregnancy and the Unborn.* Cambridge, Mass.: Harvard University Press.

Dudley, Emilius. 1902. *The Principles and Practice of Gynecology for Students and Practitioners.* Philadelphia: Lea Bros.

Duran, Jane. 1991. *Toward a Feminist Epistemology.* Lanham, Md.: Rowman and Littlefield.

Duster, Troy. 1990. *Backdoor to Eugenics.* New York: Routledge.

Dworkin, Gerald. 1988. *The Theory and Practice of Autonomy.* Cambridge: Cambridge University Press.

Dyck, Isabel. 1995. "Human Geographies: The Changing Lifeworlds of Women with Multiple Sclerosis." *Social Science and Medicine* 40(3): 307–20.

Eakin, J. M., A. Robertson, B. Poland, D. Coburn, and R. Edwards. 1996. "Towards a Critical Science Perspective on Health Promotion Research." *Health Promotion International* 11(2): 157–65.

Easlea, Brian. 1981. *Science and Sexual Oppression: Patriarchy's Confrontation with Woman and Nature.* London: Weidenfeld and Nicolson.

Edemikpong, Ntiense Ben. 1992. "We Shall Not Fold Our Arms and Wait: Female Genital Mutilation." In *Imprinting Our Image: An International Anthology by Women with Diabilities,* ed. Diane Driedger and Susan Gray. Charlottetown, P.E.I.: Gynergy Books.

Ehrenreich, Barbara. 1973. *Complaints and Disorders: The Sexual Politics of Sickness.* New York: Old Westbury.

Ehrenreich, Barbara, and Annette Fuentes. 1981. "Life on the Global Assembly Line." *MS* 9(7): 52–59.

Ehrenreich, Barbara, and Deirdre English. 1972. *Witches, Midwives, and Nurses: A History of Women Healers.* Glass Mountain Pamphlet, no. 1. Old Westbury, N.Y.: The Feminist Press.

———. 1979. *For Her Own Good: Two Hundred Fifty Years of the Experts' Advice to Women.* London: Pluto Press.

Ehrhardt, Julie, and Bernice Sandler. 1990. *Rx for Success: Improving the Climate for Women in Medical Schools and Teaching Hospitals.* Washington, D.C.: Project on the Status and Education of Women.

Eichler, Margrit. 1993. "Frankenstein Meets Kafka: The Royal Commission on

New Reproductive Technologies." In *Misconceptions: The Social Construction of Choice and the New Reproductive Technologies,* ed. G. Basen, M. Eichler, and A. Lippman. Prescott, Ont.: Voyageur Publishing.

Elliott, B. A., and M.M.P. Johnson. 1995. "Domestic Violence in a Primary Care Setting." *Archives of Family Medicine* 4:113–19.

Elston, Mary Ann. 1981. "Medicine as 'Old Husbands' Tales': The Impact of Feminism." In *Men's Studies Modified: The Impact of Feminism on the Academic Disciplines,* ed. Dale Spender. New York: Pergamon Press.

Englehardt, H. T. 1996. *The Foundations of Bioethics,* 2d ed. Oxford: Oxford University Press.

Epstein, C. J. 1997. "ASHG Presidential Address: Toward the 21st Century." *American Journal of Human Genetics* 60:1–9.

Eto, Jun. 1979. "The Breakdown of Motherhood Is Wrecking Our Children." *Japan Echo* 6:102–9.

Evans, Robert G., Morris L. Barer, and Theodore R. Marmor, eds. 1994. *Why Are Some People Healthy and Others Not? The Determinants of the Health of Populations.* New York: A. de Gruyter.

Faden, Ruth, Nancy Kass, and Deven McGraw. 1996. "Women as Vessels and Vectors: Lessons from the HIV Epidemic." In *Feminism and Bioethics: Beyond Reproduction,* ed. Susan M. Wolf. New York: Oxford University Press.

Farge, B., and B. Rahder. 1991. *Police Response to Incidents of Wife Assault.* Toronto: Assaulted Women's Helpline.

Farquhar, Dion. 1996. *The Other Machine: Discourse and Reproductive Technologies.* New York: Routledge.

Fausto-Sterling, Anne. 1985. *Myths of Gender: Biological Theories About Women and Men.* New York: Basic Books.

Featherstone, Mike, and Mike Hepworth. 1991. "The Mask of Ageing and the Postmodern Life Course." In *The Body: Social Process and Cultural Theory,* ed. M. Featherstone, M. Hepworth, and B. S. Turner. London: Sage.

Fee, Elizabeth. 1979. "Nineteenth-Century Craniology: The Study of the Female Skull." *Bulletin of the History of Medicine* 53:415–33.

———. ed. 1983. *Women and Health: The Politics of Sex in Medicine.* Amityville, N.Y.: Baywood.

Fee, Elizabeth, and Nancy Krieger. 1993. "Understanding AIDS: Historical Interpretations and the Limits of Biomedical Individualism." *American Journal of Public Health* 83:1477–86.

———, eds. 1994. *Women's Health, Politics, and Power: Essays on Sex/Gender, Medicine, and Public Health.* Amityville, N.Y.: Baywood.

Fellman, Anita Clair, and Michael Fellman. 1981. *Making Sense of the Self: Medical Advice Literature in Late Nineteenth-Century America.* Philadelphia: University of Pennsylvania Press.

Felstiner, William, and Austin Sarat. 1992. "Enactments of Power: Negotiating Reality and Responsibility in Lawyer-Client Interactions." *Cornell Law Review* 77:1447–1511.

Ferraro, K. J. 1996. "The Dance of Dependency: A Genealogy of Domestic Violence." *Discourse* 11(4): 77–91.

Ferris, L. E. 1994. "Canadian Family Physicians' and General Practitioners' Perceptions of Their Effectiveness in Identifying and Treating Wife Abuse." *Medical Care* 32(12): 1163–72.

Ferris, L. E., and F. Tudiver. 1992. "Family Physicians' Approach to Wife Abuse: A Study of Ontario, Canada, Practices." *Family Medicine* 24:276–82.

Fiedler, Deborah Cordero. 1996. "Authoritative Knowledge and Birth Territories in Contemporary Japan." *Medical Anthropology Quarterly (Special Issue on Authoritative Knowledge)* 10(2): 195–212.

Fine, Michelle, and Adrienne Asch, eds. 1988. *Women with Disabilities: Essays in Psychology, Culture, and Politics.* Philadelphia: Temple University Press.

Finger, Anne. 1984. "Claiming *All* of Our Bodies: Reproductive Rights and Disability." In *Test-Tube Women: What Future for Motherhood?* ed. Rita Arditti, Renate Duelli Klein, and Shelley Minden. London: Pandora Press. Reprinted in *Families in the U.S.: Kinship and Domestic Politics,* ed. Karen V. Hansen and Anita Ilta Garey. Philadelphia: Temple University Press, 1998.

Finkelhor, D., R. J. Gelles, G. T. Hotaling, and M. A. Straus, eds. 1983. *The Dark Side of Families: Current Family Violence Research.* Beverly Hills, Calif.: Sage.

Fisher, Sue. 1986. *In the Patient's Best Interests: Women and the Politics of Medical Decisions.* New Brunswick, N.J.: Rutgers University Press.

Fisher, Sue, and Alexandra Todd, eds. 1983. *The Social Organization of Doctor Patient Communication.* Washington, D.C.: Center for Applied Linguistics.

Fitzgerald, F. T. 1994. "The Tyranny of Health." *New England Journal of Medicine* 331:196–98.

Flitcraft, A. 1991. *AMA Scientific Statement.* American Medical Association, Chicago.

Foucault, Michel. 1965. *Madness and Civilization.* New York: Random House.

———. 1973. *The Birth of the Clinic.* New York: Vintage.

———. 1979. *Discipline and Punish.* New York: Vintage.

———. 1980a. *The History of Sexuality.* Vol. 1. New York: Vintage.

———. 1980b. *Power/Knowledge.* Ed. Colin Gordon. Brighton, Eng.: Harvester.

———. 1991. "Governmentality." In *The Foucault Effect: Studies in Governmentality,* ed. G. Burchell, C. Gordon, and P. Miller. Hemel Hempstead, Eng.: Harvester Wheatsheaf.

Fox, Renée C. 1977. "The Medicalization and Demedicalization of American Society." *Deadalus* 106:9–22.

Frankel, Richard M. 1983. "The Laying On of Hands: Aspects of the Organization of Gaze, Touch, and Talk in a Medical Encounter." In *The Social Organization of Doctor-Patient Communications,* ed. Sue Fisher and Alexandra Todd. Washington, D.C.: Center for Applied Linguistics.

Frankenberg, Ruth. 1993a. *The Social Contruction of Whiteness: White Women, Race Matters.* Minneapolis: University of Minnesota Press.

————. 1993b. "Anthropological and Epidemiological Narratives of Prevention." In *Knowledge, Power, and Practice: The Anthropology of Medicine and Everyday Life,* ed. S. Lindenbaum and M. Lock. Berkeley and Los Angeles: University of California Press.

Frederick, Sue. 1994. "Dr. Susan Love: Making Patients Medical Partners." In *Women's Health: Readings on Social, Economic, and Political Issues,* 2d ed., ed. Nancy Worcester and Mariamne H. Whatley. Dubuque, Iowa: Kendall/Hunt.

Freidan, Betty. 1993. *The Fountain of Age.* New York: Simon and Schuster.

Frenk, Julio, José Luis Bobadilla, Claudio Stern, Tomas Frejka, and Rafael Lozano. 1991. "Elements for a Theory of the Health Transition." *Health Transition Review: The Cultural, Social and Behavioural Determinants of Health* 1(1): 21–38.

Friedson, Eliot. 1970. *Profession of Medicine: A Study of the Sociology of Applied Knowledge.* New York: Dodd, Mead.

————. 1968. "The Impurity of Professional Authority." In *Institutions and the Person,* ed. H. Becker, D. Geer, and R. Weiss. Chicago: Aldine.

Frye, Marilyn. 1975. "Male Chauvinism: A Conceptual Analysis." In *Philosophy and Sex,* ed. R. Baker and F. Elliston. Buffalo, N.Y.: Prometheus Books.

Fuchs, Victor. 1974. *Who Shall Die? Health, Economics and Social Choice.* New York: Basic Books.

Fugh-Berman, Adriane. 1992. "Tales Out of Medical School." *The Nation,* January 20:37, 54–56.

Fujin Hakusho. 1989. *Kōrei sha fukushi,* ed. Nihon Fujin and Dantai-Rengōkai. Tokyo: Horupu Shuppan.

Gajerski-Cauley, Anne, ed. 1989. *Women, Development, and Disability.* Winnipeg: Coalition of Provincial Organizations of the Handicapped.

Gallagher, Catherine, and Thomas Laqueur, eds. 1987. *The Making of the Modern Body.* Berkeley and Los Angeles: University of California Press.

Gamble, Vanessa Northington, and Bonnie Ellen Blustein. 1994. "Racial Differentials in Medical Care: Implications for Research on Women." In *Women and Health Research: Ethical and Legal Issues of Including Women in Clinical Studies,* vol. 2, ed. Anna C. Mastroianni, Ruth Faden, and Daniel Federman. Washington, D.C.: National Academy Press.

Gardener, Katy. 1981. "Well Woman Clinics." In *Women, Health, and Reproduction,* ed. Helen Roberts. London: Routledge and Kegan Paul.

Gardiner, Judith Kegan. 1995. *Provoking Agents: Gender and Agency in Theory and Practice.* Chicago: University of Illinois Press.

Ghent, W. R., N. P. Da Sylva, and M. E. Farren. 1985. "Family Violence: Guidelines for Recognition and Management." *Canadian Medical Association Journal* 132:541–63.

Giachello, Aida L. 1995. "Cultural Diversity and Institutional Inequality." In

Health Issues for Women of Color: A Cultural Diversity Perspective, ed. Diane L. Adams. Thousand Oaks, Calif.: Sage.

Gill, Carol F. 1996. "Cultivating Common Ground: Women with Disabilities." In *Man-Made Medicine: Women's Health, Public Policy, and Reform*, ed. Kary L. Moss. Durham, N.C.: Duke University Press.

Gillick, M. R. 1984. "Health Promotion, Jogging, and the Pursuit of the Moral Life." *Journal of Health Politics, Policy and Law* 9:369–87.

Gilligan, Carol. 1982. *In a Different Voice: Psychological Theory and Women's Moral Development*. Cambridge, Mass.: Harvard University Press.

Gilman, Sander. 1985. *Difference and Pathology: Stereotyping of Sexuality, Race and Madness*. Ithaca, N.Y.: Cornell University Press.

———. 1988. *Disease and Representation: Images of Illness from Madness to AIDS*. Ithaca, N.Y.: Cornell University Press.

Ginsberg, Faye, and Anna Lowenhaupt Tsing. 1990. *Uncertain Terms: Negotiating Gender in American Culture*. Boston: Beacon Press.

Ginsberg, Faye, and Rayna Rapp. 1991. "The Politics of Reproduction." *Annual Review of Anthropology* 20:311–43.

———. eds. 1995. *Conceiving the New World Order: The Global Politics of Reproduction*. Berkeley and Los Angeles: University of California Press.

Goldberg, Marcel. 1982. "Cet obscur objet de l'épidémiologie." *Sciences sociales et santé* 1:55–122.

Gondolf, E., and E. Fisher. 1989. *Battered Women as Survivors*. Lexington, Mass: Lexington Books.

Gordon, Linda. 1975. "The Politics of Birth Control, 1920–1940: The Impact of Professionals." In *Women and Health: The Politics of Sex in Medicine*, ed. Elizabeth Fee. Farmingdale, N.Y.: Baywood.

———. 1976. *Women's Body, Woman's Right: A Social History of Birth Control in America*. New York: Penguin.

———. 1988. *Heroes of Their Own Lives: The Politics and History of Family Violence*. New York: Penguin Books.

Gosden, R. G. 1985. *The Biology of Menopause: The Causes and Consequences of Ovarian Aging*. London: Academic Press.

Gostin, L. 1991. "Gender Discrimination: The Use of Genetically Based Diagnostic and Prognostic Tests by Employers and Insurers." *American Journal of Law and Medicine* 17:109–44.

Graham, Hilary. 1985. "Providers, Negotiators, and Mediators." In *Women, Health, and Healing*, ed. Ellen Lewin and Virginia Olesen. London: Tavistock.

Graham, Hilary, and Ann Oakley. 1981. "Competing Ideologies of Reproduction: Medical and Maternal Perspectives on Pregnancy and Childbirth." In *Women, Health, and Reproduction*, ed. Helen Roberts. London: Routledge and Kegan Paul.

Graham, Wendy J., and Oona M. R. Campbell. 1992. "Maternal Health and the Measurement Trap." *Social Science and Medicine* 35(8): 967–77.

Grant, Nicole J. 1992. *The Selling of Contraception: The Dalkon Shield Case, Sexuality, and Women's Anatomy*. Columbus: Ohio State University Press.

Graves, William. 1929. *Gynecology*. Philadelphia: W. B. Saunders.

Greaves, Lorraine. 1995. "Women and Health: A Feminist Perspective on Tobacco Control." In *Changing Methods: Feminists Transforming Practice*, ed. Sandra Burt and Lorraine Code. Peterborough, Ont.: Broadview Press.

Green, Harvey. 1986. *Fit for America: Health Fitness, Sport, and American Society, 1830–1940*. New York: Pantheon.

Greenblatt, R. B. 1972. "Hormonal Management of the Menopause." *Medical Counter-Point* 4:19.

Greenblatt, R. B., and A. Z. Teran. 1987. "Advice to Post-Menopausal Women." In *The Climacteric and Beyond*, ed. L. Zichella, M. Whitehead, and P. A. Van Keep. Park Ridge, N.J.: Parthenon Publishing Group.

Greenhalgh, Susan, and Hiali Li. 1996. "Engendering Reproductive Policy and Practice in Peasant China: For a Feminist Demography of Reproduction." In *Gender and Scientific Authority*, ed. Barbara Laslett, Sally Gregory Kohlstedt, Helen Longino, and Evelynn Hammonds. Chicago: University of Chicago Press.

Greer, Germaine. 1991. *The Change: Women, Aging, and the Menopause*. London: Hamish Hamilton.

Grodin, M. 1992. *The Nazi Doctors and the Nuremberg Code: Human Rights in Human Experimentation*. New York: Oxford University Press.

Groesser, Antoinette. 1972. "Is Gynecology for Women?" In *The Witch's Os*, ed. M. Alleyn. Stamford, Conn.: New Moon Publications.

Gross, Amy, and Dee Ito. 1991. *Women Talk About Gynecological Surgery: From Diagnosis to Recovery*. New York: Clarkson Potter Publishers.

Grosz, Elizabeth. 1994. *Volatile Bodies: Toward a Corporeal Feminism*. Bloomington: Indiana University Press.

Guttmacher, Sally. 1997. "Whole in Body, Mind, and Spirit: Holistic Health and the Limits of Medicine." *The Hastings Center* 9(2): 15–21.

Habermas, Jurgen. 1981. *The Theory of Communicative Action*. Vol. 1, *Reason and the Rationalization of Society*. Trans. by Thomas McCarthy. Boston: Beacon Press.

Haga, Noboru. 1990. *Ryōsai kenbo* (Good wives and wise mothers). Tokyo: Yusankaku.

Hagan, Kay Leigh. 1993. "Codependency and the Myth of Recovery." In *Fugitive Information: Essays from a Feminist Hothead*. San Francisco: Pandora/ Harper San Francisco.

Haire, Doris B. 1972. *The Cultural Warping of Childbirth*. Milwaukee, Wisc.: International Childbirth Education Association.

Hall, Winfield Scott. 1917. *Sexual Knowledge*. Toronto: McClellan and Stewart.

Haller, John S. Jr. 1971. "Neurasthenia: The Medical Profession and the 'New Woman' of the Late Nineteenth Century," *New York State Journal of Medicine* 71 (February 15): 473–82.

Haller, John S. Jr., and Robin Haller. 1974. *The Physician and Sexuality in Victorian America*. Chicago: University of Illinois Press.

Hamilton, J. A. 1996. "Women and Health Policy: On the Inclusion of Females in Clinical Trials." In *Gender and Health: An International Perspective*, ed. Carolyn Sargent and Caroline Brettell. Upper Saddle River, N.J.: Prentice Hall.

Hamilton, N., and T. Bhatti. 1996. *Population Health Promotion: An Integrated Model of Population Health and Health Promotion*. Ottawa: Health Promotion Development Division.

Hancock, T. 1993. "Health, Human Development, and the Community Ecosystem: Three Ecological Models." *Health Promotion International* 8:41–47.

Handwerker, L. 1994. "Medical Risk: Implications for Poor Pregnant Women." *Social Sciences and Medicine* 38:665–71.

Handwerker, W. Penn, ed. 1990. *Births and Power: Social Change, and the Politics of Reproduction*. Boulder, Colo.: Westview Press.

Hannaford, Susan. 1985. *Living Outside Inside: A Disabled Woman's Experience. Towards a Social and Political Perspective*. Berkeley, Calif.: Canterbury Press.

Hanvey, L., and D. Kinnon. 1993. "The Health Care Sector's Response to Woman Abuse." Discussion paper for the Family Violence Division, Health Canada, National Clearinghouse on Family Violence, Ottawa, June.

Haraway, Donna. 1989. *Primate Visions: Gender, Race, and Nature in the World of Modern Science*. New York: Routledge.

———. 1991. "Situated Knowledges: The Science Question in Feminism and the Privilege of Partial Perspectives." In *Simians, Cyborgs, and Women*. New York: Routledge.

Harding, Sandra. 1991. *Whose Science? Whose Knowledge? Thinking from Women's Lives*. Ithaca, N.Y.: Cornell University Press.

———. 1993. "Rethinking Standpoint Epistemology: 'What Is Strong Objectivity'?" In *Feminist Epistemologies*, ed. Linda Alcoff and Elizabeth Potter. New York: Routledge.

———, ed. 1993. *The "Racial" Economy of Science*. Bloomington: Indiana University Press.

Harrington, Charlene, Robert J. Newcomer, Carroll L. Estes, et al. 1985. *Long Term Care of the Elderly*. Beverley Hills, Calif.: Sage.

Hartman, Betsy. 1987. *Reproductive Rights and Wrongs: The Global Politics of Population Control and Contraceptive Choice*. New York: Harper and Row.

Harvey, Elizabeth, and Kathleen Okruhlik, eds. 1992. *Women and Reason*. Ann Arbor: University of Michigan Press.

Haspels, Ary A., and Pieter A. van Keep. 1979. "Endocrinology and Management of the Peri-Menopause." In *Psycho-somatics in Peri-Menopause*, ed. Ary A. Haspels and H. Musaph. Baltimore, Md.: University Park Press.

Hausman, Bernice. 1995. *Changing Sex: Transsexualism, Technology, and Ideas of Gender*. Durham, N.C.: Duke University Press.

Hawksworth, Mary E. 1996. "Knowers, Knowing, Known: Feminist Theory and Claims of Truth." In *Gender and Scientific Authority*, ed. Barbara Laslett,

Sally Gregory Kohlstedt, Helen Longino, and Evelynn Hammonds. Chicago: University of Chicago Press.

Head, C., and A. Taft. 1995. "Improving General Practitioner Management of a Woman Experiencing Domestic Violence: A Study of the Beliefs and Experiences of Women Victims/Survivors and of GP's." Report prepared for Commonwealth General Practitioner Evaluation Program, Australia.

Health Services Directorate, Health and Welfare Canada. 1991. *Health Care Related to Abuse, Assault, Neglect, and Family Violence: Guidelines for Establishing Standards.* 2d ed. Ottawa: Health Services Directorate, Health and Welfare Canada.

Healy, B. 1991. "The Yentl Syndrome." *New England Journal of Medicine* 325(4): 274–76.

Heise, L. 1993a. "Violence Against Women: The Hidden Health Burden. *World Health Statistics Quarterly* 46(1): 185–91.

———. 1993b. "Violence Against Women: The Missing Agenda." In *The Health of Women: A Global Perspective*, ed. Marge Koblinsky, Judith Timyan, and Jill Gay. Boulder, Colo.: Westview Press.

Held, Virginia. 1993. *Feminist Morality: Transforming Culture, Society, and Politics.* Chicago: University of Chicago Press.

Hendricks-Matthews, Marybeth. 1992. "Preface" and "Violence, the Silent Epidemic." In *Violence Education: Towards a Solution*, ed. Marybeth Hendricks-Matthews. Kansas City: The Society of Teachers of Family Medicine.

———. 1993. "Survivors of Abuse: Health Care Issues." *Primary Care* 20(2): 391–406.

Herbert, C. 1991. "Family Violence and Family Physicians." *Canadian Family Physician* 37: 385–90.

Heriot, M. Jean. 1996. "Fetal Rights Versus the Female Body: Contested Domains." *Medical Anthropology Quarterly* 10(2): 176–84.

Herman, J. 1991. "The Numbers Game." *Journal of Clinical Epidemiology* 44: 207–9.

Higuchi, Keiko. 1985. "Women at Home." *Japan Echo* 12:51–57.

Hilliard, Marion. 1957. *A Woman Doctor Looks at Love and Life.* Garden City, N.Y.: Doubleday.

Hillyer, Barbara. 1993. *Feminism and Disability.* Norman and London: University of Oklahoma Press.

Ho, David D. 1997. "It's AIDS, Not Tuskegee." *Time Magazine* September 29, 63.

Hoagland, Sarah Lucia. 1992. "Lesbian Ethics and Female Agency." In *Explorations in Feminist Ethics: Theory and Practice*, ed. Susan Browning Cole and Susan Coultrap-McQuin. Bloomington: Indiana University Press.

Hoangmai, Pham, Phyllis Freeman, and Nancy Kohn. 1992. *Understanding the Second Epidemic: The Status of Research on Women and AIDS in the United States.* Washington, D.C.: Center for Women Policy Studies.

Hoff, L. A. 1991. "An Anthropological Perspective of Wife Battering." In *Vio-*

lence Against Women: Nursing Research, Education, and Practice Issues, ed. C. Sampselle. New York: Hemisphere.

Hoff, L. A., and L. Rosenbaum. 1994. "A Victimization Assessment Tool: Instrument Development and Clinical Implications." *Journal of Advanced Nursing* 20:627–34.

Hoffman, B. F., D. Sinclair, D. W. Currie, and P. Jaffee.1990. "Wife Assault: Understanding and Helping the Woman, Man, and the Children." *Ontario Medical Review* 57(7): 36–44.

Holtzman, N. A. 1989. *Proceed with Caution.* Baltimore, Md.: Johns Hopkins University Press.

Hooks, Bell. 1989. *Talking Back: Thinking Feminist, Thinking Black.* Boston: South End Press.

———. 1990. *Yearning: Race, Gender, and Cultural Politics.* Toronto: Between the Lines.

Houlihan, Inez. 1984. "The Image of Women in *Chatelaine* Editorials, 1928–1977." Master's thesis, University of Toronto.

Hubbard, Ruth. 1990. *The Politics of Women's Biology.* New Brunswick, N.J.: Rutgers University Press.

Hubbard, Ruth, and Elijah Wald. 1993. *Exploding the Gene Myth.* Boston: Beacon Press.

Hughes, M. R., and C. T. Caskey. 1991. "Medical Genetics." *Journal of the American Medical Association* 265:3132–34.

Illich, Ivan. 1976. *Medical Nemesis: The Expropriation of Health.* New York: Pantheon.

———. 1992. *In the Mirror of the Past: Lectures and Addresses, 1978–1990.* New York: Marion Boyars.

Imber, Jonathan. 1988. "The Impact of Doctors on the Definition of the Abortion Issue in the U.S.," Presentation at the Social Sciences Look at Medical Ethics Conference, McGill University, Montreal, June 12–14.

International League of Societies for Persons with Mental Handicap. 1994. *Just Technology? From Principles to Practice in Bio-Ethical Issues.* Toronto: Roehrer Institute.

Irvine, Janice M. 1990. *Disorders of Desire: Sex and Gender in Modern American Sexology.* Philadelphia: Temple University Press.

Isaac, N. E., and R. L. Sanchez. 1993. "Emergency Department Response to Battered Women in Massachusetts." *Harvard Injury Control Center,* reprint no. 47/1/54060.

Jackson, Margaret. 1987. "'Facts of Life;' or, The Eroticization of Women's Oppression? Sexology and the Social Construction of Heterosexuality." In *The Cultural Construction of Sexuality,* ed. Pat Caplan. New York: Tavistock.

Jacobson, Jodi L. 1993. "Women's Health: The Price of Poverty." In *The Health of Women: A Global Perspective,* ed. Marge Koblinsky, Judith Timyan, and Jill Gay. Boulder, Colo.: Westview Press.

Jacobus, Mary, Evelyn Fox Keller, and Sally Shuttleworth, eds. 1990. *Body/Politics: Women and the Discourses of Science*. New York: Routledge.

Jaffre, Yannick, and Alain Prual. 1994. "Midwives in Niger: An Uncomfortable Position Between Social Behaviours and Health Care Constraints." *Social Science and Medicine* 38(8): 1069–73.

Jane [pseud.]. 1990. "Just Call 'Jane.' " In *From Abortion to Reproductive Freedom: Transforming a Movement*, ed. Marlene Gerber Fried. Boston: South End Press.

Janzen, John. 1981. "The Need for a Taxonomy of Health in the Study of African Therapeutics." *Social Science and Medicine* 15B:185–94.

Japan Pharmaceutical Manufacturers Association. 1990. *Data Book, 1989*. Tokyo: Japan Pharmaceutical Manufacturers Association.

Johnson, H. 1996. *Dangerous Domains: Violence Against Women in Canada*. Toronto: Nelson Canada.

Jones, J. H. 1981. *Bad Blood: The Tuskegee Syphilis Experiment: A Tragedy of Race and Medicine*. New York: The Free Press (Collier Macmillan).

Jones, Kathleen. 1988. "On Authority, or, Why Women Are Not Entitled to Speak." In *Feminism and Foucault: Reflections on Resistance*, ed. Irene Diamond and Lee Quinby. Boston: Northeastern University Press.

Jonsen, A. R. and S. Toulmin. 1988. *The Abuse of Casuistry: A History of Reasoning*. Berkeley and Los Angeles: University of California Press.

Jordan, B. 1987. "The Hut and the Hospital: Information, Power, and Symbolism in the Artifacts of Birth." *Birth* 14(1): 181–216.

———. 1992. "Technology and Social Interaction: Notes on the Achievement of Authoritative Knowledge in Complex Settings." Technical Report IRL 92–0027. Institute for Research on Learning, Palo Alto, Calif.

——— (1978) 1993. *Birth in Four Cultures: A Cross-Cultural Investigation of Childbirth in Yucatan, Holland, Sweden, and the United States*. 4th ed. Prospect Heights, Ill.: Waveland Press.

Jordan, B., and S. Irwin. 1989. "The Ultimate Failure: Court-Ordered Caesarean Section." In *New Approaches to Human Reproduction: Social and Ethical Dimensions*, ed. Linda Whiteford and Marilyn M. Poland. Boulder, Colo.: Westview Press.

Jordanova, Ludmilla. 1989. *Sexual Visions: Images of Gender in Science and Medicine Between the Eighteenth and Twentieth Centuries*. Brighton, Eng.: Harvester Wheatsheaf.

Jose-Kampfner, Christine. 1995. "Health Care on the Inside." In *Health Issues for Women of Color: A Cultural Diversity Perspective*, ed. Diane L. Adams. Thousand Oaks, Calif: Sage.

Kahn, P. 1996. "Coming to Grips with Genes and Risk." *Science* 274:496–98.

Karl, Marile. 1995. *Women and Empowerment*. London: Zed Books.

Kasl, Charlotte Davis. 1992. *Many Roads, One Journey: Moving Beyond the Twelve Steps*. New York: HarperCollins.

Kass, Leon. 1975. "Regarding the End of Medicine and the Pursuit of Health." *Public Interest* 40 (summer): 38–39.

Katz, Jay, ed. 1972. *Experimentation with Human Beings: The Authority of the Investigator, Subject, Professions, and State in the Human Experimentation Process.* New York: Russell Sage Foundation.

Kaufert, Patricia. 1994. "Through Women's Eyes: The Case for a Feminist Epidemiology." In *On Women Healthsharing,* ed. Enakshi Dua, Maureen FitzGerald, Linda Gardner, Darien Taylor, and Lisa Wyndels. Toronto: The Women's Press.

———. 1996. "Women and the Debate over Mammography: An Economic, Political and Moral History." In *Gender and Health: An International Perspective,* ed. Carolyn Sargent and Caroline Brettell. Upper Saddle River, N.J.: Prentice Hall.

———, et al. 1988. "Menopause as Process or Event: The Creation of Definitions in Biomedicine." In *Biomedicine Examined,* ed. Margaret Lock and Deborah Gordon. Dordrecht, Holland: Kluwer Academic Publishers.

Kaufert, Patricia, and Sonja McKinlay. 1985. "Estrogen-Replacement Therapy: The Production of Medical Knowledge and the Emergence of Policy." In *Women, Health, and Healing: Toward a New Perspective,* ed. Ellen Lewin and Virginia Olesen. London: Tavistock.

Kaufert, Patricia, Penny Gilbert, and Tom Hassard. 1988. "Researching the Symptoms of Menopause: An Exercise in Methodology." *Maturitas* 10:117–31.

Kaufert, Patricia, and John O'Neil. 1990. "Cooptation and Control: The Reconstruction of Inuit Birth." *Medical Anthropology Quarterly* 4(4): 427–42.

———. 1993. "Analysis of a Dialogue on Risks in Childbirth." In *Knowledge, Power, and Practice: The Anthropology of Medicine and Everyday Life,* ed. Shirley Lindenbaum and Margaret Lock. Berkeley and Los Angeles: University of California Press.

Keat, Russell. 1986. "The Human Body in Social Theory: Reich, Foucault, and the Repressive Hypothesis." *Radical Philosophy* 42:24–32.

Keizai Kikaku Chōhen. 1982. *Nisen nen no Nihon.* Tokyo: Government printing office.

Keller, Evelyn Fox. 1995. "Fractured Images of Science, Language, and Power: A Postmodern Optic or Just Bad Eyesight?" In *Biopolitics: A Feminist and Ecological Reader on Biotechnology,* ed. Vandana Shiva and Ingunn Moser. London and Penang, Malaysia: Zed Books and the Third World Network.

Kennedy, David. 1970. *Birth Control in America: The Career of Margaret Sanger.* New Haven, Conn.: Yale University Press.

Kern, Stephen. 1975. *Anatomy and Destiny: A Cultural History of the Human Body.* Indianapolis, Ind.: Bobbs-Merrill.

Kerns, Virginia, and Judith K. Brown, eds. 1985. *In Her Prime: A New View of Middle-Aged Women.* South Hadley, Mass.: Bergin and Garvey.

Kessler, Susanne J. 1996. "The Medical Construction of Gender: Case Management of Intersexed Infants." In *Gender and Scientific Authority,* ed. Barbara

Laslett, Sally Gregory Kohlstedt, Helen Longino, and Evelynn Hammonds. Chicago: University of Chicago Press.

Kevles, Daniel J. 1992. "Out of Eugenics: The Historical Politics of the Human Genome." In *The Code of Codes: Scientific and Social Issues in the Human Genome Project.* ed. Daniel J. Kevles and Leroy Hood. Cambridge, Mass.: Harvard University Press.

Khoury, M. J., and the Genetics Working Group. 1996. "From Genes to Public Health: The Applications of Genetic Technology in Disease Prevention." *American Journal of Public Health* 86:1717–22.

Klein, Bonnie Sherr. 1992. "We Are Who You Are: Feminism and Disability." *Ms.* 3(3): 70–74.

Klein-Mathews, Yvonne. 1979. "How They Saw Us: Images of Women in National Film Board films of the 1940s and 1950s." *Atlantis* 4(2): 20–33.

Koblinsky, Marge, Oona M. R. Campbell, and Sioban D. Harlow. 1993. "Mother and More: A Broader Perspective on Women's Health." in *The Health of Women: A Global Perspective,* ed. Marge Koblinsky, Judith Timyan and Jill Gay. Boulder, Colo: Westview Press.

Koblinsky, Marge, Judith Timyan, and Jill Gay, eds. 1993. *The Health of Women: A Global Perspective.* Boulder, Colo: Westview Press.

Kohlberg, L. 1984. *Essays on Moral Development.* Vol. 2: *The Psychology of Moral Development: The Nature and Validity of Moral Stages.* San Francisco: Harper and Row.

Kolata, G. 1997. "Advent of Testing for Breast Cancer Genes Leads to Fears of Disclosure and Discrimination." *New York Times,* February 4, sec. C.

Komaromy, Miriam, A. B. Bindman, R. J. Haber, and M. A. Sande. 1993. "Sexual Harassment in Medical Training." *New England Journal of Medicine* 328(5): 322–26.

Komesaroff, Paul A. 1995. "From Bioethics to Microethics: Ethical Debate and Clinical Medicine." In *Troubled Bodies: Critical Perspectives on Postmodernism, Medical Ethics, and the Body,* ed. Paul A. Komesaroff. Durham, N.C.: Duke University Press.

———. ed. 1995. *Troubled Bodies: Critical Perspectives on Postmodernism, Medical Ethics, and the Body.* Durham, N.C.: Duke University Press.

Kōsei Hakusho. 1989. *Arata na kōreishazō to katsuryoku aru chōju fukushi shakai o mezashite.* Tokyo: Kōseishō.

Krieger, Nancy. 1994. "Man-Made Medicine and Women's Health: The BioPolitics of Sex/Gender and Race/Ethnicity." In *Women's Health, Politics, and Power: Essays on Sex/Gender, Medicine, and Public Health,* ed. Elizabeth Fee and Nancy Krieger. Amityville, N.Y.: Baywood.

Kurz, D. 1987. "Responses to Battered Women: Resistance to Medicalization." *Social Problems* 34:501–13.

Kurz, D., and E. Stark. 1988. "Not-So-Benign Neglect: The Medical Response to Battering." In *Feminist Perspectives on Wife Abuse,* ed. K. Yllö and M. Bograd. Newbury Park, Calif: Sage.

Labonte, R. 1995. "Population Health and Health Promotion: What Do They Have to Say to Each Other?" *Canadian Journal of Public Health* 86:165–68.

Labonte, R., and A. Robertson. 1996. "Delivering the Goods, Showing our Stuff: The Case for a Constructivist Paradigm for Health Promotion Research and Practice." *Health Education Quarterly* 23:431–47.

Laforce, Helene. 1990. "The Different Stages of the Elimination of Midwives in Quebec." In *Delivering Motherhood*, ed. Katherine Arnup, Andrée Lévesque, and Ruth Roach Pierson. Toronto: University of Toronto Press.

Lalonde, Marc. 1974. *A New Perspective on the Health of Canadians: A Working Document*. Ottawa: Minister of National Health and Welfare.

Lapham, E. V., C. Kozma, and J. O. Weiss. 1996. "Genetic Discrimination: Perspectives of Consumers." *Science* 274:621–24.

Laqueur, Thomas. 1990. *Making Sex: Body and Gender from the Greeks to Freud*. Cambridge, Mass.: Harvard University Press.

Laurence, Leslie, and Beth Weinhouse. 1994. *Outrageous Practices: The Alarming Truth about How Medicine Mistreats Women*. New York: Fawcett Columbine.

Leavitt, Judith Waltzer. 1980. "Birthing and Anaesthesia: The Debate over Twilight Sleep." *Signs* 6:147–64.

———. 1986. *Brought to Bed: Women and Childbearing in America, 1750–1950*. New York: Oxford University Press.

———. 1995. "'A Worrying Profession': The Domestic Environment of Medical Practice in Mid-Nineteenth-Century America." *Bulletin of the History of Medicine* 69(1): 1–29.

Leavitt, Judith Waltzer, and Whitney Walton. 1984. "'Down to Death's Door': Women's Perceptions of Childbirth in America." In *Women and Health in America*, ed. Judith Walzer Leavitt. Madison: University of Wisconsin Press.

Lebra, Takie. 1984. *Japanese Women: Constraint and Fulfillment*. Honolulu: University of Hawaii Press.

Le Breton, David. 1995. *La sociologie du risque*. Paris: Presses Universitaires du France, Que sais-je, 3016.

Leidy, L. E. 1994. "Biological Aspects of Menopause: Across the Lifespan." *Annual Reviews in Anthropology* 23:231–53.

Lenton R.A. 1995. "Power Versus Feminist Theories of Wife Abuse." *Canadian Journal of Criminology* 37(3): 305–30.

Lewontin, R. C. 1991. *Biology as Ideology: The Doctrine of DNA*. Concord, Ont.: House of Anansi Press.

Lex, Barbara W., and Janice Racine Norris. 1994. "Health Status of American Indian and Alaska Native Women." In *Women and Health Research: Ethical and legal Issues of Including Women in Clinical Studies*, vol. 2, ed. Anna C. Mastroianni, Ruth Faden, Daniel Federman, Institute of Medicine. Washington, D.C.: National Academy Press.

Lindenbaum, Shirley and Margaret Lock, eds. 1993. *Knowledge, Power, and Practice: The Anthropology of Medicine and Everyday Life*. Berkeley and Los Angeles: University of California Press.

Lippman, Abby. 1989. "Prenatal Diagnosis: Reproductive Choice? Reproductive Control?" In *The Future of Human Reproduction,* ed. Christine Overall. Toronto: The Women's Press.

———. 1991. "Prenatal Genetic Testing and Screening: Constructing Needs and Reinforcing Inequities." *American Journal of Law and Medicine* 17:15–50.

———. 1993. "Worrying—and Worrying About—the Geneticization of Reproduction and Health." In *Misconceptions: The Social Construction of Choice and the New Reproductive and Genetic Technologies,* ed. Gwynne Basen, Margrit Eichler, Abby Lippman. Prescott, Ont.: Voyageur Publishing.

———. Forthcoming. "The Gendered Nature of Geneticization." In *Implications of the New Genetics for Primary Care,* ed. Mary Briody Mahowald.

Litoff, Judy. 1978. *American Midwives, 1860 to the Present.* Westport, Conn.: Greenwood Press.

Lloyd, E. A. 1994. "Normality and Variations: The Human Genome Project and the Ideal Human Type." In *Are Genes Us? The Social Consequences of the New Genetics,* ed. Carl Cranor. New Brunswick, N.J.: Rutgers University Press.

Lloyd, Genevieve. 1993. *The Man of Reason: "Male" and "Female" in Western Philosophy.* 2d ed. Minneapolis: University of Minnesota Press.

Lock, Margaret. 1980. *East Asian Medicine in Urban Japan: Varieties of Medical Experience.* Berkeley and Los Angeles: University of California Press.

———. 1985. "Models and Practice in Medicine: Menopause as Syndrome or Life Transition?" In *Physicians of Western Medicine,* ed. R. A. Hahn and A. D. Gaines. Dordrecht, Holland: D. Reidel.

———. 1986. "Ambiguities of Aging: Japanese Experience and Perceptions of Menopause." In *Culture, Medicine, and Psychiatry,* ed. A. Kleinman. Dordrecht, Holland: D. Reidel.

———. 1988a. "A Nation at Risk: Interpretations of School Refusal in Japan." In *Biomedicine Examined,* ed. M. Lock and D. R. Gordon. Dordrecht, Holland: Kluwer Academic Publishers.

———. 1988b. "New Japanese Mythologies: Faltering Discipline and the Ailing Housewife in Japan." *American Ethnologist* 15:43–61.

———. 1990. "On Being Ethnic: The Politics of Identity Breaking and Making in Canada, or, *Nevra* on Sunday." *Culture, Medicine, and Psychiatry* 14:237–52.

———. 1993a. *Encounters with Aging: Mythologies of Menopause in Japan and North America.* Berkeley and Los Angeles: University of California Press.

———. 1993b. "Ideology, Female Midlife, and the Greying of Japan." *Journal of Japanese Studies* 19:43–78.

———. 1995. "Contesting the Natural in Japan: Moral Dilemmas and Technologies of Dying." *Culture, Medicine and Psychiatry* 19:1–38.

———. 1996. "Social and Cultural Issues in Connection with Breast Cancer Testing and Screening." Paper presented at symposium "Genetic Testing for Breast Cancer Susceptibility: The Science, The Ethics, The Future," International Bioethics Conference, San Francisco, November.

Lock, Margaret. Forthcoming. "Menopause: Lessons from Anthropology." *The Journal of Psychosomatic Medicine.*

Lock, Margaret, Patricia Kaufert, and Penny Gilbert. 1988. "Cultural Construction of the Menopausal Syndrome: The Japanese Case." *Maturitas* 10:317–32.

London, Steve, and Charles Hammond. 1986. "The Climacteric." In *Obstetrics and Gynecology,* ed. D. Danforth and J. Scott. Philadelphia: J. B. Lippincott.

Longino, H. E. 1990. *Science as Social Knowledge: Values and Objectivity in Scientific Inquiry.* Princeton, N.J.: Princeton University Press.

———. 1993. "Feminist Standpoint Theory and the Problems of Knowledge: Review Essay." *Signs* 19:201–12.

Lorde, Audre. 1980. *The Cancer Journals.* Argyle, N.Y.: Spinsters, Ink.

Love, Susan. 1990. *Dr. Susan Love's Breast Book.* Reading, Mass.: Addison-Wesley.

———. 1997. *Dr. Susan Love's Hormone Book: Making Informed Choices About Menopause.* New York: Random House.

Lowe, Marion. 1982. "Social Bodies: The Interaction of Culture and Women's Biology." In *Biological Woman—The Convenient Myth: A Collection of Feminist Essays and a Comprehensive Bibliography,* ed. Ruth Hubbard, Mary Sue Henifin, and Barbara Fried. Cambridge, Mass.: Schenkman.

———. 1983. "The Dialectic of Biology and Culture." In *Woman's Nature: Rationalizations of Inequality,* ed. Marion Lowe and Ruth Hubbard. New York: Pergamon Press.

Lowy, Fredrick H. 1994. "Memorandum to 'Those Interested in Research Involving Humans in Canada.'" Issued as Chair, Tri-Council Working Group, Toronto, November 16.

Lufkin, Edward C., and Steven Ory. 1989. "Estrogen Replacement Therapy for the Prevention of Osteoporosis." *American Family Physician* 40:205–12.

Lupton, Deborah. 1995. *The Imperative of Health: Public Health and the Regulated Body.* London: Sage.

MacIntyre, Sally. 1977. "Childbirth: The Myth of the Golden Age." *World Medicine,* June 15, 17–22.

Mack, T. M., and R. K. Ross. 1989. "Risks and Benefits of Long-Term Treatment with Estrogens." *Schweiz.med.Wschr* 119:1811–20.

MacLeod, L. 1980. *Wife Battering in Canada: A Vicious Circle.* Ottawa: Canadian Advisory Council on the Status of Women.

———. 1989. *Wife Battering and the Web of Hope: Progress, Dilemmas and Visions of Prevention.* Ottawa: Health and Welfare Canada, National Clearinghouse on Family Violence.

MacPherson, Kathleen L. 1981. "Menopause as Disease: The Social Construction of a Metaphor." *Advances in Nursing Science* 3(2): 95–113.

Mahoney M. 1994. "Victimization or Oppression? Women's Lives, Violence, and Agency." In *The Public Nature of Private Violence,* ed. M. Fineman and R. Mykitiuk. New York: Routledge.

Mahowald, Mary Briody. 1993. *Women and Children in Health Care: An Unequal Majority.* New York: Oxford University Press.

Mainichi Daily News. 1987. "Pill Researcher." Interview with Takuro Kobayashi, Tokyo, February 23

Mairs, Nancy. 1987. "On Being a Cripple." In *With Wings: An Anthology of Literature by and About Women with Disabilities,* eds. Marsha Saxton and Florence Howe. New York: The Feminist Press at the City University of New York.

Malloch, Lesley. 1989. "Indian Medicine, Indian Health: Study Between Red and White Medicine." *Canadian Women Studies* 10(2&3): 23–31.

Malterud, Kirsti. 1992. "Strategies for Empowering Women's Voices in the Medical Culture." Paper presented at the 5th International Congress on Women's Health Issues, Copenhagen, Denmark, August 25–28.

Mann, Charles. 1995. "Women's Health Research Blossoms." *Science* 269(5225) (August 11): 766–70

Markel, H. 1992. "The Stigma of Disease: Implications of Genetic Screening." *American Journal of Medicine* 93:209–15.

Martin, D., and J. Mosher. 1995. "Unkept Promises: Experiences of Immigrant Women with the Neo-Criminalization of Wife Abuse." *Canadian Journal of Women and the Law* 8(1): 3–44.

Martin, Emily. 1987. *The Woman in the Body: A Cultural Analysis of Reproduction.* Boston: Beacon Press.

———. 1990. "The Ideology of Reproduction: The Reproduction of Ideology." In *Uncertain Terms: Negotiating Gender in American Culture,* ed. Faye Ginsberg and Anna Lowenhaupt Tsing. Boston: Beacon Press.

———. 1991. "The Egg and the Sperm: How Science has Constructed a Romance Based on Stereotypical Male-Female Roles." *Signs: Journal of Women in Society* 16(3): 485–501.

———. 1994. *Flexible Bodies: Tracking Immunity in American Culture from the Days of Polio to the Age of AIDS.* Boston: Beacon Press.

Martin, Jane Roland. 1994. "Methodological Essentialism, False Difference, and Other Dangerous Traps." *Signs* 19(3): 630–57.

Martindale, Kathleen. 1996. "Stop Feeling or You'll Never Be Normal Again: My Life with Cancer Since Lump Day." In *Pushing Limits: Disabled Dykes Produce Culture,* ed. Shelley Tremain. Toronto: Women's College Press.

Mason, Jutta. 1988. "Midwifery in Canada." In *The Midwife Challenge,* ed. Sheila Kitzinger. London: Pandora Press.

Mastroianni, Anna C., Ruth Faden, and Daniel Federman, eds. 1994. *Women and Health Research: Ethical and Legal Issues of Including Women in Clinical Studies.* 2 vols. Washington, D.C.: National Academy Press.

Matthews, Gwyneth Ferguson. 1983. *Voices from the Shadows: Women with Disabilities Speak Out.* Toronto: The Women's Press.

Mawhood, Rhonda. 1989. "Advertisements for Beauty Products in Canada, 1901–1941." Master's thesis, McGill University.

McAnally, L. E., C. R. Corn, and S. F. Hamilton. 1992. "Aspirin for the Prevention of Vascular Death in Women." *Annals of Pharmacotherapy* 26: 1530–34.

McClure, Regan. 1994. *Lesbian Health Guide*. Toronto: Queer Press.

McFarlane J., B. Parker, K. Soeken, L. Bullock. 1992. "Assessing for Abuse During Pregnancy: Severity and Frequency of Injuries and Associated Entry into Prenatal Care." *JAMA* 267(23): 3176–78.

McLaren, Angus. 1986. "The Creation of a Haven for 'Human Thorough-breds': The Sterilization of the Feeble-Minded and the Mentally Ill in British Columbia." *Canadian Historical Review* 67(2): 127–50.

McLaren, Angus, and Arlene Tigar McLaren. 1986. *The Bedroom and the State: The Changing Practices and Politics of Contraception and Abortion in Canada.* Toronto: McClelland and Stewart.

McLeer, S. V., and A. H. Anwar. 1987. "The Role of the Emergency Physician in the Prevention of Domestic Violence." *Annals of Emergency Medicine* 16:107–13.

McNaughton, Janet. 1989. "The Role of the Midwife in the Traditional Health Care of Newfoundland Women." Ph.D. diss., Memorial University.

McPhedran, Marilou, Harvey Armstrong, Rachel Edney, Pat Marshall, Roz Roach, Briar Long, and Bonnie Homeniuk. 1991. *Task Force on Sexual Abuse of Patients: The Final Report.* Toronto: College of Physicians and Surgeons of Ontario.

Mellow, Gail O. 1989. "Sustaining Our Organizations: Feminist Health Activism in an Age of Technology." In *Healing Technology: Feminist Perspectives,* ed. Kathryn Strother Ratcliff, Myra Marx Ferree, Gail O. Mellow, Barbara Drygulski Wright, Glenda D. Price, Kim Yanoshik, and Margie S. Freston. Ann Arbor: University of Michigan Press.

Mendelsohn, Robert. 1981. *Male Practice: How Doctors Manipulate Women.* Chicago: Contemporary Books.

Merleau-Ponty, Maurice. 1962. *The Phenomenology of Perception.* Trans. by Colin Smith. London: Routledge and Kegan Paul.

Merton, Vanessa. 1994. "Review Essay: Women and Health Research." *Journal of Law Medicine and Ethics* 22(3): 272–79.

Messing, K. 1991. *Occupational Health and Safety Concerns of Canadian Women: A Review.* Ottawa: Labour Canada.

———. 1995. "Don't Use a Wrench to Peel Potatoes: Biological Science Constructed on Male Model Systems Is a Risk to Women Worker's Health." In *Changing Methods: Feminists Transforming Practice,* ed. S. Burt and L. Code. Peterborough, Ont.: Broadview Press.

Messing, K., and D. Mergler. 1995. "The Rat Couldn't Speak but We Can: Inhumanity in Occupational Health Research." In *Re-Inventing Biology,* ed. Ruth Hubbard and Lynda Birke. Bloomington: Indiana University Press.

Messing, K., Ghislaine Doniol-Shaw, and Chantal Haentjens. 1994. "Sugar and Spice and Everything Nice: Health Effects of the Sexual Division of Labor Among Train Cleaners." In *Women's Health, Politics, and Power: Essays on Sex/Gender, Medicine, and Public Health,* ed. Elizabeth Fee and Nancy Krieger. Amityville, NY: Baywood.

Meyers, Diana T. 1989. *Self, Society, and Personal Choice.* New York: Columbia University Press.

Ministère de la Santé. 1993. *Statistiques sanitaires année 1992.* Cotonou, Benin.

———. 1994. *Statistiques sanitaires année 1993.* Cotonou, Benin.

Ministère du Plan et de la Restructuration Économique. 1994. *Deuxième recensement général de la population et de l'habitation, tome 2: Dynamique de la population.* Cotonou, Benin.

Minnich, E. K. 1990. *Transforming Knowledge.* Philadelphia: Temple University Press.

Mitchinson, Wendy. 1982. "Canadian Medical History: Diagnosis and Prognosis," *Acadiensis* 12(1): 125–35.

———. 1990. "The Health of Medical History," *Acadiensis* 20(1): 253–63.

———. 1991. *The Nature of Their Bodies: Women and Their Doctors in Victorian Canada.* Toronto: University of Toronto Press.

———. 1993. "The Medical Treatment of Women." In *Changing Patterns: Women in Canada.* Toronto: Stewart, McLelland.

Mitchinson, Wendy, and Janice Dickin McGinnis, eds. 1988. *Essays in the History of Canadian Medicine.* Toronto: McClelland and Stewart.

Mitsuda, Kyōko. 1985. "Kindaiteki Boseikan no Juyō to Kenkei: Kyōiku Suru Hahaoya Kara Ryōsai Kenbo e" (The importance and transformation of the condition of modern motherhood: From Education Mother to Good Wife and Wise Mother). In *Bosei o tou* (What is motherhood?), ed. H. Wakita. Kyoto: Jinbunshoin.

Mochida, Takeshi. 1980. "Focus on the Family." *Japan Echo* 3:75–76.

Modlin, John, and Alfred Saah. 1991. "Public Health and Clinical Aspects of HIV Infection and Disease in Women and Children in the United States." In *AIDS, Women and the Next Generation: Towards a Morally Acceptable Public Policy for HIV Testing of Pregnant Women and Newborns,* eds. Ruth Faden, Gail Geller, and Madison Powers. New York: Oxford University Press.

Mohanty, Chandra Talpade. 1991. "Under Western Eyes: Feminist Scholarship and Colonial Discourses." In *Third World Women and the Politics of Feminism,* ed. Chandra Mohanty, Ann Russo, and Lourdes Torres. Bloomington: Indiana University Press.

Morantz-Sanchez, Regina. 1984. "The Menopause." *International Journal of Psychoanalysis* 65(pt. 1): 55–62.

———. 1985. *Sympathy and Science: Women Physicians in American Medicine.* New York: Oxford University Press.

More, E. S. 1994. "Empathy Enters the Profession of Medicine." In *The Empathetic Practitioner: Empathy, Gender, and Medicine,* ed. E. Singer More and M. A. Milligan. New Brunswick, N.J.: Rutgers University Press.

More, E. S., and M. Milligan, eds. 1994. "Introduction." *The Empathic Practitioner.* New Brunswick, N.J.: Rutgers University Press

Morgan, Kathryn Pauly. 1979. "In Praise of Older Women: An Analysis of Aging." *National Action Committee, Status of Women Journal,* March, 1–4.

———. 1987. "Women and Moral Madness." In *Science, Morality, and Feminist*

Theory, ed. Marsha Hanen and Kai Nielsen. *Canadian Journal of Philosophy* 13 (supplementary vol.): 201–26.

———. 1991. "Women and the Knife: Cosmetic Surgery and the Colonization of Women's Bodies." *Hypatia* 6(3): 25–53.

———. 1995. "We've Come to See the Wizard! Revelations of the Enlightenment Epistemology." In *Philosophy of Education*, ed. Alven Neiman. Urbana: Philosophy of Education Society, University of Illinois at Urbana-Champaign.

———. 1996a. "Rites and Rights: The Biopolitics of Beauty and Fertility." In *Philosophical Perspectives in Bioethics*, ed. L. W. Sumner and J. Boyle. Toronto: University of Toronto Press.

———. 1996b. "Sexism." In *The Encyclopedia of Philosophy, Supplement*, ed. Donald M. Borchert. New York: Simon and Schuster Macmillian.

———. 1998. "Sexualized Doctor-Patient Relationships: 'Therapeutic' Erections or (Acts of) Eroto-Terrorism?" In *Interpersonal Violence*, ed. S. French. Toronto: McGraw-Hill-Ryerson.

Morris, Colin. 1980. "Individualism in Twelfth-Century Religion: Some Further Reflections." *Journal of Ecclesiastical History* 31(2): 195–206.

Morris, Jenny, ed. 1989. *Able Lives: Women's Experience of Paralysis*. London: The Women's Press.

Morsy, Soheir A. 1995. "Deadly Reproduction Among Egyptian Women: Maternal Mortality and the Medicalization of Population Control." In *Conceiving the New World Order: The Global Politics of Reproduction*, ed. Faye D. Ginsburg and Rayna Rapp. Berkeley and Los Angeles: University of California Press.

———. 1997. "Biotechnology and the Taming of Women's Bodies." In *Processed Lives: Gender and Technology in Everyday Life*, ed. Jennifer Terry and Melodie Calvert. New York: Routledge.

Mort, Frank. 1987. *Dangerous Sexualities: Medico-Moral Politics in England Since 1830*. London: Routledge and Kegan Paul.

Moscarello, R. J., K. J. Margittai, and M. Rossi. 1994. "Difference in Abuse Reported by Female and Male Canadian Medical Students." *Canadian Medical Association Journal* 150(3): 357–63.

Moss, Kary L., ed. 1996. *Man-Made Medicine: Women's Health, Public Policy, and Reform*. Durham, N.C.: Duke University Press.

Mullings, Leith. 1995. "Households Headed by Women: The Politics of Race, Class, and Gender." In *Conceiving the New World Order: The Global Politics of Reproduction*, ed. Faye D. Ginsburg and Rayna Rapp. Berkeley and Los Angeles: University of California Press.

Munro Kerr, J., R. N. Johnstone, James Young, et al. 1933. *Combined Textbook of Obstetrics and Gynaecology for Students and Medical Practitioners*. Edinburgh: E. & S. Livingstone.

Nash, Theresa. 1982. "Images of Women in National Film Board of Canada Films During World War II and the Postwar Years, 1939–1949." Ph.D. diss., McGill University.

National Defense Council for Victims of Karōshi. 1990. *Karōshi* (Death from overwork). Tokyo: Madosha.

National Women's Health Network. 1989. *Taking Hormones and Women's Health.* Washington, D.C.: National Women's Health Network.

Nations-Unies. 1994. Conférence internationale sur la population et le développement. Le Cairo, Egypt, September 5–13, 1994, A/conf. 171/13.

Nechas, Eileen, and Denise Foley. 1994. *Unequal Treatment: What You Don't Know About How Women are Mistreated by the Medical Community.* New York: Simon and Schuster.

Nedelsky, Jennifer. 1989. "Reconceiving Autonomy." *Yale Journal of Law and Feminism* 1(1): 7–36.

Nelkin, D. and M. S. Lindee. 1995. *The DNA Mystique: The Gene as a Cultural Icon.* New York: W. H. Freeman.

Nelson, Lynn Hankinson. 1990. *Who Knows: From Quine to Feminist Empiricism.* Philadelphia: Temple University Press.

———. 1993. "Epistemological Communities." In *Feminist Epistemologies,* ed. Linda Alcoff and Elizabeth Potter. New York: Routledge.

Newberger, E. H., S. E. Barkan, E. S. Lieberman, M. C. McCormick, K. Yllö, L. T. Gary, and S. Schechter. 1992. "Abuse of Pregnant Women and Adverse Birth Outcome: Current Knowledge and Implications for Practice." *JAMA* 267(17): 2370–72.

Nishimura, Hideo. 1981. *Josei to Kanpō* (Women and herbal medicine). Osaka: Sōgensha.

Nolte, Sharon, and Sally Ann Hastings. 1991. "The Meiji State's Policy." In *Recreating Japanese Women, 1600-1945,* ed. Gail Lee Bernstein. Berkeley and Los Angeles: University of California Press.

Norsigian, Judy. 1996. "The Women's Health Movement in The United States." In *Man-Made Medicine: Women's Health, Public Policy, and Reform,* ed. Kary L. Moss. Durham, N.C.: Duke University Press.

Nuttall S. E., L. J. Greaves, and B. Lent. 1985. "Wife Battering: An Emerging Problem in Public Health." *Canadian Journal of Public Health* 76:297–99.

Oakley, Ann. 1976. "Wisewoman and Medicine Man: Changes in the Management of Childbirth." In *The Rights and Wrongs of Women,* ed. Juliet Mitchell and Ann Oakley. Harmondsworth, Eng.: Penguin.

———. 1980. *Women Confined: Towards a Sociology of Childbirth.* London: Martin Robertson.

———. 1984. *The Captured Womb: A History of the Medical Care of Pregnant Women.* Oxford: Basil Blackwell.

Ōgawa, Naohiro. 1988. "Population Aging and Medical Demand: The Case of Japan." In *Economic and Social Implications of Population Aging.* Proceedings of the International Symposium on Population Structure and Development, Tokyo. New York: United Nations.

O'Neil, John, and Patricia Leyland Kaufert. 1995. "Irniktakpunga! Sex Determination and the Inuit Struggle for Birthing Rights in Northern Canada." In

Conceiving the New World Order: The Global Politics of Reproduction, ed. Faye D. Ginsburg and Rayna Rapp. Berkeley and Los Angeles: University of California Press.

Ontario Medical Association, Special Committee on Wife Assault. 1985. "Curbing Wife Assault: Role of the Physician." *Ontario Medical Review* 52:181–82.

Ontario Medical Association, Committee on Wife Assault, endorsed by the Canadian Medical Association. 1991. *Reports on Wife Assault*. Ottawa: Department of National Health and Welfare and National Clearinghouse on Family Violence.

Ontario Native Women's Association. 1989. *Breaking Free: A Proposal for Change to Aboriginal Family Violence*. Thunder Bay: Ontario Native Women's Association.

Oosterbaan, Margaret M., and Maria V. Barreto da Costa. 1995. "Guinea-Bissau: What Women Know About the Risks: An Anthropological Study in WHO." *World Health Statistics Quarterly*, Safe Motherhood: Selected Research Results, 48(1): 39–43.

Oppenheimer, Jo. 1983. "Childbirth in Ontario: The Transition from Home to Hospital in the Early Twentieth Century," *Ontario History* 75(1): 36–61.

Oudshoorn, Nelly. 1990. "On the Making of Sex Hormones: Research Materials and the Production of Knowledge." *Social Studies of Science* 20:5–33.

————. 1994. *Beyond the Natural Body: An Archeology of Sex Hormones*. New York: Routledge.

Overall, Christine, and William P. Zion, eds. 1991. *Perspectives on AIDS: Ethical and Social Issues*. New York: Oxford Univesity Press.

Paltiel, Freda. 1993. "Women's Mental Health: A Global Perspective." In *The Health of Women: A Global Perspective*, ed. Marge Koblinsky, Judith Timyan, and Jill Gay. Boulder, Colo.: Westview Press.

Parsons, Gail. 1977. "Equal Treatment for All: American Medical Remedies for Male Sexual Problems, 1850–1900." *Journal of the History of Medicine* 32:55–71.

Passot, Bernard. 1993. *Le Bénin*. Paris: L'Harmattan.

Peccei, Jocelyn Scott. 1995. "A Hypothesis for the Origin and Evolution of Menopause." *Maturitas* 21:83–89.

Pellegrino, E., and D. C. Thomasma. 1988. *For the Patient's Good: The Restoration of Beneficience in Health Care*. New York: Oxford University Press.

————. 1993. *The Virtues in Medical Practice*. Oxford: Oxford University Press.

Pence, E., and M. Paymar. 1986. *Power and Control: Tactics of Men Who Batter*. Duluth: Minnesota Program Development, Inc.

Perales, Cesar A., and Lauren S. Young, eds. 1988. *Too Little, Too Late: Dealing with the Health Needs of Women in Poverty*. New York: Harrington Park Press.

Petchesky, Rosalind Pollack. 1987. "Foetal Images: The Power of Visual Culture in the Politics of Reproduction." In *Reproductive Technologies: Gender, Motherhood, and Medicine*, ed. Michelle Stanworth. Minneapolis: University of Minnesota Press.

————. 1995. "The Body as Property: A Feminist Re-vision." In *Conceiving the*

New World Order: The Global Politics of Reproduction, ed. Faye D. Ginsburg and Rayna Rapp. Berkeley and Los Angeles: University of California Press.

Petchesky, Rosalind Pollack, and Jennifer Weiner. 1990. *Global Feminist Perspectives on Reproductive Rights and Reproductive Health.* New York: Reproductive Rights Education Project, Hunter College.

Piantadosi, P., and J. Wittes. 1993. "Politically Correct Clinical Trials" (letter to the editor.) *Controlled Clinical Trials* 14:562–67.

Pirie, Marion. 1988. "Women and the Illness Role: Rethinking Feminist Theory." *Canadian Review of Sociology and Anthropology* 25(4): 628–48.

Plath, David. 1980. *Long Engagements.* Stanford: Stanford University Press.

Plato. 1950. *The Republic.* Translated by J. L. Davies and D. J. Vaughan. London: Macmillan.

Posner, Judith. 1979. "It's All in Your Head: Feminist and Medical Models of Menopause (Stange Bedfellows)." *Sex Roles* 5:179–90.

Prevention of Maternal Mortality Network. 1995. "Situation Analyses of Emergency Obstetric Care: Examples from Eleven Operations Research Projects in West Africa." *Social Science and Medicine* 40(5): 657–67.

Ptacek, James. 1988. "Why Do Men Batter Their Wives?" In *Feminist Perspectives on Wife Abuse,* ed. K. Yllö and M. Bograd. London: Sage.

Purdy, Laura. 1996a. *Reproducing Persons.* Ithaca, N.Y.: Cornell University Press.

———. 1996b. "A Feminist View of Health." In *Feminism and Bioethics: Beyond Reproduction,* ed. Susan M. Wolf. New York: Oxford University Press.

Quéniart, Anne. 1988. *Le corps paradoxal: Regards de femmes sur la maternité.* Montreal: Éditions Saint-Martin.

Rabinow, Paul. 1992. "Artificiality and Enlightenment: From Sociology to Biosociology." In *Incorporations,* ed. J. Crary and S. Kwinter. New York: Urzone.

Rackauckas, Teresa M. 1991. *Empowering Women in Medicine.* Report of the Feminist Majority Foundation and American Women's Medical Association (AMWA). Washington, D.C.: AMWA.

Rapp, Rayna. 1989. "Chromosomes and Communication: The Discourse of Genetic Counseling." In *New Approaches to Human Reproduction: Social and Ethical Dimensions,* ed. Linda M. Whiteford and Marilyn L. Poland. Boulder, Colo: Westview.

———. 1990. "Constructing Amniocentesis: Maternal and Medical Discourses." In *Uncertain Terms: Negotiating Gender in American Culture,* ed. Faye Ginsberg and Anna Lowenhaupt Tsing. Boston: Beacon Press.

Ratcliff, Kathryn Strother, Myra Marx Feree, Gail O. Mellow, Barbara Drygulski Wright, Glenda D. Price, Kim Yanoshik, and Margie S. Freston. 1989. *Healing Technologies: Feminist Perspectives.* Ann Arbor: University of Michigan Press.

Raymond, Janice. 1979. *The Transsexual Empire.* Boston: Beacon Press.

———. 1982, "Medicine as Patriarchal Religion." *Journal of Medicine and Philosophy* 7(2): 197–216;

———. 1993. *Women as Wombs: Reproductive Technologies and the Battle over Women's Freedom*. San Francisco: Harper San Francisco.

Raymond, Jocelyn Motyer. 1991. *The Nursery World of Dr. Blatz*. Toronto: University of Toronto Press.

Reed, James. 1978. *The Birth Control Movement and American Society: From Private Vice to Public Virtue*. Princeton, N.J.: Princeton University Press.

Regina v. Lavallee 1990. 55 C.C.C. (3d) 97 (S.C.C.).

Reid, Robert L. 1988. "Menopause: Part I: Hormonal Replacement." *Bulletin: Society of Obstetricians and Gynecologists* 10:25–34.

Reissman, Catherine Kohler. 1983. "Women and Medicalization: A New Perspective." *Social Policy* 14 (summer): 3–18.

Rhodes, Lorna. 1990. "Studying Biomedicine as a Cultural System." In *Medical Anthropology: A Handbook of Theory and Method*, ed. T. Johnson, C. Sargent. Westport, Conn: Greenwood Press.

Rich, Adrienne. 1980. "Compulsory Heterosexuality and Lesbian Existence." *Signs* 5(4): 630–60.

———. 1985. *Of Woman Born: Motherhood as Experience and Institution*. New York: W.W. Norton.

Richie, B. E., and V. Kanuha. 1993. "Battered Women of Color in Public Health Care Systems: Racism, Sexism, and Violence." In *Wings of Gauze: Women of Color and the Experience of Health and Illness*, ed. B. Bair and S. E. Cayleff. Detroit: Wayne State University Press.

Roberts, Dorothy E. 1996. "Reconstructing the Patient: Starting with Women of Color." In *Feminism and Bioethics: Beyond Reproduction*, ed. Susan M. Wolf. New York: Oxford University Press.

Robertson, A. 1990. "The Politics of Alzheimer's Disease: A Case Study in Apocalyptic Demography." *International Journal of Health Services* 20:429–42.

Rock, Melanie. 1996. "Knowing the Body: A Critical Analysis of Efforts to Map and Protect the Human Genome." Paper delivered at the conference "Incorporating the Antibody: Women, History and Medical Discourse," University of Western Ontario, October.

Rock, Patricia. 1996. "Eugenics and Euthanasia: A Cause for Concern for Disabled People, Particularly Disabled Women." *Disability and Society* 11(1): 121–27.

Rodgers, Karen. 1994. "Wife Assault: The Findings of a National Survey." *Juristat* 14(9): 1–21.

Romain, Jules. [1927?]. *Knock; ou, Le triomphe de la médecine*. New York: Appleton-Century-Crofts.

Rosenberger, Nancy. 1992. "The Process of Discourse: Usages of a Japanese Medical Term." *Social Science and Medicine* 34(3): 237–47.

Rosenfield, Allan, and Deborah Maine. 1985. "Maternal Mortality—A Neglected Tragedy: Where Is the M in MCH?" *The Lancet* 2(8446): 83–85.

Ross, Elizabeth, and Judith Sachs. 1996. *Healing the Female Heart: A Holistic Approach to Prevention and Recovery from Heart Disease*. New York: Pocket Books.

Ross, Philip D., Hiromichi Norimatsu, James W. Davis, Katsuhiko Yano,

Richard D. Wasnick, Saeko Fukiwara, Yutaka Hosoda, and L. Hoseph Melton. 1991. "A Comparison of Hip Facture Incidence Among Native Japanese, Japanese Americans, and American Caucasians." *American Journal of Epidemiology* 133:801–9.

Rosser, Sue V. 1994. *Women's Health: Missing from U.S. Medicine.* Bloomington: Indiana University Press

Rothman, Barbara Katz. 1982. *In Labour: Women and Power in the Birthplace.* London: Junction Books.

———. 1984. "The Meanings of Choice in Reproductive Technology." In *Test-Tube Women: What Future for Motherhood?* ed. R. Arditti, R. Duelli Klein, S. Minden. London: Pandora Press.

———. 1986. *The Tentative Pregnancy: Prenatal Diagnosis and the Future of Motherhood.* New York: Viking Press.

Rowland, Robyn. 1992. *Living Laboratories: Women and Reproductive Technologies.* Bloomington: Indiana University Press.

Russet, Cynthia Eagle. 1989. *Sexual Science: The Victorian Construction of Womanhood.* Cambridge, Mass.: Harvard University Press.

Ruth, Barbara. 1996. "Lament to the Medical-Industrial Division of the Capitalist Patriarchal Complex." In *Pushing Limits: Disabled Dykes Produce Culture,* ed. Shelley Tremain. Toronto: Women's College Press.

Ruzek, Sheryl Burt. 1978. *The Women's Health Movement: Feminist Alternatives to Medical Control.* New York: Praeger.

Ruzek, Sheryl Burt, and Jessica Hill. N.d. "Positive Approaches to Promoting Women's Health." Manuscript prepared for Women's Directorate, Ontario.

Ryberg, Percy E. 1942. *Health, Sex, and Birth Control.* Toronto: Anchor Press.

Saillant, Francine, and Michel O'Neill, eds. 1987. *Accoucher autrement: Repères historiques, sociaux et culturels de la grossesse et de l'accouchement au Québec.* Montreal: Éditions Saint-Martin.

Sandelowski, Margarete. 1984. *Pain, Pleasure, and American Childbirth: From the Twilight Sleep to the Read Method, 1914–1960.* Westport, Conn.: Greenwood Press.

Santow, Gigi. 1995. "Social Roles and Physical Health: The Case of Female Disadvantage in Poor Countries." *Social Science and Medicine* 40(2): 147–61.

Sargent, Carolyn. 1989. *Maternity, Medicine, and Power: Reproductive Decisions in Urban Benin.* Berkeley and Los Angeles: University of California Press.

Sargent, Carolyn, and Caroline Brettell. 1996. *Gender and Health: An International Perspective.* Upper Saddle River, N.J.: Prentice Hall.

Sargent, Carolyn, and Grace Bascope. 1996. "Ways of Knowing About Birth in Three Cultures." *Medical Anthropology Quarterly* (Special Issue on Authoritative Knowledge) 10(2): 213–36.

Sas, G. R., J. B. Brown, and B. Lent. 1994. "Detecting Woman Abuse in Family Practice." *Canadian Family Physician* 40:861–64.

Sassetti, M. 1992. "Battered Women." In *Violence Education: Towards a Solution,* ed. M. Hendricks-Matthews. Kansas City: Society of Teachers of Family Medicine.

————. 1993. "Domestic Violence, Family Violence, and Abusive Relationships." *Primary Care; Clinics in Office Practices* 20(2): 289–305.

Saxton, Marsha. 1984. "Born and Unborn: The Implications of Reproductive Technologies for People with Disabilities." In *Test-Tube Women: What Future for Motherhood?* ed. Rita Arditti, Renate Duelli Klein, Shelley Minden. London: Pandora Press.

Saxton, Marsha, and Florence Howe, eds. 1987. *With Wings: An Anthology of Literature by and About Women with Disabilities.* New York: The Feminist Press at the City University of New York.

Scheman, Naomi. 1983. "Individualism and the Objects of Psychology." In *Discovering Reality: Feminist Pespectives on Epistemology, Metaphysics, Methodology, and Philosophy of Science,* ed. Sandra Harding and Merril B. Hintikka. Dordrecht, Holland: D. Reidel.

————. 1993. *Engenderings: Constructions of Knowldge, Authority, and Privilege.* New York: Routledge.

Schiebinger, Londa. 1987. "Skeletons in the Closet: The First Illustrations of the Female Skeleton in Eighteenth-Century Anatomy." In *The Making of the Modern Body,* ed. Catherine Gallagher and Thomas Laqueur. Berkeley and Los Angeles: University of California Press.

————. 1989. *The Mind Has No Sex? Women in the Origins of Modern Science.* Cambridge, Mass.: Harvard University Press.

————. 1993. *Nature's Body: Gender in the Making of Modern Science.* Boston: Beacon Press.

Scott, J. W. 1990. "Deconstructing Equality-vs.-Differences; or, The Uses of Poststructuralist Theory for Feminism." In *Conflicts in Feminism,* ed. M. Hirsch and E. Fox Keller. New York: Routledge.

Scully, Diana. 1980. *Men Who Control Women's Health: The Miseducation of Obstetrician-Gynecologists.* Boston: Houghton Mifflin.

Scully, Diana, and Pauline Bart. 1973. "A Funny Thing Happened on My Way to the Orifice; Woman in Gynaecology Textbooks." *American Journal of Sociology* 78:1045–50.

Seaman, Barbara. 1969. *The Doctors' Case Against the Pill.* New York: Avon.

Seaman, Barbara, and Gideon Seaman. 1977. *Women and the Crisis in Sex Hormones.* New York: Rawson Associates.

Secker, Barbara. Forthcoming. "Labelling Patient (In) Competence: A Feminist Analysis of Medico-Legal Discourse." *The Journal of Social Philosophy.*

Shanner, Laura. 1996. "Bioethics Through the Back Door: Phenomenology, Narratives, and Insights into Infertility." In *Philosophical Perspectives on Bioethics,* ed. L. W. Sumner and Joseph Boyle. Toronto: University of Toronto Press.

Shaw, Barret, ed. 1994. *The Ragged Edge: The Disability Experience from the Pages of the First fifteen Years of the "Disability Rag."* Louisville, Ky: Avocado Press.

Shaw, Nancy Stoller. 1974. *Forced Labour: Maternity Care in the United States.* London: Pergamon Press.

Sheehan, Donald. 1936. "Discovery of the Autonomic Nervous System." *AMA Archives of Neurology and Psychiatry* 35:1081–115.

Sheehy, Gail. 1991. "The Silent Passage: Menopause." *Vanity Fair,* October, 222–63.

Sheeran M. 1996. "Massachusetts DSS Protects Children by Protecting Mothers." *Synergy* 2(1): 6–8.

Sherwin, Susan. 1992. *No Longer Patient: Feminist Ethics and Health Care.* Philadelphia: Temple University Press.

———. 1994. Women in Clinical Studies: A Feminist View." In *Women and Health Research: Ethcal and Legal Issues of Including Women in Clinical Studies,* ed. A. Mastrioanni, R. Faden, and D. Federman. Washington, D.C.: National Academy Press.

———. 1996a. "Cancer and Women: Some Feminist Ethics Concerns." In *Gender and Health: An International Perspective,* ed. Carolyn Sargent and Caroline Brettell. Upper Saddle River, N.J.: Prentice Hall.

———. 1996b. "Theory versus Practice in Ethics: A Feminist Perspective on Justice in Health Care." In *Philosophical Perspectives on Bioethics,* ed. L. W. Sumner and Joseph Boyle. Toronto: University of Toronto Press.

Shin, Maria Y. 1991. "Immigrant and Racial Minority Women Organize." *Canadian Woman Studies/Les Cahiers de La Femme* 12(1): 55–57.

Shiva, V. 1995. "Democratizing Biology: Reinventing Biology from a Feminist, Ecological, and Third World Perspective." In *Reinventing Biology: Respect for Life and the Creation of Knowledge,* ed. L. Birke and R. Hubbard. Bloomington: Indiana University Press.

Shorr, Ephraim. 1940. "The Menopause." *Bulletin of the New York Academy of Medicine* 16:453–74.

Shorter, Edward. 1982. *A History of Women's Bodies.* New York: Basic Books.

Shortt, S.E.D. 1981. "Medical Professionalization: Pitfalls and Promise in the Historiography." *Journal of the History of Canadian Science, Technology and Medicine* 5(3): 210–19.

Showalter, Elaine. 1985. *The Female Malady: Women, Madness, and English Culture.* New York: Pantheon Books.

Siemiatycki, J., R. Dewar, R. Lakhani, L. Nadon, L. Richardson, and M. Gerin. 1989. "Cancer Risks Associated with Ten Organic Dusts: Results from a Case-control Study in Montreal." *American Journal of Industrial Medicine* 16:547–67.

Silvera, Mikeda. 1994. "Black Women Organize for Health." Interview with Erica Mercer. In *On Women Healthsharing,* ed. Enakshi Dua, Maureen FitzGerald, Linda Gardner, Darien Taylor, and Lisa Wyndels. Toronto: Toronto Women's Press.

Silvers, Anita. 1994. "'Defective' Agents: Equality, Difference, and the Tyranny of the Normal." *Journal of Social Philosophy* 25:154–75.

———. 1995. "Reconciling Equality to Difference: Caring (f)or Justice for People with Disabilities." *Hypatia: A Journal of Feminist Philosophy* 10(1): 30–55.

———. Forthcoming. "Whose Lives Are Worth Living?" In *Implications of the New Genetics for Primary Care*, ed. Mary Briody Mahowald.

Sinclair D. 1985. *Understanding Wife Assault: A Training Manual for Counsellors and Advocates*. Toronto: Government Bookstore.

Singer, P. 1993. *Practical Ethics*. 2d ed. Cambridge: Cambridge University Press.

Smith, Dorothy. 1990. *The Conceptual Practices of Power*. Toronto: University of Toronto Press.

Smith, Janet Farrell. 1996. "Communicative Ethics in Medicine: The Physician-Patient Relationship." In *Feminism and Bioethics: Beyond Reproduction*, ed. Susan Wolf. New York: Oxford University Press.

Smith, Robert. 1974. *Ancestor Worship in Contemporary Japan*. Stanford: Stanford University Press.

Somers, Anne. 1971. *Health Care in Transition: Directions for the Future*. Chicago: Hospital Research and Educational Trust.

Spanier, Bonnie. 1995. *Im/Partial Science: Gender Ideology in Molecular Biology*. Bloomington: Indiana University Press.

Spelman, Elizabeth. 1988. *Inessential Woman: Problems of Exclusion in Feminist Thought*. Boston: Beacon Press.

Stallybras, Peter. 1986. "Patriarchial Territories: The Body Enclosed." In *Rewriting the Renaissance: The Discourses of Sexual Difference in Early Modern Europe*, ed. Margaret W. Ferguson, Maureen Quilligan, and Nancy J. Vickers. Chicago: University of Chicago Press.

Stark, E., and A. Flitcraft. 1982 "Medical Therapy as Repression: The Case of the Battered Woman." *Health and Medicine*, summer/fall, 29–32.

———. 1991. "Spouse Abuse." In *Violence in America: A Public Health Approach*, ed. M. L. Rosenberg and M. A. Fenley. New York: Oxford University Press.

Stark, E., A. Flitcraft, and W. Frazier. 1979. *International Journal of Health Services* 9(3): 461–93.

———. 1994. "Medicine and Patriarchal Violence: The Social Construction of a 'Private' Event." In *Women's Health, Politics, and Power: Essays on Sex/Gender, Medicine, and Public Health*, ed. Elizabeth Fee and Nancy Krieger. Amityville, N.Y.: Baywood.

Statistics Canada. 1994. *Wife Assault: The Findings of a National Survey*. Juristat Service Bulletin. Ottawa: Statistics Canada. March.

Steinmetz, S. 1977–78. "The Battered Husband Syndrome." *Victimology: An International Journal* 2:499–509.

Stevens, Patricia E., and Joanne M. Hall. 1994. "A Critical Historical Analysis of the Medical Construction of Lesbianism." In *Women's Health, Politics, and Power: Essays on Sex/Gender, Medicine and Public Health*, ed. Elizabeth Fee and Nancy Krieger. Amityville, N.Y.: Baywood.

Stewart, D., and A. Cecutti. 1993. "Physical Abuse in Pregnancy." *Canadian Medical Association Journal* 149(9): 1257–63.

Stewart, Houston, Beth Percival, and Elizabeth R. Epperly, eds. 1992. *The More We Get Together: Women and Disability*. Charlottetown, P.E.I: Gynergy Books.

Stewart, M., J. Belle Brown, W. W. Weston, I. McWhinney, Carol L. McWilliam, and Thomas R. Freeman. 1995. *Patient-Centered Medicine: Transforming the Clinical Method.* London: Sage.

Strathern, Marilyn. 1992. *Reproducing the Future: Anthropology, Kinship, and the New Reproductive Technologies.* New York: Rouledge.

Strohman, R. 1994. "Epigenesis: The Missing Beat in Biotechnology?" *Bio/Technology* 12:156–64.

Strong-Boag, Veronica, and Kathryn McPherson. 1986. "The Confinement of Women: Childbirth and Hospitalization in Vancouver, 1919–1939." *BC Studies* 69–70:142–75.

Sugg, N. K., and T. Inui. 1992. "Primary Care Physicians' Response to Domestic Violence." *JAMA* 267(23): 3157–60.

Sumner, L.W., and Joseph Boyle, eds. 1996. *Philosophical Perspectives on Bioethics.* Toronto: University of Toronto Press.

Sundari, T. K. 1994. "The Untold Story: How the Health Care Systems in Developing Countries Contribute to Maternal Mortality." In *Women's Health, Politics, and Power: Essays on Sex/Gender, Medicine, and Public Health,* ed. Elizabeth Fee and Nancy Krieger. Amityville, N.Y.: Baywood.

Tavris, Carol. 1992. *The Mismeasure of Women.* New York: Simon and Schuster.

Tesh, S. N. 1988. *Hidden Arguments: Political Ideology and Disease Prevention Policy.* New Brunswick, N.J.: Rutgers University Press.

Tew, Marjorie. 1990. *Safer Childbirth: A Critical History of Maternity Care.* London: Chapman & Hall.

"The Human Laboratory: Experimenting on Women in the Third World—Good Science or Gross Exploitation?" 1995. Documentary aired on the series *Witness,* Canadian Broadcasting Company, Fall. Videocassette.

Theriot, Nancy M. 1993. "Women's Voices in Nineteenth-Century Medical Discourse: A Step Toward Deconstructing Science." *Signs* 19(1): 1–31.

Thompson, Anne. 1995. "Notes on the Use of Routine Episiotomy," draft FHE/MSM, WHO, Geneva.

Thompson, Becky. 1994. *A Hunger So Wide and So Deep: American Women Speak Out on Eating Problems.* Minneapolis: University of Minnesota Press.

Thomson, Rosemarie Garland. 1994. "Redrawing the Boundaries of Feminist Disability Studies." *Feminist Studies* 20:583–95.

———. 1997. "Feminist Theory, the Body, and the Disabled Figure." In *The Disability Studies Reader,* ed. Lennard Davis. New York: Routledge.

Tiefer, Leonore. 1995. *Sex Is Not a Natural Act and Other Essays.* Boulder, Colo.: Westview Press.

Tilden V. P., T. A. Schmidt, J. Limandri, G. T. Chiodo, M. S. Garland, and P. A. Loveless. 1994. "Factors That Influence Clinicians' Assessment and Management of Family Violence." *American Journal of Public Health* 84:628–33.

Tinker, Anne, and Marjorie A. Koblinsky. 1993. *Vers une maternité sans risque.* Documents de synthèse de la Banque Mondiale. Washington, D.C.: Banque Mondiale.

Todd, Alexandra Dundas. 1989. *Intimate Adversaries: Cultural Conflict Between Doctors and Women Patients*. Philadelphia: University of Pennsylvania Press.

Tokyo Shinbun. 1990. "Rōjin Kaigo Josei ni Zusshiri" (Nursing of the elderly lands on women). September 13.

Tong, Rosemarie. 1996. "Feminist Approaches to Bioethics." In *Feminism and Bioethics: Beyond Reproduction*, ed. Susan M. Wolf. New York: Oxford University Press.

Toronto Advisory Committee on Cultural Approaches to Violence Against Women and Children. 1992. "Our Ways: Anti-Racist and Culturally Appropriate Approaches to Combatting Women Assault." Toronto: Toronto Advisory Committee on Cultural Approaches to Violence Against Women and Children.

Tremain, Shelley, ed. 1996. *Pushing Limits: Disabled Dykes Produce Culture*. Toronto: Women's College Press.

Tremblay, Celine. 1990. "Les particularités et les difficultés de l'intervention preventive dans le domaine de la santé et de la sécurité des femmes en milieu de travail." Paper presented at the 58th Annual Meeting of the Association canadienne-francaise pour l'avancement des sciences, Université Laval, Quebec City, May 14. Cited in Messing 1995.

Triechler, Paula A. 1988. "AIDS, Gender, and Biomedical Discourse: Current Contests for Meaning." In *AIDS: The Burdens of History*, ed. Elizabeth Fee and Daniel M. Fox. Berkeley and Los Angeles: University of California Press.

Trott, Ellen Joyce. 1984. "Attitudes Towards Birth Control: Canada, 1885–1935." Master's thesis, Carleton University, Ottawa.

Trute B., P. Sarsfield, and D. A. Mackenzie. 1988. "Medical Response to Wife Abuse: A Survey of Physicians' Attitudes and Practices." *Canadian Journal of Community Mental Health* 7(2): 61–71.

Tuana, Nancy. 1989. "The Weaker Seed: The Sexist Bias of Reproductive Theory." In *Feminism and Science*, ed. Nancy Tuana. Bloomington: Indiana University Press.

———. 1993. *The Less Noble Sex: Scientific, Religious, and Philosophical Conceptions of Women's Nature*. Bloomington: Indiana University Press.

———. 1997. "Revaluing Science: Starting from the Practices of Women." In *Feminism, Science, and the Philosophy of Science*, ed. Lynn Hankison Nelson and Jack Nelson. Boston: Kluwer Academic Publishers.

———, ed. 1989. *Feminism and Science*. Bloomington: Indiana University Press.

Türmen, Tomris. 1994. "The Burden of Maternal Mortality and Morbidity." Speech given at the Rockefeller Foundation, New York, September.

UNICEF (United Nations International Children's Emergency Fund). 1996. *The Progress of Nations*. New York.

Valverde, Clara, and Connie Clement. 1994. "Nurturing Politics and Health: Centre de Sante des Femmes du Quartier." In *On Women Healthsharing*, ed. Enakshi Dua, Maureen FitzGerald, Linda Gardner, Darien Taylor, and Lisa Wyndels. Toronto: The Women's Press.

Valverde, M., L. MacLead, and K. Johnson. 1995. *Wife Assault and the Criminal Justice System.* Toronto: University of Toronto, Centre of Criminology.

Vayda, Eugene. 1978. "Keeping People Well: A New Approach to Medicine" *Human Nature* 1(7): 64–71.

Vertinsky, Patricia Anne. 1990. *The Eternally Wounded Woman: Women, Doctors, and Exercise in the Late Nineteenth Century.* Manchester: Manchester University Press.

Vlassof, Carol. 1994. "Gender Inequalities in Health in the Third World: Uncharted Grounds." *Social Science and Medicine* 39(9): 1249–59.

Vliet, Elizabeth. 1995. *Screaming to Be Heard: Hormonal Connection Women Suspect . . . and Doctors Ignore.* New York: M. Evans and Co.

Von Staden, Heinrich. 1992. "The Discovery of the Body: Human Dissection and Its Cultural Contexts in Ancient Greece." *Yale Journal of Biology and Medicine* 65:223–41.

Walker, Leonore. 1984. *The Battered Woman Syndrome.* New York: Springer Publishing.

Wallis, Lila A. 1994. "Why a Curriculum on Women's Health." In *Reframing Women's Health: Multidisciplinary Research and Practice,* ed. Alice J. Dan. London: Sage.

Wane, Defa. 1992. "L'information des femmes quant à leur santé reproductive: Le cas du centre de P.M.I. de Diourbel au Sénégal. Master's thesis, Université Laval, Quebec.

Warshaw, Carol. 1989. "Limitations of the Medical Model in the Care of Battered Women." *Gender and Society* 3(4): 506–17.

———. 1994. "Domestic Violence: Challenges to Medical Practice." In *Reframing Women's Health,* ed. A. J. Dan. Thousand Oaks, Calif.: Sage.

Waxman, B. F. Forthcoming. "Up Against Eugenics: Disabled Women's Challenge to Receive Reproductive Health Services." *Sexuality and Disability.* Cited in Gill 1996.

Wear, Delese. 1997. *Privilege in the Medical Academy: A Feminist Examines Gender, Race, and Power.* New York: Teachers College Press.

Weinstein, Milton, and Anna Tosteson. 1990. "Cost Effectiveness of Hormone Replacement." In *Multi-Disciplinary Perspectives on Menopause: Annals of the New York Academy of Sciences,* vol. 592, ed. M. Flint, F. Kronenberg, and W. Utian. New York: New York Academy of Sciences.

Weiss, Kay. 1977. "What Medical Students Learn About Women." In *Seizing Our Bodies,* ed. Claudia Dreifus. New York: Vintage Books.

Wendell, Susan. 1990. "Oppression and Victimization: Choice and Responsibility." *Hypatia* 5(3): 15–46.

———. 1996. *The Rejected Body: Feminist Philosophical Reflections on Disability.* New York, N.Y.: Routledge.

Wenger, N. K., L. Speroff, and B. Packard. 1993. "Cardiovascular Health and Disease in Women." *New England Journal of Medicine* 329(4): 247.

Wentz, Anne Colston. 1988. "Management of the Menopause." In *Novak's Text-*

book of Gynecology, ed. H. W. Jones, A. C. Wentz, L. S. Burnett, 11th ed. Baltimore: Williams & Wilkins.

Wertz, Dorothy. 1981. "Man-Midwifery and the Rise in Technology." In *Birth Control and Controlling Birth: Women Centered Perspectives,* ed. Helen B. Holmes, Betty B. Hoskins, and Michael Gross. Clifton, N.J.: Humana Press.

West, Candace. 1984. *Routine Complications: Troubles with Talk Between Doctors and Patients.* Bloomington: Indiana University Press.

Westlund, Andrea. 1997. "Pre-Modern and Modern Power: Foucault and the Case of Domestic Violence." Paper presented to the Candian Society for Women in Philosophy, Dalhousie University.

Whateley, Mariamne, and Nancy Worcester. 1989. "The Role of Technology in the Cooptation of the Women's Health Movement: The Cases of Osteoporosis and Breast Cancer Screening." In *Healing Technology: Feminist Perspectives,* ed. Kathryn Strother Ratcliff, Myra Marx Ferree, Gail O. Mellow, Barbara Drygulski Wright, Glenda D. Price, Kim Yanoshik, and Margie S. Freston. Ann Arbor: University of Michigan Press.

White, D. G. 1991. "Wearing a Wife-Assault-Prevention Button: Impact on a Family Practice." *Canadian Medical Association Journal* 145(8): 1005–12.

White, Evelyn C., ed. 1990. *The Black Women's Health Book: Speaking for Ourselves.* Seattle, Wash.: Seal Press.

Whiteford, Linda. 1996. "Political Economy, Gender, and the Social Production of Health and Illness." In *Gender and Health: An International Perspective,* ed. Carolyn F. Sargent and Caroline B. Brettell. Upper Saddle River, N.J.: Prentice-Hall.

WHO (World Health Organization). 1990. *World Health Statistics Annual.* Geneva: WHO.

———. 1995a. *Mother Baby Package: Implementing Safe Motherhood in Countries,* Geneva: WHO.

———. 1995b. *Women's Health: Improve Our Health, Improve the World,* Geneva: WHO.

———. 1995c. *World Health: Statistics Quarterly,* "Safe Motherhood: Selected Research Results," 48.

———. 1996, *Research on the Menopause in the 1990s.* WHO Technical Report Series. Geneva: WHO

Whorton, James C. 1982. *Crusaders for Fitness: The History of American Health Reformers.* Princeton, N.J.: Princeton University Press.

Wilkins, K., and E. Mark. 1992. "Potential Years of Life Lost, Canada, 1990." *Chronic Disease in Canada* 13(6): 111–13.

Williams, Penelope. 1996. "Sick of Dying: Neglect, Misinformation, and Gender Bias have Festered Unchecked in Women's Health Care." *Homemaker's Magazine,* November/December, 46–54.

Wilson, Susannah. 1977. "The Changing Image of Women in Canadian Mass Circulating Magazines, 1930–1970." *Atlantis* 2(2): 33–45.

Winston, R. 1996. "Designer Babies? Not in My Lab," *Times* (London), September 12.

Wolf, Susan M. 1994. "Beyond 'Genetic Discrimination': Toward the Broader Harm of Geneticism." *Journal of Law and Medical Ethics* 23:345–53.

———, ed. 1996. *Feminism and Bioethics: Beyond Reproduction*. New York: Oxford University Press.

Women's Counselling Referral and Education Center. 1985. *Helping Ourselves: A Handbook for Women Starting Groups*. Toronto: The Women's Press.

Worcester, Nancy, and Mariamne H. Whatley. 1994. "The Selling of HRT: Playing on the Fear Factor." In *Women's Health: Readings on Social, Economic, and Political Issues*, ed. Nancy Worcester and Mariamne H. Whatley. 2d ed. Dubuque, Iowa: Kendall/Hunt.

Working Group on Ethics Guidelines for Research with Human Subjects. 1994. Minutes of meeting, Toronto, June 30.

Working Group on the Montreal Declaration. 1996. "A Meeting of Ideals: Declaration of Intent for Research in Health Promotion and Population Health." Document prepared for the 4th Canadian Congress on Health Promotion, Montreal, June.

World Bank. 1993. *World Development Report: Investing in Health*. New York: Oxford University Press.

Yeatman, Anna. 1993. "Voice and Representation in the Politics of Difference." In *Feminism and the Politics of Difference*, ed. Sneja Gunew and Anna Yeatman. Halifax: Fernwood Publishing.

Ylvisaker, Miriam. 1987. "Significant Others." In *With Wings: An Anthology of Literature by and About Women with Disabilities*, ed. Marsha Saxton and Florence Howe. New York: The Feminist Press at the City University of New York.

Young, Iris Marion. 1990. *Justice and the Politics of Difference*. Princeton, N.J.: Princeton University Press.

Zambrana, Ruth, and Marsha Hurst. 1994. "The Interactive Effect of Health Status on Work Patterns Among Urban Puerto Rican Women." In *Women's Health, Politics, and Power: Essays on Sex/Gender, Medicine, and Public Health*, ed. Elizabeth Fee and Nancy Krieger. Amityville, N.Y.: Baywood.

Zita, Jacquelyn. 1989. "The Premenstrual Syndrome: 'Dis-easing' the Female Cycle." In *Feminism and Science*, ed. Nancy Tuana. Bloomington: Indiana University Press.

———. 1993. "Heresy in the Female Body: The Rhetorics of Menopause." In *Menopause: A Midlife Passage*, ed. Joan C. Callahan. Bloomington: Indiana University Press.

Zola, Irving Kenneth. 1978. "Medicine as an Institution of Social Control." In *The Cultural Crisis of Modern Medicine*, ed. John Ehrenreich. New York: Monthly Review Press.

———. 1993. "Self, Identity, and the Naming Question: Reflections on the Language of Disability." *Social Science and Medicine* 36(2): 167–73

About the Authors

Françoise Baylis

One relevant factor in my personal trajectory is the development of a deep-seated objection to labeling. In my world view, a label is a tag we attach to people (or people attach to themselves), on the basis of which we feel free, or, rather, justified, in making assumptions about the person tagged. Far better that we should get to know a person through her spoken or written word than we should assume that we know the person because of her political, social, religious, or other affiliations.

Françoise Baylis received her Ph.D. in philosophy with a specialization in biomedical ethics in 1989 from the University of Western Ontario. She is currently an associate professor in the Office of Bioethics Education and Research and in the Philosophy Department at Dalhousie University. Prior to this she worked at the Westminster Institute for Ethics and Human Values in London, Ontario, the Hospital for Sick Children in Toronto, and the University of Tennessee in Knoxville. Françoise Baylis has a long-standing interest in ethical issues in reproduction, women's health, pediatrics, and research. She has lectured extensively on assisted reproductive technologies, research involving human subjects, and informed choice.

Marilynne Bell

Tentatively exploring my sexuality as an adolescent in the sixties, I quickly learned about dating violence. Date rape back then was "the girl's fault," a consequence of poor moral character. I was the "bad girl," outcast from adolescent culture. It was a tough lesson. The

boys got away with it. As a feminist university student in 1967 I

became a member of the transition house movement, identifying

women in abusive relationships, hearing about the daily threat these

women faced, experiencing the resistance of the "establishment" to

acknowledge woman abuse and the resistance of local and provincial

government to accepting a role in prevention, treatment, or care. My

work in this field has never ceased, only the focus of my efforts.

Marilynne Bell became interested in the situation of women in abusive relationships while working in a Women's Center in Guelph, Ontario. Hearing women's individual stories about the violence in their lives and the collective realities they faced when they sought assistance or services became the foundation for her early community and political activism. Following her medical training at McMaster University, she moved to the Maritimes to complete a residency in family medicine. Her medical practice in the Halifax community continued to underscore the relative lack of services providing safety for these women. At present Marilynne Bell is an assistant professor teaching both undergraduate medical students and residents in family medicine. The focus of her activism has switched to medical education. She has integrated topics on violence— woman abuse, sexual abuse in childhood, sexual assault in adulthood, and sexual harassment—into the curricula of both programs.

Maria De Koninck

I came to focus on health, then on reproductive health, and finally

more specifically on childbirth because maternity (I refer to the

physiological, psychological, and social experience) appears to me as

the locus of the "difference" at all levels, including its "institution-

alization" (reading Adrienne Rich's Of Woman Born *has been very*

important to me).

Maria De Koninck is a professor in the Département de médecine sociale et préventive at l'Université Laval in Quebec. She received her Ph.D. in sociology in 1988; the topic of her thesis was cesarean childbirth. She was named first chair of Women's Studies at l'Université

Laval in 1988 and occupied that position until 1992. Prior to this she worked as a research officer at Social Services of the Quebec government. Recently she has been principal investigator in projects on women physicians in Quebec, on conciliation of pregnancy and work, and on women, health, and environment in Sahelian countries of western Africa, and she participated to the evaluation of midwives' practice in Quebec. In the past twenty years, she has widely published and lectured on different issues in women's health.

Jocelyn Downie

> *The few feminists I met while I was in high school were violently and vocally anti-male and anti-heterosexuality and seemed to me to be extreme on a number of issues. They attributed all of this to feminism. I looked at them and said that if that is what feminism is, then I am not a feminist. Thus, I became part of the large group of women of my generation who would say they live as feminists but reject the label of feminist. While in graduate school, however, I became interested in the concept of personhood. My research led me to the feminist literature on personhood and this then led me to the feminist literature more generally. My interest and involvement in feminism grew but, given my early impressions of feminists, remained largely academic for a number of years. Finally, in first-year law school, I was exposed to racism, homophobia, and sexism, the likes of which I had never before seen. I responded by becoming politicized and I embraced the label of feminist and the responsibility to fight against all forms of oppression.*

Jocelyn Downie is the director of the Health Law Institute and an assistant professor in the faculties of law and medicine at Dalhousie University. Prior to taking up this position, she completed a B.A. and M.A. in philosophy at Queen's University and an M.Litt. in philosophy at the University of Cambridge. She then worked for two years as a research associate at the Westminster Institute for Ethics and Human Values, completed an LL.B. at the University of Toronto, clerked for Chief Justice Antonio Lamer at the Supreme Court of Canada, and went to the University of Michigan at Ann Arbor for an LL.M. She is currently writing a doctoral dissertation on assisted death in Canada. Her research interests lie at the intersection of law, health care, and ethics. Issues considered recently include assisted death, research involving human subjects, and the state intervention in the lives of pregnant women.

Abby Lippman

As with many of my generation/age, I got my training in most important things, feminism included (though it was not called that then), from the street, especially from doing things in the U.S. civil rights and antiwar movements of the sixties and seventies with groups of women. So, when I went back to school as a "mature" student, my past made me unable to disentangle theory and political practice, academics and activism. Action had preceded theory in my life, and it remains a feature of how I work even now. It never occurred to me then that the standard scholarly mask of (disembodied) objectivity was other than an absurd notion, because things just didn't work that way on the streets. This lesson learned empirically continues to drive my efforts in and outside of the university to ensure that health is possible for all women.

Abby Lippman graduated from Cornell University with a B.A. in comparative literature in 1960 and received a Ph.D. from McGill University in biology (human genetics) in 1978. The intervening nonstudent years were divided between the paid work force, community activism, and caring for her children. She is now a full professor in Joint Departments of Epidemiology and Biostatistics and of Occupational Health at McGill University, with cross appointments in the Departments of Human Genetics and Social Studies of Medicine (McGill) and the Département de médecine sociale et préventive at Université de Montréal. Combining activism with research, she was also co-chair of the Human Genetics Committee of the United States–based Council for Responsible Genetics for many years and is now president of the board of a community organization, Head & Hands/A deux mains, that works with youth and young adults. Her current research agenda includes feminist studies of applied genetic technologies, a qualitative participatory investigation of women living with a diagnosis of breast cancer, and explorations of the relationships among social change (particularly health "reforms"), policy development, and women's health.

Margaret Lock

The People's Park fiasco of the early 1970s in California, culmination

of the student movement as it was played out on the Berkeley

campus, was a revelation to me, especially since it came after years

of vital, sometimes dangerous, anti–Vietnam War activities on my

part. I understood then that politics are rarely simply black or white,

left or right, good or bad. A total of more than eight years spent

intermittently in Kyoto and Tokyo doing research also taught me to

respect ambiguities, contradictions, gray zones—in other words, to

be wary of easy answers. Living in the midst of Quebec politics

for the past twenty years has amply confirmed this insight. I am

adamant that nationalisms and a politics of essential difference have

no place in the world today, and that women are particularly at risk

in such a climate.

Margaret Lock is a professor in the Department of Social Studies of Medicine and the Department of Anthropology at McGill University. She is the author of *East Asian Medicine in Urban Japan: Varieties of Medical Experience* (1980) and *Encounters with Aging: Mythologies of Menopause in Japan and North America* (1993), which won the J. I. Staley Prize, School of American Research, the Eileen Basker Memorial Prize, the Canada-Japan Book Award, and the Berkeley Award and was a finalist for the Hiromi Arisawa Award. Both books were published by the University of California Press and are translated into Japanese. She has edited five other books and written over one hundred scholarly articles. She was the recipient of Canada Council Izaak Killiam Fellowship for 1993–1995 and is a Fellow of the Royal Society of Canada and a member of the Canadian Institute of Advanced Research, Population Program. Margaret Lock's current interests are in the relationships among culture, technology, and body politics.

Wendy Mitchinson

The older I get, the more I appreciate the strength and independence of

my mother. Certainly by all appearances a "traditional" woman, she

represents how statistics on women do not tell the complete story of

women's lives. Her life as she has lived it is resonant with informal

agency. This, no doubt, has influenced the way I see women in the past.

Wendy Mitchinson is a professor of history at the University of Water-loo. She has written widely on women and reform in Canada and is one of the co-authors of *Canadian Women: A History* (Toronto: University of Toronto Press, 1996). Her work on women and health resulted in the publication of *The Nature of Their Bodies: Women and Their Doctors in Victorian Canada* (Toronto: University of Toronto Press, 1991). She is currently writing a similar study focusing on the first half of the twentieth century.

Kathryn Pauly Morgan

I was the first-born and only daughter of an American Catholic

doctor and doctor's wife in a family of five children. By all accounts, I

was a plump, sassy, terminally shy girl. Leaving aside roller-coaster

dieting years, I guess I've grown up into a plump, witty, terminally

shy woman. "My Father was a Doctor." While he was still alive, I

can remember writing an essay in seventh or eighth grade about his

hands. I saw his hands—somewhat short and stocky like my own—as

capable of diagnosing, healing, and caring. When my father died, the

health care workers from the two hospitals where he had privileges all

came to the wake. Patients lined up around the block at the funeral

home to pay their respects to our family and to share their own sense

of loss. I knew that my father's hands were educated hands, and I felt,

as I was finishing high school, that I wanted to be a doctor, too

(although I thought, given my shyness, it was probably better if I

tried to become a pathologist!). So, I went to Career Day only to be told, by one of my father's closest medical friends, "You don't really

want to be a doctor. Why not try becoming a nurse or a laboratory

technician? Then you can help your father." Thus is the heart

diverted. And thus is the heart betrayed when I found out that my

father was not the prototype for all male physicians.

Kathryn Pauly Morgan received her B.A. in philosophy from Alverno College and her M.A. and Ph.D. in philosophy from Johns Hopkins University. She also completed a M.Ed. degree in educational foundations at the University of Alberta and has pursued additional graduate work in women's health through the "Women, Health, and Healing" graduate program at the University of California, San Francisco. She is currently a professor of philosophy at the University of Toronto, holding cross-appointments to the Women's Studies Program and the Joint Center for Bioethics. Having learned to speak to living human beings, she was awarded an Ontario Council of University Faculty Associations Award for Excellence in Teaching. She has written extensively in the areas of feminist ethics, philosophy of the body, feminist bioethics, gender and technology (sexuality, reproduction, cosmetic surgery), feminist pedagogy, and philosophy of sexuality. She is co-author, with Diller, Houston, and Ayim, of *The Gender Question in Education: Theory, Pedagogy, and Politics* (Boulder, Colo.: Westview, 1996) and is currently at work on a book tentatively entitled "Revisiting Frankenstein: Gender, Bio-Technology, and the Creation of Human Artifacts."

Janet Mosher

I have long identified myself as a "feminist"—grade seven is my

earliest remembrance of publicly calling myself a feminist. And I

remember wearing my "WHY NOT" pin in grade nine, and thinking

that I could play trumpet much better than any guy I knew (indeed

feeling rather proud when at a stage band competition one of the

judges remarked that our all-female trumpet section was the

"ballsiest" in the competition!). I was certainly a "liberal feminist" in

those days. I also vividly remember my mother's comments being

published in an Atlantic magazine in an article on the occupations of men and women. She was quoted as saying that it would be fine if her

daughter became a doctor (which one did) or if her son became a

nurse (which neither did, nor might I add, did they pursue any sort of

"female" occupation). My experience until law school was basically

just that I, and the other girls, later women, I knew were on equal

footing with "the guys." Law school was my first experience of being

silenced.

Janet Mosher received her LL.M. from the University of Toronto, her LL.B. from Queen's University, and her M.Mus.A. from the University of Western Ontario. She is an associate professor at the University of Toronto, cross-appointed between the faculties of Law and Social Work, and is the director of the combined LL.B./M.S.W. program. Her research interests and political commitments lie in the areas of violence against women, legal ethics, and the impact of legal processes and legal services upon members of various oppressed groups.

Barbara Parish

During the sixties and seventies, when I was in grammar school and

university, feminism was never part of my picture. The battles were

pacifism, "ban the bomb," and racism to a lesser degree. I did,

however, have a reputation as a radical among other nurses and

friends. Feminism was not initially a label that I would have applied

to myself, but I realized over time that it was the label others attached

to me. I gradually came to realize that it is an honor to be so labeled,

regardless of the intention. Within this honorary title I can still be

who I want to be, whereas at first it worried me that I might have to

lop bits off to fit.

Barbara Parish is an associate professor in the Department of Obstetrics and Gynaecology at Dalhousie University. Starting her career off traveling widely as a nurse and midwife, she went on to study political science and ended up attending McMaster Medical School in an attempt to combine her political interest and social conscience with a concern and respect for the individual. After McMaster she moved to Halifax for an internship at Dalhousie University, followed by a residency in Obstetrics and Gynaecology. Her ongoing interests include general obstetrics, ethics, international women's health and medical education, and midwifery.

Susan Sherwin

> *As far back as I can remember, I have been deeply committed to social justice and I have been appalled by instances of social injustice. As a graduate student in 1969, I joined a consciousness-raising group out of a sense that I had personally suffered little from sexism but felt I had a responsibility to get involved to help the many less fortunate women of the world. Slowly, I began to understand how I was indeed affected by sexism. I learned to see the ways in which it had been directed against me and also how I had internalized many of the attitudes and values that support sexism (and racism and all the other social causes that concerned me). Yet, I have always been uncomfortable discussing my own sense of oppression, since gender is the only category of oppression on which I fall on the disadvantaged side of the dichotomy and my privilege in other categories largely mitigates the harms I am personally exposed to as a woman. But I distrust my tendency to adopt a feminism for "other women," i.e., those who are worse off than myself; I think it is important to understand my personal investment in social reform that will challenge many of my existing privileges while correcting the social injustice I abhor.*

Susan Sherwin completed her undergraduate studies in philosophy and mathematics at York University, Toronto, and then did a doctorate in philosophy at Stanford University; her dissertation is entitled "The Moral Foundations of Feminism." She spent a year on a postdoctoral fellowship in the Moral Problems in Medicine Project at Case Western Reserve University, where she worked on the first major anthology of philosophical approaches to medical ethics (*Moral Problems in Medicine*, ed. Samuel Gorovitz et al. [Englewood Cliffs, N.J.: Prentice Hall, 1976; 2d ed., 1983]). She has been at Dalhousie University since 1974 and she is now a professor of philosophy and women's studies (currently co-ordinator of women's studies). Most of her research activity has been in the area of feminist health care ethics. She is the author of *No Longer Patient: Feminist Ethics and Health Care* (Philadelphia: Temple University Press, 1992).

Index

abortion, 27, 32, 79n. 9, 83, 113, 151; physician's complicity in, 134–35, 136

abuse, woman (wife) (*see also* feminism; violence), 4, 10, 11, *and* Chapter 9; legal responses to, 220–25, 231n. 15; medicalization of, 16–17, 30, 206; medical responses to, 213–14, 218–21; and rape, 83; responsibility for, 209–11, 215–16; role of protocols and guidelines in, 16, 205, 218–23, 225, 227–30; treatment sources for, 211–12

Adams, Diane, 112

Africa, West (Benin), 8, 15, *and* Chapter 7

agency, 14, 41, 47nn. 22, 23, 147n. 15, 216, 247; collective, 127; defined, 32–33; in health, 50, 66, *and* Chapter 6; medicalized, 96–97; of physicians, 123; of women, 11–13, 17, 84, 109–13, 204, 225–30

aging: and men, 184–85, 201, 203–4; and women, 15–16, 40–41, 59, 152, 238, *and* Chapter 8

AIDS, 7, 58, 60, 110, 238–40, 244

alternative therapies, 88, 128, 169–71, 189; within medicine, 30, 91, 111–12, 138–40, 144, 201, 231n. 10

Aristotle, 102

autonomy, 11–13, 19, 175, 179, 202, 204, 206, 227; constitutive elements of, 35; feminist analysis of, Chapter 2, *esp.* 19, 37; our own, 255–56; principle of respect for, 19–25, 32; relational, 12–13, 17, 37–44, 92, 104, 256–57; relation of, to oppression, 25–27, 32–39, 240, 245, 256; role of, in health care, 20, 84; role of, in research, 246–47; skills for, 36–37, 40, 42; traditional interpretations of, 6, 20, 21

Babbitt, Susan, 36–37, 46n. 13

Backhouse, Constance, 83–84, 91

Bartky, Sandra Lee, 62

Benhabib, Seyla, 208

Bhayana, Bhooma, 112

bioethics. *See* ethics, health care

biology: and diversity, 182; and individual and differences, 74; as local, 16, 137, 182, 200–203; as malleable, 181

biomedicine (*see also* alternative therapies; medicalization), 3, 9; challenges to, Chapter 5; as dominant model, 11, 30–31; history of, Chapter 6; individualistic focus of (*see* individualism); relation of, to health, 3, 12; role of, in oppression, 3, 14

birth control. *See* fertility

Block, Gladys, 242

body, female, 14, 59, 124–25, 203; as deviant, 125, 185, 242; as pathological, 102–3, 107–8; as signifier, 178,